The Nexus between Nursing and Patient Safety

Cynthia A. Oster • Jane S. Braaten

Editors

The Nexus between Nursing and Patient Safety

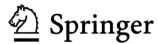 Springer

Editors
Cynthia A. Oster
Nursing and Professional Development
CommonSpirit Health – Mountain Region
Centennial, CO, USA

Jane S. Braaten
Quality and Patient Safety
AdventHealth Parker
Parker, CO, USA

ISBN 978-3-031-53157-6   ISBN 978-3-031-53158-3   (eBook)
https://doi.org/10.1007/978-3-031-53158-3

This Springer imprint is published by the registered company Springer Nature Switzerland AG
The registered company address is: Gewerbestrasse 11, 6330 Cham, Switzerland

If disposing of this product, please recycle the paper.

Contents

Contributors

Jennifer T. Alderman, PhD, MSN, RN, CNL, CNE, CHSE University of North Carolina at Chapel Hill, Chapel Hill, NC, USA

Gail Armstrong, PhD, DNP, ACNS-BC, RN, CNE, FAAN University of Colorado Anschutz Medical Campus, College of Nursing, Aurora, CO, USA

Stephanie Bennett, PhD, MBA, RN Patient- and Family-Centered Care and Education, Emory Healthcare, Atlanta, GA, USA

Nell Hodgson Woodruff School of Nursing, Emory University, Atlanta, GA, USA

Jane S. Braaten, PhD, APRN, CNS, ANP, CPPS, CPHQ Quality and Patient Safety, AdventHealth Parker, Parker, CO, USA

Jane M. Carrington, PhD, RN, FAAN, FAMIA Department of Family, Community and Health System Science, University of Florida College of Nursing, Gainesville, FL, USA

University of Florida, College of Nursing, Gainesville, FL, USA

Health Care Quality, Gainesville, FL, USA

Aurora Davis, MSN, RN, OCN, CCPS University of Colorado Hospital, UCHealth, Aurora, CO, USA

Lori Lynn Fewster-Thuente, PhD, RN Rosalind Franklin University of Medicine and Science, College of Nursing, College of Health Professions, North Chicago, IL, USA

Paige R. Gannon, MPH, BSN, RN Emory University School of Medicine, Emory Healthcare, Atlanta, GA, USA

William E. Gordon, DMin, MDiv, BS Rosalind Franklin University of Medicine and Science, College of Health Professions, North Chicago, IL, USA

Marissa B. Jamarik, DNP, RN, NEA-BC Roper St. Francis Healthcare, Charleston, SC, USA

Kelley Kovar, DNP, RN, NE-BC AdventHealth Littleton, Littleton, CO, USA

Patricia McGaffigan, MS, RN, CPPS Institute for Healthcare Improvement (IHI), Boston, MA, USA

Molly McNett, PhD, RN, CNRN, FNCS, FAAN Helene Fuld Health Trust National Institute for Evidence-based Practice for Nursing and Healthcare, College of Nursing, The Ohio State University, Columbus, OH, USA

Joel Mumma, PhD Healthcare Human Factors Lab, Division of Infectious Diseases, Emory University School of Medicine, Atlanta, GA, USA

Armando Nahum H2Pi and Patient Safety Activist, Smyrna, GA, USA

Andréa Narvaez, DNP, MHA, RN, NE-BC AdventHealth Parker, Parker, CO, USA

Christine W. Nibbelink, PhD, RN University of San Diego, School of Nursing, San Diego, CA, USA

Cynthia A. Oster, PhD, APRN, MBA, ACNS-BC, FAAN Nursing and Professional Development, CommonSpirit Health – Mountain Region, Centennial, CO, USA

Kristen A. Oster, DNP, APRN, ACNS-BC, CNOR, CNS-CP Mountain Region, CommonSpirit Health, Centennial, CO, USA

Marian Savage, PhD, RN, NEA-BC, CPHQ, PMP Quality and Patient Experience, Roper St. Francis Healthcare System, Charleston, SC, USA

Gwen Sherwood, PhD, RN, FAAN, ANEF University of North Carolina at Chapel Hill, Chapel Hill, NC, USA

Sharon Tucker, PhD, APRN-CNS, EBP-C, FNAP, FAAN Helene Fuld Health Trust National Institute for Evidence-based Practice for Nursing and Healthcare, College of Nursing, The Ohio State University, Columbus, OH, USA

Mary T. Walsh, PsyD Mountain Division, CommonSpirit Health, Centennial, CO, USA

Bradley W. Weaver, PhD Division of Infectious Diseases, Emory University School of Medicine, Emory Healthcare, Atlanta, GA, USA

Kelly Wild, MS, RN, ACCNS-AG, CCRN AdventHealth Parker, Parker, CO, USA

Part I
Foundations of Patient Safety

Patient Safety: History, Current Models, and Future Directions for Improvement

Jane S. Braaten

1 Introduction

Patient safety is a term echoed daily throughout the halls of hospitals, clinics, ambulatory healthcare agencies, and anywhere where healthcare is delivered. It is a non-arguable fact that we, as healthcare professionals, should keep those who are in receipt of our care, safe from harm. Even Florence Nightingale [1] asserted that hospitals at the very least should do the sick no harm. However, achieving the goal of reliable and consistent safety is not as easy as Nightingale's declaration. Patient safety today is complex, multifaceted with technology and social factors intertwined. As commonplace as the term "patient safety" is used, it is still somewhat elusive and misunderstood at many levels. Patient safety deserves a new understanding and actions to move forward to achieve the outcomes that Nightingale envisioned.

1.1 Definition of Patient Safety

The World Health Organization (WHO) defines patient safety as follows: "Patient Safety is a health care discipline that emerged with the evolving complexity in health care systems and the resulting rise of patient harm in health care facilities. It aims to prevent and reduce risks, errors and harm that occur to patients during provision of health care. A cornerstone of the discipline is continuous improvement based on learning from errors and adverse events" [2]. The WHO has declared patient safety as a global health priority and states that the occurrence of adverse

J. S. Braaten (✉)
AdventHealth Parker, Parker, CO, USA
e-mail: jane.braaten@adventhealth.com

© The Author(s), under exclusive license to Springer Nature
Switzerland AG 2024
C. A. Oster, J. S. Braaten (eds.), *The Nexus between Nursing and Patient Safety*,
https://doi.org/10.1007/978-3-031-53158-3_1

events due to unsafe care is likely one of the ten leading causes of death and disability across the world. Furthermore, the issues that are most concerning in patient safety include:

- Medication errors
- Health care associated infections
- Unsafe surgical care procedures and complications from surgery
- Unsafe injection practices that transmit infections
- Diagnostic errors
- Unsafe transfusion practices exposing patients to adverse reactions and transmission of infections
- Sepsis
- Radiation errors
- Venous thromboembolism [2]

The significance of patient safety cannot be overstated. The measurement, understanding of how errors occur, and how to improve patient safety is a continual challenge. For example, patient safety is measured in various ways with limitations that leave us with an incomplete picture of harm from preventable mistakes. Clinical measurement of patient harm includes retrospective chart reviews which focus on identifying "triggers" that may suggest an adverse event; voluntary error reporting systems, electronic surveillance that detects triggers of adverse events, administrative data which is used to detect coded events of harm and patient reports of harm [3]. This type of measurement is quantifiable and easily understood with patient safety defined as the absence of adverse events. However, patient safety is much more than just metrics.

The discipline of nursing is at the frontline of preventing harm in healthcare. As the care providers who spend the most time with patients, nurses need to not only be clinical experts but also experts on how harm occurs and how to prevent harm. This chapter will provide a lens for which nurses can view and make sense of patient safety through first, an introduction to the history of patient safety and the current state of healthcare harm. The next section will discuss current models used to understand error and prevention with a distinct focus on frontline care. The chapter will conclude with a discussion of future directions that inform the roles of all healthcare providers, specifically clinical nurses who intentionally and visibly protect those in our care from harm and serve as frontline leaders for patient safety.

2   History of Patient Safety and Current State

2.1   To Err Is Human

As mentioned earlier, keeping patients safe and free from medical errors is not a recent concept. Accounts of unintentional errors and harm go back for decades [4]. However, when safety historians are asked what started the patient safety movement, most agree that the report by the Institute of Medicine (IOM), *To Err is Human*, published in 2000 [5], caused a burning platform that began a force for change [6]. This report highlighted preventable medical errors that caused harm. The authors stated that 44,000–98,000 humans were killed every year due to medical errors and more than a million more people were injured. They equated this to a jumbo jet crash every day. This connection was frightening and made headlines nationally and internationally.

An article published at the time [7] discussed why, after many years of mistakes and unintended outcomes, the IOM report caused such an uproar. The simple answer is that the report was designed to create a public demand to increase safety in healthcare. The jumbo jet comparison probably was intended to make headlines to create a quote to lead the change. The report included stories of individuals who had died from medical errors. Wears and Sutcliffe [6] state, despite many criticisms and inaccuracies, the report achieved status because it played upon the fears of the public toward a trusted profession. The use of the word "error" in the IOM report created a victim (the patient) and a perpetrator (the healthcare system). It also made clear the imperative that the healthcare community needed to "fix this problem." This report and its controversial jumbo jet comparison created the perfect message for journalists to disseminate. The public and professional recognition of the problem called for nothing other than a commitment to improvement from the medical community. Although the patient safety movement existed long before this report, the public attention to patient safety began in earnest.

Stelfox et al. [8] noted a substantial increase in publications on the topic of patient safety after this report was published. More attention was focused on patient safety than ever before. Patient safety began to become a part of national dialogue as well as embedded and institutionalized into healthcare organizations. Efforts also included adopting safety interventions from national organizations and other fields, measuring patient safety with metrics, and creating improved information technology [9]. Examples of campaigns, programs, and movements that came after the IOM report and their respective websites are below:

- The Institute for Healthcare Improvement (IHI) launches the 100,000 lives campaign, a massive campaign to improve safety in hospitals as well as a follow-up campaign with a broader safety goal, to save five million lives. (Overview | IHI—Institute for Healthcare Improvement)
- Patient safety specialists, patient safety officers, created as well as a certification for patient safety expertise, the Certified Professional in Patient Safety (CPPS). (CPPS: Certified Professional in Patient Safety | IHI—Institute for Healthcare Improvement)
- The National Patient Safety Foundation (NPSF) creates the Lucian Leape Institute to promote patient safety. (IHI Lucian Leape Institute | IHI—Institute for Healthcare Improvement)
- The AHRQ releases the Hospital Survey on Patient Safety Culture (HSOPS). (Surveys on Patient Safety Culture (SOPS) | Agency for Healthcare Research and Quality (ahrq.gov)

- The Josie King Foundation created to prevent harm from medical errors. (Landing—Josie King Foundation)
- Patient safety indicators introduced to reliably measure patient harm from a variety of causes. (AHRQ QI: Patient Safety Indicators Overview)
- The Joint Commission introduces annual patient safety goals to guide care and raise awareness. (National Patient Safety Goals | The Joint Commission)

This is, of course, not a complete list, but examples of the work that commenced after the IOM report and continues to take place in the world of patient safety. So does all this activity equate to real safety? Are we now safe in healthcare? The jury remains out on these questions due to variation in measurement over the years. Clinical measurement of harm has not been consistent, so it is difficult to clearly show improvement. Also, reporting and acknowledgment of adverse events have increased dramatically so it is difficult to know if we are just reporting and noticing these events more often or if they are more prevalent.

3   Are We Safer?

Thirteen years after the IOM report, James [10] used a trigger tool to identify harm in healthcare and found that more patients died per year than originally cited in the IOM report. He estimated that up to 400,000 patients die each year due to medical harm rather than 98,000. Pangioti et al. [11] found that in various medical settings, 1 in 20 patients experience harm. More recently, 23 years after the IOM report, Bates et al. [12] found that up to 25% of patients in a hospital setting experience an adverse event and that a fourth of those events are preventable. In the publication, *Still Not Safe*, [6], the authors list 17 studies from 2004 through 2016 that found safety had not improved as anticipated and as expected. As noted earlier, the variation in measuring "error" and "harm" is not consistent and the complexity of healthcare is not the same as it was in 1999, so it is difficult to measure progress in any standardized method [13]. However, despite all the action and programs directed at patient safety, it appears that healthcare is still not as safe as it could or should be.

As explanation for the lack of improvement, Donald Berwick stated in an editorial, that safety has taken a back seat to other issues in healthcare [13]. Wears and Sutcliffe [6] discuss conditions that may explain why patient safety has not improved much over the years:

- Patient safety has become institutionalized in healthcare with a system that has become more bureaucratic than anything else with measuring and monitoring as the focus.
- Safety science from other fields has largely not been translated to healthcare.
- Framing medical harm and adverse events as "error" places the onus on the individual at the frontline to change and not the organization that supports the frontline.

The authors compare the difference between healthcare's advancement of safety to the airline industry:

> Aviation safety was not advanced by pilots working on "safety projects, but rather by partnership between subject matter experts (pilots, air traffic controllers, mechanic etc.) and safety scientists (psychologists, engineers, communication scientist etc.) [6, p. 197]

In other words, aviation safety advanced due to knowledge and experience from the frontline and collaboration between safety scientists and the frontline experts. This collaboration has not occurred as readily in healthcare.

Others have reflected on the progress or lack of progress. A recent inquiry [14] asked 13 hospital and healthcare executives for their opinion on why healthcare safety has not improved. The interviewees all acknowledge the difficulty in measuring progress in error and harm reduction. They also identified many areas that have improved such as anesthesia care, reduction of hospital acquired infections, transparency of harm, and high reliability organization culture change. On the other hand, the interviewees cite that patient safety suffers from the following:

- Lack of proactivity
- Lack of real system change
- Lack of innovative thinking
- Lack of transformation within the context of current healthcare reality (financial constraint, staffing shortages)
- Lack of robust measurement
- Lack of patient input on patient safety
- Lack of usage of safety science engineers
- Lack of learning from near misses and close calls as well as successful cases

Adding to that challenge is the difficult landscape we have been navigating through, during and after the pandemic. Preventable hospital acquired infections that had shown great improvement regressed during the post pandemic time period [15].

In summary, patient safety is a dynamic challenge for healthcare. It is dependent on collaboration between clinicians/patients with safety science to understand and prevent errors and should be focused on how to support the frontline as the complexity of healthcare is growing exponentially. The understanding of how patient safety is realized in healthcare is still somewhat elusive and is focused more on metrics than how safety is created by systems and individuals. The next section will discuss the safety models relevant to frontline clinicians as means to understand and prevent error as we place patient safety into a context that nurses can and do apply every day.

4 Useful Models of Safety

4.1 Swiss Cheese Model (SCM): A Simple, Well-Known Model for Understanding of Error

The Swiss Cheese Model (SCM) created by James Reason [16] is one of the most widely known and used models to understand how accidents and errors occur. In this model, accident-causing conditions move through several weak layers in a system and finally result in a harm causing event. The simple explanation is that each layer of cheese represents a barrier to an accident. When the barrier is weak as compared to a piece of Swiss cheese with holes, the error continues through the block of cheese until it meets a barrier that is solid which stops the error. If no barriers are solid and without holes or weaknesses, the error finally gets through the cheese or system and causes harm.

This model explains errors that are caused by active and latent factors. These factors have also been described as "sharp end" or "blunt end" errors [17]. The latent factors or blunt end errors occur within the system and often are not realized until harm occurs. Currently, these latent contributors can include organizational culture, leadership and supervisory factors, equipment issues, staffing issues, policies that do not work at the frontline, production pressure, and many more. An active or sharp end error is one that happens nearest to the harm and is often experienced by an individual. These are usually caused by three types of human error as shown in Table 1. Skill based, rule based, and knowledge based errors are originally described by Jens Rasmussen [18].

There are many critiques of the SCM which include that it is too simplistic, linear, and static [19] so that it does not assist in the dynamic environment in which healthcare is practiced. However, a key contribution of this model is that it identifies two ways that accidents and errors occur: from acts by individuals and by issues within an organization or system which may be contributing factors. The model has practical power and makes sense to healthcare for the following reasons:

- It visually explains a basis for accidents that makes sense.
- It explains that accidents do not just occur because of an individual making a mistake: many factors contribute.

Table 1 Types of human errors

	Skill-based error	Rule-based error	Knowledge-based error
Definition	Lapse, slip, misstep	Failure to follow a process or procedure	"Figuring it out" Failure to obtain guidance when in an unfamiliar situation
Cause	Usually occurs while doing routine processes. Can be caused by inattention and or distraction	Process wasn't known, available, clear, or able to easily follow	Pride, illusion of competence, culture doesn't support asking questions

- It acknowledges that contributors to accidents are within the systems we create and exist long before an accident occurs. These contributors need to be corrected in order to prevent reoccurrence of an accident.
- The model emphasizes that even though we believe we have safeguards to errors in place, there may be weaknesses in the implementation of those safeguards that allow an error to progress.
- It subtly depicts that an error can be prevented or averted by one action that "plugs" up a Swiss cheese hole. However, acknowledging that this may prevent one accident from progressing but may not prevent the next one.

Weigmann and colleagues [20] give a great example of the practical application of the model. They recall the old story of the Dutch boy who noticed a leak in the dam and plugged the dam up with his finger, saving the city from flooding. The leak was an error that was noticed and corrected immediately by a person at the frontline, thus preventing harm. However, the factors that led to the leak needed to be addressed or the hero would have been stuck with his finger in the dam for days. This is a simple application of how latent factors contribute to errors that can be corrected quickly by an attentive frontline but need to be addressed at a higher level.

Let's apply this to an understanding of a common error involving clinicians working within a medical system: the medication error. The example in Fig. 1. illustrates the error within the SCM.

Specifically in this model, an error does not cause harm immediately. The error typically goes through several layers of barriers until it gets to a patient to cause harm. Several factors within each step of the error can be effectively examined within this model. Note that in each step of the process, there may be active failures as well as latent conditions as shown in Table 2.

This model, as any model, has strengths and weaknesses. Still, the main points are strong and practical.

- Errors in a complex system will go through many layers prior to causing actual harm. Healthcare providers are the frontline of defense who can recognize red flags of failure and stop the error from progressing.
- There are many factors at a system level that contribute to errors that are not recognized or addressed.

1.Error starts	2.Error continues	3.Error continues	4.Error continues	5.Harm to patient
Physician keys in wrong medication dose.	Phamacy rushed and doesn't notice	Nurse is new, short staffed and does not question	Patient does not question the dose	Patient receives incorrect dose

Fig. 1 Application of SCM to medication error

Table 2 Active failures and latent conditions in a medication error

	Active failure	Latent condition	Active solution that would've prevented error from progressing	Latent solution
Physician keys in wrong medication dose	Doesn't double check the dose entered	Physician is pressured to see more patients. No ability to review orders before filing	Physician realizes he is distracted. Double checks and corrects the error.	Adding a visual double check summary of order prior to submitting
Pharmacy rushed and doesn't notice error	Distracted and defers to physician	Supervising many new staff and no ability to easily contact physician for questions	Pharmacy notices a higher dose and questions the order	Electronic alert when dose is higher than normal. Examination of staffing level and effect on workload
Nurse new, short staffed and doesn't question dose	Assumes the dose is correct. "It's gone through two check points"	No ability to easily locate medication resource in order to question order	Nurse calls pharmacy and questions the order	Easily accessible medication references. Expectation to question orders that do not make sense
Patient does not question the dose	Assumes dose is correct. "Nurse knows their job"	Patient has no prompt to ask questions of healthcare providers	Patient tells nurse that the dose is higher than normal	Prompt in patient information to ask questions about medications and procedures

In order to promote safety, we must assure that frontline staff are empowered to notice and stop errors in the moment and that systems provide resources to examine the system contribution to the error before it occurs again and causes harm. The next model that complements and helps understanding of failures in the SCM model is human factors.

4.2   Human Factors and Patient Safety

A field of study that pertains widely to safety in healthcare and nursing is human factors and ergonomics. The definition of human factors as adopted by the Human Factors and Ergonomics Society (HFES) is:

> Ergonomics (or human factors) is the scientific discipline concerned with the understanding of interactions among humans and other elements of a system, and the profession that applies theory, principles, data, and methods to design in order to optimize human well-being and overall system performance. Ergonomists contribute to the design and evaluation of tasks, jobs, products, environments, and systems in order to make them compatible with the needs, abilities, and limitations of people [21]

In other words, human factors study how humans and the system interact in order to produce outcomes. Human factors work focuses on how to optimize human performance within the context that human beings work and live. Human performance is fraught with frailties. Human factors science appreciates this and attempts to optimize the systems with which humans interact in order to account for these frailties.

As noted in Table 1, there are three types of human errors: skill based, rule based, and knowledge based. Additionally, the field of aviation has identified 12 common human factors that lead to these types of errors and has coined them the "dirty dozen" [22].

1. Lack of communication
2. Distraction
3. Complacency
4. Stress
5. Lack of resources
6. Lack of teamwork
7. Pressure
8. Lack of awareness
9. Lack of knowledge
10. Lack of assertiveness
11. Fatigue
12. Norms

Human factors account for these types of errors and attempts to identify system, process, or workflow design in order to mitigate these errors. Considering how this is seen from the SCM, human factors attempt to correct the latent failures within a system by making them more noticeable or stoppable at the point of human contact.

The application of a human factors lens is important because healthcare is a complex sociotechnical system. This is a system that is interconnected, cannot be easily reduced to individual parts, and is a balance between social (humans) and technology (machines/devices/computers). Two main tenants of a sociotechnical system are as follows:

1. The interaction between the social and the technical aspects of work is paramount to the success or nonsuccess of the work product.
2. An overemphasis on either the social or technical focus can lead to an imbalance and defects in the other category [23].

Thus, the goal of a sociotechnical system is termed "joint optimization" of the social and technical aspects of work [24]. This is the basis of application of human factors science to healthcare. Optimization means to design systems and processes that make it easier for humans to do the right thing and more difficult to do the wrong thing. For example:

A new medication dispensing cabinet has been installed on the nursing unit. This new unit promises to increase productivity, decrease medication errors, manage medication inventory, and allow dispensing of medications more quickly by allowing nurses to type in the first letter of the medication for a "pick list" display that the nurse can use to quickly select the medication. Nurses become used to quickness of the system and have selected incorrect medications when getting interrupted or distracted (skill-based human error). The pick list also comes up with many different strengths of the same medication, so dosage errors have occurred. The system is designed to bring up the medication and dosage that is most selected as the first on the pick list. It is very easy to select the wrong medication and administer to a patient without noticing, especially if there is poor environmental lighting or the nurse is busy, distracted, or fatigued.

Looking at this issue through a human factors lens, it appears that the dispensing cabinet and the frontline staff who access the cabinet have an imbalance in joint optimization. Perhaps the installation was intended to increase productivity and increase speed of dispensing; however, the initial analysis was only focused on the technology. Focusing on how the frontline staff member interacts with the cabinet within the context of the busy nursing unit would lead to the discovery of many processes that could fail. Mitigation of these processes such as a "no interruption zone" while at the cabinet or hard stops that do not allow high-risk medications to be removed without an additional verification considers human factors and could prevent error. However, these interventions that consider human factors may not necessarily save time as the installation of the cabinet was intended to do.

Human factors science is incredibly important to nursing in healthcare today as technology innovations are abundant and always changing how we do our work. Focusing our lens on how technology and human beings can interact to produce outcomes while not allowing technology to take over is one of the most important safety challenges currently, and of the future. The current popularity of artificial intelligence poses an interesting new challenge in how to optimize the technology without allowing it to dominate. The presence of human factors scientists is rare within the current healthcare landscape but as more and more technology and artificial intelligence emerges, the use of these scientists will be critical.

4.3   High Reliability, Complexity, and a Resilient System

Furthering the work on the importance of sociotechnical optimization, the human factor, and system causes and barriers of and to error is the model of highly reliable organizations (HRO). This model is based on the concepts of anticipation of error and the ability to mitigate or catch errors before they make it through the system (recall the SCM) to harm a patient. Highly reliable organizations are those that are high risk, complex, and potentially dangerous, but have very few errors [25].

The concept of highly reliable organizations began early in the 1990s, however, it became more widespread in healthcare, with the publication of *Managing the Unexpected: Assuring High Performance in an Age of Complexity* [25]. Weick and Sutcliffe studied organizations with a record of high risk and few errors and found that these organizations have characteristics in common that were quite different and even groundbreaking when applied to a healthcare setting. Table 3 describes the five characteristics:

Highly reliability theory states that errors and error-producing conditions in highly complex systems cannot be completely eradicated. However, they can be anticipated and caught by astute human beings prior to the error causing harm. Thus, error-producing factors are always present; however, individuals and systems that are alert to red flags can mitigate the error so harm does not occur or is minimal. HRO theory focuses on what is called mindful organizing [26]. Mindful organizing in this context is the ability to pay attention so unexpected deviations are noticed and dealt with prior to a harm causing event. For example:

- HROs do not simply follow protocols and check off tasks on a checklist.
- HROs practice continuous monitoring of situations for red flags that might indicate potential failure.

Table 3 Characteristics of Highly Reliable Organizations (HROs) [26]

	Practical definition	Mind set	Example	Absence
Preoccupation with failure	HROs always anticipate failures in a proactive manner	See small failures as "red flags" or the beginnings of a larger failure	Encouraging discussion of the possibility of failure with each process	Avoiding or discouraging discussion of possible failure points
Reluctance to simplify	HROs take error producing situations seriously even if they don't cause harm	Investigating events that do not cause harm as intensely as those that do	Investigating close calls and near misses for system changes	"No harm, no foul" failure to investigate events unless they have caused harm
Sensitivity to operations	Paying attention to how processes really work at the frontline	Testing a process to examine for failures with the staff who perform the work	Management observing processes at the frontline and asking about workarounds	Expecting "top down" protocols to succeed without input from the frontline
Deference to expertise	HROs shift decisions away from formal authority toward expertise and experience	"Who is the most knowledgeable about this topic?"	Including variety and diversity to decisions made	All decisions come from the top
Commitment to resilience	HROs pay close attention to their capability to improvise, adapt and act	"How can we assist our frontline to make decisions in urgent situations?"	Allowing those at the frontline the resources available to adapt to changing situations	Hierarchy of control that stalls decision making at the frontline

- HROs practice collaboration, communication, and expertise to develop on the spot options to prevent harmful situations from escalating out of control.
- HROs deal proactively to red flags of errors that are about to occur instead of reactively after the event occurs [26].

The opportunity here is one that is often missed in healthcare: identifying and acting on weak signals of failure prior to the "weak signal" escalating of out control. Consider the following examples of weak signals in healthcare today:

- "We have only new nurses with less than 1 year of experience working on the nightshift."
- "This patient has been off of the ordered telemetry monitor for an hour and no one is placing her back on."
- "This piece of equipment has failed two times. Thankfully, it did not harm a patient yet."

These are only a few examples that come up often in healthcare. Early detection and mitigation of these small failures could avert a large failure that causes harm. However, small failures that do not cause harm in the moment are often not corrected. Near misses such as the examples mentioned should be considered priorities that need correction instead of successes because they did not cause harm. Small failures are not easily identified but are much easier to correct than large failures.

A key factor in mindful organizing for a more emergent situation is sensemaking. Sensemaking is about assessing a situation while it is in progress and determining action from the constant and changing assessment [27]. A team focus is important in identifying concerning conditions, making sense of the potential of danger, and finding options for solutions while in the moment. An example of this in healthcare is the team response during a resuscitation event.

- A 72-year-old female patient is on the way to the bathroom when she suddenly falls to the ground. This is noticed by the telemetry observer who notices that the cardiac rhythm is slowing. The telemetry observer calls the nurse. The nurse responds first to witness the patient on the floor and helps her back up to the bed. She calls the emergency response team. The team responds and notes the bradycardia, discusses current medications the patient is on, and places the patient on an external pacemaker. Patient is transferred to the intensive care unit, and medications are adjusted. She is discharged in stable condition 3 days later.
- What were the keys to the successful outcome of this situation in a HRO?
  - Sensemaking and identification of red flag: The slowing of the cardiac rhythm clued the telemetry observer that something was not right.
  - Acting on a red flag: Calling the emergency response team, brainstorming the cause from patient information and recognizing the patient was on medications that might lower her heart rate.
  - Team discussion: Allowed for a variety of opinions from the local experts (frontline staff) on the current and changing condition.

In this situation, the outcome might have been different if the red flag was not noticed or not acknowledged. Listening to the telemetry observer's concern, considering the context of the low heart rate and a new medication and calling for other opinions contributed to the positive outcome. Sensemaking is an active process and involves listening to subtle cues, asking for a variety of opinion, considering all aspects of the situation and changing course on the spot to create a positive outcome [27]. These factors all contribute to adaptability in the face of changing conditions which is a hallmark of an HRO.

5   Safety II: Learning from Success

All models discussed previously in this chapter are different but build on each other and provide direction for nursing and patient safety as they explain how harm can occur and be avoided as shown in Fig. 2.

The Swiss Cheese Model views errors as beginning higher up within the system, making their way through weak barriers to cause harm at the frontline of care. Human factors science views errors as occurring because there is a mismatch between the system and how humans typically work within the system. High reliability views errors as occurring because of a lack of adaptability in the system and individual to unexpected situations. The common denominators within these models include humans, systems, adaptability, and failures. The last model that will be discussed focuses on all those factors, except failure.

Our final model of safety complements our prior discussion on error models but flips the mindset. Eric Hollengal [28] introduced the concept of Safety II or

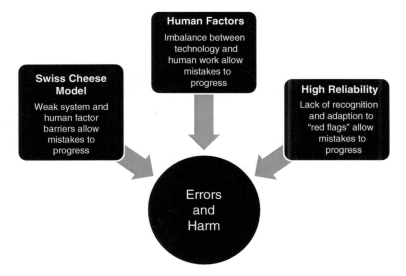

Fig. 2 Summary of how errors and harm occur from the lens of current safety models

focusing our efforts on learning how we achieve success and not how we fail. It is similar to the concept of appreciative inquiry [29], learning from a lens of capability or strength as opposed to deficit and failure. This is a change of focus for most patient safety programs as we currently begin our work when a failure occurs and not the opposite.

A key difference in Safety II is the lens in which we view people and safety. Traditionally, errors and failures get attributed to a human error by not following protocol or deviation from a set standard. Safety II realizes that people are not problems to control tightly with standards. People are problem solvers who adapt to emergent situations for which there exists no standard [30].

Hollengal compares Safety II to the traditional field of safety in which we currently operate which he calls Safety I [28]. Safety I focuses on what goes wrong and finding the cause of that failure and fixing it. Key principles of looking at safety through a Safety I lens include the following [31]:

- Safety is an absence of adverse events.
- An adverse event triggers an investigation.
- Adverse events occur because of a failure in a linear process.
- There is a root cause for every failure that can be found and corrected.
- Safety can be achieved by anticipating all expected conditions of work and adhering to standard protocols and procedures that exist for all conditions.
- Processes create safety and people should operate within existing processes.

These principles reflect a somewhat reactive process designed for use when an error occurs and remains dormant when error free. Our current safety systems traditionally measure outcomes and therefore, safety, in these terms. For example:

- "We have had 5 patient falls with injury this month"—find and fix the causes. We are not safe.
- "We have had no indwelling catheter urinary tract infections this month"—no need for action. We are safe.

Safety I has been a useful philosophy and has led to improvements such as the use of the Root Cause Analysis (RCA) and 5 Why's methods for investigation and improvement in standardizing and assuring compliance with standard processes [17]. The SCM is an example of a Safety 1 theory for which root causes lie within the layers of Swiss cheese and one only must ask "why" five times to get to the root cause. However, as critics of the SCM will state, achieving safety is not that linear or simple within a complex sociotechnical system where the unexpected is the norm and not the exception. It is impossible to anticipate all emergent conditions that might arise in our current systems and creating a system where frontline staff only have tools to deal with expected conditions is a system that is destined for failures. So, what is needed to deal with this gap?

Safety II attempts to fill this gap by recognizing that human beings at the frontline often must adapt and adjust in the moment dependent on ever-changing conditions. Variability, flexibility, and improvisation are needed when dealing with the unexpected to create positive outcomes. In comparison with Safety I, Safety II attempts to study how this adaptation is created at the frontline to learn the skills and conditions necessary to "make things go right" despite the absence of perfect conditions. Whereas traditional safety or Safety I has somewhat rigid rules and standards and does not allow for creative deviation. This leaves a gap for the unexpected events when the rules do not exist.

The main principles of Safety II include [31]:

- Safety is the presence of positive adaptations that lead to success despite adverse conditions.
- Near misses or close calls trigger an investigation.
- Adverse events can occur due to a failure of adaptation to emergent/unexpected conditions.
- There is never just one root cause of an event in a complex system.
- People at the frontline create safety by adapting to current conditions.
- Existing processes do not work for every situation.

Safety II emphasizes the positive and is proactive. Theoretically, much more can be learned from positive opportunities than negative because the former occurs more often than the latter. Dekker [32] wrote about a process which resulted in an error that was investigated. Common causes for the errors were workarounds, miscalculations, not following standards, and other common human behaviors. The solutions included the traditional reinforcement of the standards and avoidance of workarounds. Alternatively, the same process was investigated, many times it was completed without an error and surprisingly, the same human behaviors were found, including the workaround and not following standards. The point of Dekker's story was that the same issues caused failure or success, however, he did find differences in the two investigations. The successful process had several more social/cultural characteristics that the error process did not. For example:

- Variety of opinion and the ability to speak up or disagree
- Discussing risk at all times; not taking routine tasks for granted
- Ability to stop the process or stop the line for a safety issue
- Deference to expertise or deferring to the person with the most knowledge
- No barriers between disciplines, departments, or traditional hierarchy
- Creativity to adapt a process
- Pride in workmanship and the product

Notably these characteristics are similar to those found in HROs. The focus for success is not learning how people cause failures but how they create success. The key to this approach is recognizing that studying how human beings work to create safety is just as important as investigating process failures.

An example of Safety II in action was the response of hospitals and healthcare facilities to the global pandemic of 2020. There were no existing protocols to guide

Table 4 Work as done versus work as imagined [28, 31]

	Practical definition	Impact to safety
Work as imagined	How those outside of the frontline imagine how the work is done	Standards do not always fit to unexpected situations and when not created by those at the frontline do not fit within the complexity of work
Work as done	The work done at the frontline with adaptations to achieve expected outcomes	Adaptations can be done to create safety or can lead to shortcuts that are a detriment to safety. Contributing factors to successful adaptations need to be supported and work that cannot be adapted needs to be identified

us through this emergent situation. What we relied on was the expertise, innovation, collaboration, and resilience of teams within these facilities to create dynamic processes that worked to keep communities safe. This type of adaptation is created by empowered frontline workers acting to create safety in real time without a guideline or an existing framework to follow. Facilitating this resilience is the power of Safety II.

5.1   Work as Done Versus Work as Imagined

A focus on the work as completed at the frontline is a key concept in understanding Safety II. Traditional healthcare systems operate with an abundance of procedures and protocols to manage and control the work that is being done. However, these policies and procedures often do not match what is happening at the user interface. Policies and procedures created by designers of work specify the "work as imagined" and attempt to create a process to follow for every imagined possibility. "Work as done" is what happens when these documents meet the user at the "sharp end" and they often do not fit all the situations imagined by the designers [31]. Consequently, those at the frontline then need to adapt work to meet outcomes and deadlines successfully. Take note, that this does not mean frontline workers do not follow safety protocols; it means that they adapt to achieve safety even if the protocol does not fit perfectly as summarized in Table 4.

5.2   Implementation of Safety II Concepts

Safety II is not as radical as it seems and may be already something that exists but needs intentionality to create change. Suggestions to implement Safety II concepts include the following:

- Ask different questions [33]
  - Instead of always asking what went wrong, ask about near misses and how an error was avoided.
  - Ask staff how they adapt to production pressure or high turnover times to assure safe care in the allotted time frame.

- Practice a true deference to expertise [33]
  - Review and match workplace standards and policies to the actual way the work is done to identify imbalance and mitigate risks.
  - Test processes and revise with input by frontline staff prior to implementation.
  - Ask for a variety of opinion for every situation and assure all voices are heard.
- Review successful or simulated high-risk cases and point out strengths to be promoted and reinforced [34]
  - Focus on how anticipation of failure, situational awareness, and questioning attitude lead to success in high-risk situations.
  - Search for contributing factors to the success of a situation dependent on teamwork and communication.
- Make proactive thinking a habit [27]
  - Promote tools and practice simulation to increase situational awareness and sensemaking in real time.
  - Make anticipation of error a habit.
- Examine the idea that safety is the presence of "capacity" [30]
  - Capacity is the ability to adapt to disruptions.
  - Identify resources available in time of crisis.
  - Focus on skills that promote empowerment of those on the frontline.

Most importantly, learn from the ideas, creativity, and adaptability of those people who work on the frontline. They are the key to patient safety.

6   The Way Forward: Nurses Lead Patient Safety with the Power of Safety Science

The presence or not of safety is often illusive and not well defined. It is difficult to quantify safety in a healthcare system without discussing the metrics that we feel are an indication of safety. Consider the Leapfrog Hospital Safety Grade in the United States. The Leapfrog organization [33, 35] focuses on measuring patient safety and assigns grades to hospitals (A, B, C, D, F) based on patient safety metrics such as numbers of hospital acquired conditions and the presence of factors that enhance safety such as prioritizing hand hygiene and having certain policies focused on safety. Hospitals that receive an A grade are considered the safest hospitals for which to receive care and lower grades are accordingly not as safe in this grading system.

The measurement model of confirming safety by a safety metric is typically how we measure safety in healthcare. This is generally accepted by all in the field of healthcare; however, it can cause us to rely on these numbers to represent the presence or not of "safety" and forget that these metrics depend on processes and cultural conditions to support safety. As we have discussed in this chapter, safety in healthcare is more than a number or a grade. Safety is created by people who influence systems and processes every minute of the day in high-risk situations. Safety is created by adapting in the moment with expertise and intention. Nurses, specifically, are one of the largest groups with constant contact at the "sharp end" who create safety.

The models we have discussed range from a reactive, somewhat linear model that describes how errors can cause patient harm to a more proactive model which focuses on adaptation and resilience. All models are useful in the healthcare context for nursing. Notably, missing from these models is the effect of diversity and equality and how this contributes to safety events and safety progress. Considering all the models and information presented, nurses, as leaders of patient safety should focus on the following from each area discussed:

- History of safety and lack of sustainable progress
  - Acknowledge that true achievement of safety is not just a metric but it is in what people at the frontline do every day.
  - Thus, safety accountability lies with the systems and cultures that we create and reinforce with our actions.
  - Creation of systems and cultures that reinforce safety should be informed by collaboration with safety science.
- Swiss Cheese Model
  - Application of the SCM to understand how errors begin higher up in the system and only reach a patient to cause harm if barriers are not in place.
  - These barriers can be processes and policies but most often it is frontline staff at the "sharp end" identifying an issue and stopping the process from continuing.
- Human Factors Engineering
  - Apply theory of human factors and use human factors engineers whenever possible to assure that new projects and technology are evaluated from an end user lens.
  - Use a list of human factors when evaluating any error. Asking questions about distraction, fatigue, environmental conditions can identify contributing issues that need to be optimized.
  - Remember that technology is a machine and people are the ones who evaluate the output and make the decisions.
- Highly Reliable Organizations
  - Practice anticipation of errors by asking "What if…?" questions.
  - Look at the structure and communication in teams and identify which voices are heard and which are not. Variety of opinions and ability to ask questions is important.
  - Prepare for the unexpected by increasing capacity and ability to problem solve at the frontline.
- Safety II
  - Ask different questions to provide learning on how success is created in everyday work.
  - Create programs that support reporting near misses and close calls.

- Review and simulate high-risk situations and what processes are critical for a positive outcome.
- Review processes to assure that they can reasonably be completed at the frontline and if not, assure that safe adaptations and resources are available for unexpected situations.

7   Summary

In closing, patient safety is not in its infancy but there is still so much to be realized as to the conditions necessary to achieve safe patient care. The models discussed in this chapter give context to where patient safety began and where it needs to go for improvement. The focus on metrics and the absence of adverse events as our only measures of safety does not tell the complete story. The presence of safety is more about people, expertise, sensemaking, collaboration, freely speaking up, and adapting to situations that could not be imagined. Therefore, safety can only be realized in how we collaborate within teams and at the frontline.

Achievement of patient safety is not an objective feature that an organization has, it is more an outcome of what the organization and the individuals within it do every day and in every second to recognize and prevent error. It is an action and an intention in everything we do and cannot take a back seat to other measures. The intention of this chapter was to gain insight into the history of safety science with application to the role of nursing. The chapters contained within this book will give further examples of the role of nursing in applying this science within the scope and passion of nursing to improve outcomes worldwide.

Key Points

- Patient safety is not in its infancy but still has not achieved the potential that is needed to prevent patient harm.
- A contributing factor to this lack of improvement is a failure to use and apply safety science consistently.
- The presence of patient safety is most often defined by metrics; however, it is much more than that.
- The Swiss Cheese Model is the basic model of patient safety that describes how errors travel from system causes to human failure to cause harm unless a reliable barrier halts the process.
- Human factors engineering, highly reliable organizations theory, and Safety II are among the most robust safety science models that can be used to understand how people at the frontline problem solve to effectively create those barriers.
- Current patient safety practice focuses on failures and does not engage unless there is a failure.
- Learning from successes will give more insight on how adaptations occur and under what conditions foster positive adaptations.

- Bringing the focus back to how people interact within the complexity of a highly sociotechnical organization to adapt and adjust is imperative to safety.
- Nursing coupled with the power of their expertise and situated at the frontline of care is in a prime position to lead this journey.

References

1. Nightingale F. Notes on nursing: what it is and what it is not. London: Harrison and Sons; 1859. (Commemorative addition, 1992, Lippincott Williams and Wilkins, Philadelphia).
2. World Health Organization. (2019). Fact Sheet Patient Safety. Patient Safety (who.int).
3. AHRQ. Measurement of patient safety. Measurement of patient safety I PSNet. 2019. ahrq.gov.
4. Leape L. Error in medicine. JAMA. 1994;272(23):1851–7.
5. Institute of Medicine (US) Committee on Quality of Health Care in America. In: Kohn LT, Corrigan JM, Donaldson MS, editors. To err is human: building a safer health system. National Academies Press (US); 2000.
6. Wears R, Sutcliffe K. Still not safe: patient safety and the middle-managing of American medicine. 2019. https://doi.org/10.1093/oso/9780190271268.001.0001.
7. Millenson ML. Pushing the profession: how the news media turned patient safety into a priority. BMJ Qual Saf. 2002;11:57–63.
8. Stelfox HT, Palmisani S, Scurlock C, et al. The "to err is human" report and the patient safety literature. BMJ Qual Saf. 2006;15:174–8.
9. AAMC. 20 years of patient safety. AAMC news 20 years of patient safety I AAMC. 2019.
10. James JT. A new, evidence-based estimate of patient harms associated with hospital care. J Patient Saf. 2013;9(3):122–8. https://doi.org/10.1097/PTS.0b013e3182948a69.
11. Panagioti M, Khan K, Keers RN, Abuzour A, Phipps D, Kontopantelis E, Bower P, Campbell S, Haneef R, Avery AJ, Ashcroft DM. Prevalence, severity, and nature of preventable patient harm across medical care settings: systematic review and meta-analysis. BMJ (Clin Res Ed). 2019;366:l4185. https://doi.org/10.1136/bmj.l4185.
12. Bates DW, Levine DM, Salmasian H, Syrowatka A, Shahian DM, Lipsitz S, Zebrowski JP, Myers LC, Logan MS, Roy CG, Iannaccone C, Frits ML, Volk LA, Dulgarian S, Amato MG, Edrees HH, Sato L, Folcarelli P, Einbinder JS, Reynolds ME, Mort E. The safety of inpatient health care. N Engl J Med. 2023;388(2):142–53. https://doi.org/10.1056/NEJMsa2206117.
13. Berwick D. Constancy of purpose for improving patient safety-missing in action. NEJM. 2023;388(2). Constancy of purpose for improving patient safety—missing in action. cdn-website.com.
14. New England Journal of Medicine Catalyst. Lessons from health care leaders: rethinking and reinvesting in patient safety. NEJM Catalyst. 2023.
15. Leapfrog Group. New Leapfrog Hospital Safety Grade Reveals Significant Increase in Healthcare-Associated Infections and Worsening Patient Experience During COVID-19 Pandemic I Leapfrog; 2023. leapfroggroup.org.
16. Reason JT. Human error. Cambridge, England: Cambridge University Press; 1990.
17. Braaten JS, Nattrass L. Root cause analysis: a tool for high reliability in a complex environment. In: Oster CA, Braaten JS, editors. High reliability organizations: a healthcare handbook for patient safety & quality, 2e. McGraw Hill; 2021. https://apn.mhmedical.com/content.aspx?bookid=3152&sectionid=264987739.
18. Rasmussen J. Skills, rules, and knowledge; signals, signs, and symbols, and other distinctions in human performance models. IEEE Transactions on Systems, Man, & Cybernetics. 1983;SMC-13(3):257–66. https://doi.org/10.1109/TSMC.1983.6313160.
19. Larouzee, LaCuz. Good and bad reasons: the Swiss cheese model and its critics. Saf Sci. 2020;126(2020):104660. https://doi.org/10.1016/j.ssci.2020.104660.

20. Wiegmann DA, Wood LJ, Cohen TN, Shappell SA. Understanding the "Swiss cheese model" and its application to patient safety. J Patient Saf. 2022;18(2):119–23. https://doi.org/10.1097/PTS.0000000000000810.
21. HFES. What is Human Factors and Ergonomics | HFES. Accessed 23 Sept 2023. https://www.hfes.org/About-HFES/What-is-Human-Factors-and-Ergonomics
22. FAA The Human Factors "Dirty Dozen" | SKYbrary Aviation. https://skybrary.aero/articles/human-factors-dirty-dozen
23. Trist E, Bamforth K. Some social and psychological consequences of the long wall method of coal-getting. Hum Relat. 1951;1:3–38.
24. Maio D, (Dr.), Paola. Towards a metamodel to support the joint optimization of socio technical systems. Systems. 2014;2:273–96. https://doi.org/10.3390/systems2030273.
25. Weick KE, Sutcliffe KM. Managing the unexpected: assuring high performance in an age of complexity. San Francisco, CA: Jossey-Bass, a John Wiley & Sons; 2001.
26. Weick KE, Sutcliffe KM. Managing the unexpected: resilient performance in an age of uncertainty. 2nd ed. San Francisco: Jossey-Bass; 2007.
27. Weick KE, Sutcliffe KM. Managing the unexpected. Sustained performance in a complex world. 3rd ed. Wiley; 2015.
28. Hollnagel E. Safety-I and safety-II: the past and future of safety management. CRC Press; 2018.
29. Cooperrider D. Retrieved from on 5 July 2023 from What is Appreciative Inquiry? http://www.davidcooperrider.com/ai-process/
30. Dekker S. Safety differently: human factors for a new era. Boca Raton: CRC Press, Taylor & Francis Group; 2015.
31. Dong-Han H. Safety-II and resilience engineering in a nutshell: an introductory guide to their concepts and methods. Saf Health Work. 2020;12(1). https://www.sciencedirect.com/science/article/pii/S2093791120303619.
32. Dekker S. SafetyDifferently.com. Why do things go right? Safety differently. 2018.
33. Dekker S, Conklin T. Do safety differently. Santa Fe, NM: Pre-Accident Media; 2022.
34. Bentley SK, McNamara S, Meguerdichian M, et al. Debrief it all: a tool for inclusion of safety-II. Adv Simul. 2021;6:9. https://doi.org/10.1186/s41077-021-00163-3.
35. Leapfrog Hospital Safety Grade | Leapfrog. leapfroggroup.org.

Culture of Safety: What Is It and What It Is Not

Gail Armstrong

1 Introduction

Since the Institute of Medicine's (IOM) call to improve patient safety outcomes in 2000, there has been a variety of work to improve patient safety outcomes [1]. In 2022 data suggest that there have been notable improvements in the safe delivery of care for patients admitted to the hospital for acute myocardial infarction, hear failure, pneumonia, and major surgical procedures [2]. There has been a wide variety of interventions and studies to improve patient safety. While implementation of safety interventions and strategies based on best practices or robust evidence has been shown to be effective, the culture or context of the microsystem of care has been repeatedly found to be an important variable in improving patient safety. Safety culture not only impacts the explicitly visible elements of a clinical setting, but it also shapes the components that are not as visible, that are "not said" or reflected only in symbolic actions [3]. Creating a microsystem culture that works toward recognizing safety challenges and implementing sustainable solutions are key elements of a culture of safety [4]. This chapter will define, outline criteria for, and discuss measurement of a culture of safety in an organization.

G. Armstrong (✉)
University of Colorado Anschutz Medical Campus, College of Nursing, Aurora, CO, USA
e-mail: Gail.Armstrong@cuanschutz.edu

© The Author(s), under exclusive license to Springer Nature
Switzerland AG 2024
C. A. Oster, J. S. Braaten (eds.), *The Nexus between Nursing and Patient Safety*,
https://doi.org/10.1007/978-3-031-53158-3_2

2   Structure: Background

2.1   Definition of Culture of Safety

The idea of safety culture has been used for more than three decades, yet an agreed upon definition has been elusive. The foundation of the term "safety culture" and conceptual starting point originated from the 1988 report by the International Nuclear Advisory Safety Group (INSAG) examining the 1986 Chernobyl disaster [5]. Before IOM's clarion call for safety as a priority in healthcare, safety culture was loosely described in high-risk industries to be a corporate atmosphere where safety is collectively appreciated and accepted as the number one priority [6]. The appeal for safety culture is explicit in *To Err Is Human* [7]: "Health care organizations must develop a culture of safety such that an organization's care processes and workforce are focused on improving the reliability and safety of care for patients" (p. 14). Soon after *To Err Is Human*, a lengthy definition of safety culture was offered that included several distinguishing elements that have persisted in the literature: "Safety culture is the product of individual and group values, attitudes, perceptions, competencies, and patterns of behavior that determine the commitment to, and the style and proficiency of an organization's safety management [5, p. 12]."

A decade after *To Err Is Human*, a comprehensive review of the literature found little agreement in how safety culture is defined in healthcare. Sammer et al. offer seven subcultures that are vital to consider when improving safety culture: leadership, teamwork, evidence-base, communication, learning, justice, and patient centeredness [8]. A concurrently occurring literature review similarly found disagreement among researchers as to how safety culture is defined [9]. A more recent literature review (2019) examined the relationships and connections between patient safety, safety culture, and quality of care outcomes. These authors discovered inconsistencies in phrasing, varying use of a theoretical framework, minimal attention to validity of instruments, and significant methodological variations [10].

The most important federal agency that funds patient safety work, the Agency for Healthcare Research and Quality (AHRQ), offers specific key features that characterize an effective culture of safety. Instead of defining elements of an established safety culture, AHRQ focuses on features that contribute to the development of safety culture in healthcare. These contributors include the clear recognition of the high-risk nature of an organization's activities, a blame-free environment that encourages individuals to report errors or near misses, the support of interprofessional collaboration regardless of rank to find safety solutions and an organizational commitment of resources to address safety concerns [11].

The lack of agreement about a safety culture definition is understandable with the explosion of literature. A recent review of the volume of articles exploring safety culture identifies the earliest reference being in 1978, and 1675 articles focusing on safety culture published in 2018 [12]. Despite elusive agreement on the concept of safety culture, a 2021 review found that safety culture is commonly identified as a contributor to safety lapses in various high-risk industries yet the link between safety culture and poor safety outcomes is highly inconsistent [12]. Bisbey et al.'s model conceptualizes safety culture as being impacted by enabling factors (leadership's commitment and prioritization of safety, policies, and resources for safety, cohesion, psychological safety, safety knowledge and skills, and sense of control) and by enacting behaviors (communication and information exchange, teamwork, incident reporting and fair rewards/punishment) [12]. An update to this model (given the name, The Safer Culture Framework) further explores and refines the impact of enabling factors that create the necessary norms, values, and assumptions for a safety culture to develop, and enacting behaviors that are the consequences of safety culture, or the behaviors that individuals engage in as a result of their assumptions, values, and collective norms [13].

Recent thinking has also explored the impact of effective safety culture on healthcare costs. When the phenomenon of safety culture is considered through the lens of value-based healthcare, value-based care models can broaden the understanding of safety culture. As preventable adverse events can be increasingly avoided, so too the costs associated with safety lapses are avoided [14].

Adaptation of safety culture models to specific clinical contexts illustrates how the emphases of model elements differ, depending on the needs of that clinical setting. A recent literature review to investigate the application of safety culture to Emergency Department (ED) care identified a handful of relevant articles with similar themes. A conceptual framework specifically for safety culture in the ED identified ten significant elements, with teamwork, managerial expectations around safety and organizational learning being the three most important dimensions [15]. These conceptual elements make sense given the complex, high acuity condition of ED patients, the unpredictability and rapid pace of the ED environment, and the multidisciplinary team that experiences frequent hand-offs.

In light of the high volume of literature being published on safety culture, and the historic disagreement in models or definitions, it is vital that healthcare leaders who aspire to improve safety culture start their work with clear definitions and utilization of a well-researched model. With operational clarity in definitions and conceptual assumption, a healthcare leader is better poised for success in improving safety culture in a microsystem, mesosystem, or macrosystem.

2.2 The Impact of a Culture of Safety

With the recent significant increase in literature exploring the impact of safety culture, exemplary studies will be highlighted. Most high-risk industries (e.g., aviation, nuclear energy, and healthcare) have had a sustained interest in quantifying the impact of safety culture. A recent 2022 study examined the impact of corporate culture on accidents in high-risk industries associated with construction. Corporate cultures and workplace environments that had a clear priority on safety significantly reduced industrial accidents among workers [16]. Another study outside of healthcare examined whether psychosocial hazards are impacted by safety culture. Psychosocial hazards are occupational hazards that affect a worker's psychological state and impact their ability to safely contribute to the work. A higher level of safety culture environment improves workers' safety performance by reducing their psychosocial hazards [17].

Research specific to the impact of safety culture in healthcare reveals that safety culture offers significant benefits. A recent study across 29 units of five hospitals found that higher ratings of safety culture were associated with fewer incidents of missed nursing care, and missed nursing care was associated with falls, an important patient safety outcome [18]. Similarly enhanced safety culture has been found to be correlated with increased adherence to evidence-based practices in hemodialysis, resulting in lower infection rates and improved patient outcomes [19].

As safety culture is implemented in healthcare settings with specific clinical emphases, distinct aspects of safety culture may be highlighted. When applied in several burn units with 213 providers, the safety culture standard of no punitive responses to error was particularly important. Given the high complexity and great vulnerability of burn patients, providers emphasized the need for protection from punishment when reporting errors [20]. In the care of intrapartum patients, safety culture standards specific to teamwork were most important. In a survey of 184 providers of intrapartum patients, perceptions of effective teamwork were closely correlated to views of a unit's safety culture [21]. Similarly in a survey of perioperative healthcare teams, teamwork within the operating room (OR) was identified as correlated to safety culture. OR teams that had high teamwork scores also assessed themselves as having strong safety culture [22].

In more general care settings, understanding which interventions contribute to stronger safety culture can be helpful. A literature review examining which improvement strategies effectively improve safety culture in primary care revealed a wide array of practices. Because of the variety of improvement strategies in primary care, no clear correlation can be identified. Further research is needed to help primary care practices make an evidence-based choice for effective interventions to increase safety culture [23].

At times the larger community context is highly influential in how healthcare teams experience safety culture. In a study of 403 registered nurses, surveys assessing safety culture were completed before the COVID-19 pandemic and after the third wave of the global pandemic. Twelve dimensions of safety culture were assessed; every dimension had fewer positive responses except for teamwork within units. Although nurses experienced overall lower safety culture during the stresses of the COVID-19 pandemic, these pressures resulted in stronger teamwork within a unit [24].

3   Process: Tools for Success

Culture is a vital component when considering the effectiveness of patient safety improvements, as the context of values, beliefs, assumptions, and norms impact how improvements are perceived, accepted (or not), implemented (or not), and sustained (or not). As the Safer Culture Framework suggests enabling factors contribute to creating clear cultural norms that support the necessary practices of effective safety culture [13].

3.1 Psychological Safety

A key enabling factor contributing to safety culture is healthcare team members' experiences of hierarchy on healthcare teams. Different educational models across various disciplines, compounded by vastly different professional identity formation processes contribute to more or less reliance on hierarchy by healthcare team members. Psychological safety is a term used to describe whether there is the perception of a steep hierarchy on a team or in a system, or whether this hierarchy has been flattened. Psychological safety is how safe a person perceives the interpersonal environment to speak up if they witness an error or need to ask for help [25]. Collectively, psychological safety is a shared team belief that one will not be reprimanded, punished, or embarrassed for speaking up, sharing ideas, posing questions, raising concerns, or making mistakes [26–29]. Psychological safety is created by values and behaviors of both leaders and lateral team members. Exploration of what kind of culture contributes to psychological safety found the importance of leadership. Leadership practices such as leadership inclusiveness, trustworthiness, openness to change, and ethical leadership can promote a psychologically safe environment [30]. Team training can support psychological safe collective norms. A structured teamwork training for cardiothoracic surgery teams resulted in an increase in psychological safety [31].

What disrupts psychological safety is rude, disruptive, or aggressive (RDA) behavior. This problematic behavior often relies on one's rank in a discipline or in the healthcare hierarchy. An examination of RDA communication between physicians revealed this loss of trust is damaging behavior and experienced as a personal violation and can result in emotional distress, substance abuse, and professional demotivation [32]. Recent research supports that disruptive physician behavior damages team morale by creating a psychological unsafe working environment [33]. Because psychological safety is a foundational phenomenon for strong safety culture, it is vital to address any contributors that violate the basic trust of psychological safety.

3.2 Just Culture

Psychological safety can be a part of a system-level phenomenon of Just Culture. Historically errors have been associated with name (identifying who was involved with the error), blame (identifying who was responsible for the error), and shame (punishing those were involved with an error). This punitive model leads to healthcare workers lying about errors, secrecy about mistakes, and significant reluctance to report errors.

Sidney Dekker has long written about implementation of Just Culture in healthcare. Dekker differentiates traditional (retributive) responses to error that focus on punishment from updated Just Culture that focused on restoration. Rather than focusing on which rule was broken, or who is to blame, or how severe is the violation, a restorative approach seeks to understand who is hurt, what is needed and who is the best person to meet these needs [34]. Dekker identified clear incentives for implementing updated Just Culture models, including leadership's ability to respond to real-time data and monitor the safety of an organization [34].

Just Culture is becoming more common in health systems, where error analysis is not solely about identifying individuals at fault but prioritizes understanding how an error occurred. A just culture paradigm encourages a standard of accountability—it is neither punitive nor blame-free. Just culture shifts the focus from errors and outcomes to examining how to improve system design to avoid the recurrence of an error [35].

Just Culture is essential for strong safety culture, as being open about errors is necessary to address patient safety issues. A conceptual analysis that breaks down Just Culture identified six core dimensions necessary for just culture: balance, trust, openness of communication, quality of the event reporting process, feedback and communication about events, and overall goal of continuous improvement [36].

Just Culture is a crucial antecedent to effective safety culture. Inherent to Just Culture is the trust that data and error information will be used to improve a system and not punish the healthcare team. If trust is not reliable, there may be minimal reporting and limited discussion of errors and system gaps [37]. With inconsistent or unpredictable reporting of errors, learning opportunities are missed. Other explorations of the connections between Just Culture and safety culture identify the complexity of safety culture. Many factors contribute to safety culture; a recent narrative review of the literature prioritized the attention by leaders to establishing Just Culture as crucial for effective safety culture [38]. An analysis of Just Culture and safety culture in the perioperative environment identified Just Culture as a pillar of safety culture, and identified the necessary components as psychological safety, leadership responsibility, staff member responsibility, and staff member empowerment [39]. Similarly, a recent conceptual analysis of safety culture emphasizes the necessity of Just Culture in building organizational trust. This trust supports reporting of errors so that system gaps can be addressed [40]. With Just Culture and the uninhibited reporting of errors, healthcare teams can work toward developing a safety culture that effectively addresses gaps.

Dekker provides key points to remember when implementing Just Culture. Understanding the complex context of healthcare is vital as a single account is only a part of the picture. Dekker emphasizes how no one account provides all of the necessary details [34]. Compromise is the core of effective Just Culture. Disclosure is an important part of Just Culture as well. Once a practitioner or team discloses an error or near miss, the system is obligated to protect those individuals. Responding to an error or near miss in a proportionally appropriate manner (e.g., not overreacting) is crucial to effective Just Culture [34].

3.3   Reporting Systems

Establishing Just Culture so healthcare team members feel safe enough to be willing to report errors is a preliminary step in effective safety culture. Willingness to report errors needs to then lead to actual reporting of errors. Incident reports have the potential to provide insights into safety lapses that have led to patient harm and can facilitate the development of preventative strategies [41]. However, reporting systems, or incident reporting systems (IRS), are notoriously complex, burdensome, and not user friendly. Well-documented challenges in IRS include low engagement by staff (especially physicians), information overload due to unselective reporting, failure to generate useful improvements, and the faulty use of incident reporting data to trend safety over time [42]. Even though the aim of IRS is to promote learning and to improve patient safety, these goals are compromised by the acute variability of the data reported and low volume of incidents reported [42]. A survey of 220 radiation oncologists focused on safety culture and incident reporting systems. Even when a positive safety culture was indicated, participants were reluctant to submit incident reports because "it takes too long." Along with the complexity of multiple reporting systems, there was varied understanding of which incidents to report, and when incidents should be reported [43]. Recent research indicates that early career physicians are more likely to report safety incidents if reporting building blocks are established early in their practice as physicians. A successful curriculum with pediatric residents included providing the necessary education to identify medical errors with an emphasis on systems-based causes, modeling of error reporting by faculty, and integrating error reporting and discussion into the residents' daily activities [44]. An integrative review of more than 10,000 articles examined barriers nurses experience in reporting errors and identified several common themes. The main themes and subthemes identified were organizational barriers (poor reporting systems, lack of support by managers, and unclear definition of medication error), and professional and individual barriers (fear of blame by management and colleagues in the form of a lawsuit, and inadequate knowledge of errors) [45].

3.4   Blame-Free Reporting

Despite efforts of a clinical organization that establishes Just Culture and values safety culture, several barriers exist to incident reporting. A commonly referenced barrier to reporting safety lapses is the potential for being penalized for involvement in care that results in an error. Providers and healthcare team members worry that submission of an incident report puts them at increased risk if a patient or family takes legal action. Legal concerns that contribute to underreporting include fear of professionals being involved in lawsuits because of the lack of specific regulations that protect them, fear of being sued if information from an incident report is obtained, the threat to a professional's reputation, the perception of guilt by colleagues and fear of error analysts being summoned as witnesses to testify about the facts of a case [46]. Blame-free systems do not yet exist. Recommendations to move IRS closer to blame-free focus on systems shift to address the criminalization of medial error. Clearly distinguishing, in terms of legal definitions, between medical error and malpractice may contribute to providers feeling less concerned about legal actions. Additionally prioritizing confidentiality and strong data encryption systems may assist healthcare team members in feeling that data from IRS are less likely to be shared [46]. Similar findings were reported in a study focusing on reporting of safety incidents in nursing homes. Building an IRS that focuses on reducing system barriers and reporting obstacles would contribute to a non-punitive, more effective patient safety culture in nursing homes [47].

3.5   Encouragement to Report near Misses

Capturing data related to near-miss events offers an excellent opportunity to assess patient safety lapses. A near miss is defined as a healthcare event that might have had an adverse outcome but did not. The avoidance of harm may be because of chance, or a person or circumstance intervened [3].

Data associated with near-miss events shed a valuable spotlight on patient safety conditions. Although harm to a patient was avoided, a near miss indicates that hazardous conditions or unsafe practice persist. The no-harm nature of near-miss events often decreases healthcare professionals' sense of urgency in reporting, yet these events are ripe for significant individual, team, and system learning. Research about near-miss event reporting is particularly fertile because a recent tragedy has been averted, and with remedy, a future tragedy may be avoided [48]. Reporting of near misses may indicate a strong safety culture because members of the healthcare team voluntarily report what could have evolved into an adverse event.

3.6   Good Catch Programs

One strategy to counterbalance healthcare teams' fear of being punished for errors or near misses is to incentivize reporting near misses. Good Catch Programs reward or publicly praise a healthcare team member for reporting a near miss. Rewarding staff can encourage Good Catch submissions and provide more opportunities to improve patient safety [49]. As early as 2008 hospital systems were reporting implementation of Good Catch Programs [50]. Beyond encouraging reporting of near misses, Good Catch Programs can lead to sustainable improvement over time. In a 16 operating room inpatient/outpatient cancer center, a patient safety reporting process included Good Catch Awards. In this program, 29 patient safety hazards were identified, each of which led to a unique initiative to address the original hazard. Even after several years, more than 85% of the quality improvements have been sustained [51]. Accurate tracking of the types of near misses also improves the usability of the data collected. One hospital system divided Good Catch cases into quality improvement-based categories (processes, medication, safety, communication, and equipment) [52]. Good Catch Programs are also found to be a valuable strategy in nursing education. Incorporating a Good Catch Program into nursing education simulations lays down an early foundation for nurses to report near misses [53]. With large scope implementation, Good Catch Programs can net impressive increase in near-miss reporting. A large pediatric health care system increased the number of safety event reports from 4668 in fiscal year 2014 to 10,971 safety event reports in fiscal year 2017 [54].

3.7   Transparency

Part of the reason Good Catch Programs can be so effective in contributing to and supporting safety culture is because they make public unsafe conditions or safety concerns, which traditionally has not been encouraged. This shift to transparency is important for safety culture as it modifies the collective norms around safety gaps. In response to a surgical service suffering from preventable errors, one large academic health center reported utilizing increased transparency through quality dashboards. Surgeon-specific transparent dashboards were created to share individual surgical outcomes with each other as well as develop a financial quality incentive that would be based on clinical outcomes and are reviewed transparently on a quarterly basis [55]. With transparent sharing of quality data, providers and healthcare team members can begin to trust that safety lapses, or safety concerns will not be punished, chastised, or subjected to discipline. Safety culture is inherently built on trust, and interventions that contribute to transparency around safety data to strengthen safety culture.

Intentionally encouraging transparency within a healthcare team and system is equally important for patients and families who often feel like they are on the outside of the healthcare team. For more than a decade, evidence has been building in how disclosures about errors to patients and families are much more effective than secrecy or denial. Transparent disclosure reduces the reported likelihood of changing physicians and increases patient satisfaction, trust, and positive emotional response [56]. Similar to systematic sharing of quality data on a team to support transparency, disclosure to patients and families should occur in a systematic way that ensures honesty and transparency regarding the care that has been provided [57]. "By rejecting the old paradigm of silence and secrecy following an adverse event and making open disclosure of adverse events to patients and their families a part of the routine practice of medicine, real transparency can be promoted. Transparency is the foundation for trust between patient and provider and is also necessary for organizational learning, which is the basis for improving the safety of health care organizations for the patients they serve" [58, p. 175–176].

3.8   Safety Huddles

Another effective approach to strengthening safety culture is to adopt regularly recurring practices that are based on psychological safety, Just Culture, blame-free reporting, and transparency; safety huddles are such a practice. Although standardization of safety huddle models is lacking, there are data that safety huddles positively impact safety culture. A large study (five hospitals, 92 units) implemented daily safety huddles to discuss threats to patient safety and actions to mitigate risk. Patient safety huddles were successfully embedded in 64 units, where repeated measurement of teamwork and safety climate increased [59]. As an intervention to support safety culture, safety huddles can be implemented in a variety of practice settings. Embedding daily safety huddles was recently studied on a psychiatric inpatient unit with a multidisciplinary team. Near-miss reporting increased across time points. Patient satisfaction with staff teamwork significantly increased over time. Healthcare team member satisfaction and perception of work group communication, collaboration, and psychological safety scores are improved [60].

Due to the variability in huddle models and implementation, safety huddles are a ripe area for needed research. Although improvement work using safety huddles is promising, the evidence lacks consistency. A systematic literature review examined scheduled, multidisciplinary, hospital-based safety huddles. This review of more than 1000 articles revealed a dearth of consistent high-quality, peer-reviewed evidence about the effectiveness of hospital-wide safety huddles. There is an acute need for more research focusing on huddle program design and implementation fidelity [61].

4 Outcome

4.1 Measurement of Safety Culture

Although there are practices that support the presence of safety culture, safety culture is not tied to one specific practice or standard. Safety culture is the result of collective values, beliefs, and assumptions about patient safety as a priority within a specific practice environment. Recommendations on assessing safety culture encourage the use of reliable and valid survey tools [62]. Survey tools are the dominant methodology because of the practicality, time-efficiency, and ability to gather large amounts of data in a reliable and reproducible manner [63]. To ensure high response rates to safety culture questionnaires, key factors include mode of administration, questionnaire length, and timing of administration [64].

Assessment of safety culture focuses on capturing different facets of this phenomenon. A well-used tool that focuses on Just Culture (the Just Culture Assessment Tool) includes six subscales that measure important components of safety culture: blame-free approach with accountability, feedback and communication, openness of communication, quality of the event reporting process, continuous improvement, and trust [36].

Rather than focusing on one intervention to improve safety outcomes, measuring perception of safety culture is a common objective. A recent systematic review of 14 years of published research on measuring the perception of safety culture revealed increased interest in this assessment. Five measurement tools were predominantly used, and critical factors impacting the perception of safety culture are consistently teamwork and organizational learning [65].

4.2   Safety Culture Survey Tools

The safety culture literature clusters around five commonly used tools to measure safety culture. The Hospital Survey on Patient Safety Culture (HSOPSC) was released by the Agency for Healthcare Research and Quality (AHRQ) in 2004 to help hospitals assess the safety culture within their organization. The HSOPSC contains 42 items and is designed to measure 12 dimensions of patient safety culture [66]. The HSOPSC tool is one of the most widely used assessments for measuring safety culture in hospitals. Recent utilization of the HSOPSC in the Middle East suggests that international use of this tool requires attention to the demands of the care settings, the target population, and consideration of the national and local healthcare contexts [67]. The HSOPSC tool is available on the AHRQ website: https://www.ahrq.gov/sops/surveys/hospital/index.html.

Manchester Patient Safety Framework (MaPSaF) is another tool that measures safety culture. Originally intended to be used in primary care, it is now used in a variety of clinical settings. Nine dimensions were identified through which safety culture is expressed. These dimensions include overall commitment to quality, priority given to patient safety, perceptions of the cause of patient safety incidents, investigating patient safety incidents, organizational learning, communication about safety incidents personnel management, staff education, and teamwork. The resulting framework conceptualizes patient safety culture as multidimensional and dynamic and seems to have a high level of face validity and utility within primary care [68]. The MaPSaF tool is available on AHRQ's Patient Safety Network website: https://psnet.ahrq.gov/issue/manchester-patient-safety-framework-mapsaf

The Veterans Health Administration the largest healthcare system in the US, developed its own Patient Safety Culture Survey (VHA-PSCS). Recent re-examination of this tool reduced the questions from 34 items to 20 items, with four subscales: (1) Risk identification and just culture; (2) Error transparency and mitigation; (3) Supervisor communication and trust; (4) Team cohesion and engagement. As a large healthcare system where one of their practice pillars is safety culture, the VHA-PSCS is useful in benchmarking and comparing progress across the organization [69].

The Safety Attitudes Questionnaire (SAQ) was released in 2006 after extensive psychometric testing. The SAQ demonstrates good psychometric properties. Healthcare organizations can use the survey to measure caregiver attitudes about six patient safety-related domains (teamwork climate, safety climate, perceptions of management, job satisfaction, working conditions, and stress recognition). This tool can be used to compare a unit or system with other like organizations, to prompt interventions, to improve safety attitudes, and to measure the effectiveness of these interventions [70].

Recent research explored the value of measuring safety culture through the novel use of both the MaPSaF and the SAQ. Researchers utilized an integrative approach in administering both surveys as the MaPSaF provides an awareness of safety problems through collective discussion, while the SAQ is an individual survey. Results show that an integrated approach in evaluation of an organization's safety culture may lead to helpful data that illustrates strengths and weaknesses in safety culture at both the collective and individual levels [71].

The Safety Climate Survey was developed in connection to the Safety Culture Survey. The Safety Climate Survey and the Safety Culture Scale appear to be measuring one construct and exhibit sufficient reliability for use [72].

5   Case Study: "How to" Application

A small group of nurses on a 52 bed Med/Surg unit (2East) at an urban hospital are concerned about anecdotal buzz of an increase in concerning errors on their unit. Specifically, three adverse outcomes are being repeated in these discussions: patient falls, medication errors, and hospital-acquired infections (HAIs). There has been frequent turnover in the 2E Manager position and in the last 3 years 2E has had five managers. A new manager, Amy, has just arrived and seems to be planning on staying in this position for the next 3–5 years. Gloria is a nurse on 2E and part of this small group of concerned nurses. Gloria is in graduate school, studying to become a Clinical Nurse Specialist, and is learning about safety culture in one of her classes.

Gloria sets up a meeting with Amy to discuss concerns by the nurses, and some ideas she has to improve the status of patient safety on 2E. Amy asks Gloria to co-lead a Safety Steering Committee for 2E where they can enlist the help of other members of the healthcare team to address safety events. Gloria and Amy strategize how to recruit nurses, Physicians, Respiratory Therapists, Occupational Therapists, a Case Manager, and a Hospital Manager to this Steering Committee. Together Amy and Gloria put together elements of a strategic plan to develop with the Safety Steering Committee and the hospital Quality Department. With the eventual goal of strengthening 2E's safety culture, Amy and Gloria identify early data needs, possible training opportunities, and growth strategies.

Early Data Needs:
- Obtain data about the number of patient falls, medication administration errors, and HAIs for the last 2 years on 2E.
- Ask the Quality Department for data on incident reports on actual errors and near misses for the previous 2 years.
- Before any training occurs, collect baseline data about the safety culture on 2E. A decision has been made to use both the Manchester Patient Safety Framework and Safety Attitude Questionnaire for continuous data collection over time.

Possible Training Opportunities: After several meetings and reviewing best practices related to patient falls, medication administration errors, HAIs and safety culture, the Steering Committee suggests concurrent addressing of specific safety issues on 2E (e.g., no fall prevention protocol) while also providing training on vitals aspects of safety culture (psychological safety, Just Culture, blame-free reporting, transparency). In collaboration with 2E's healthcare team, the Steering Committee proposes a 3-year plan to begin to address specific patient safety concerns, while simultaneously establishing and strengthening strong safety culture on 2E.

Growth Strategies: As more members of the 2E's healthcare team learn more about safety culture, there are increasing opportunities to grow this microsystem's safety culture.

- Early data on reporting near misses indicates 2E team rarely reports near misses. Amy and Gloria decide to initiate a Good Catch Program on the Unit.
- There are increased inquiries about making quality and safety data more transparent. From these appeals, the hospital's Information Technology (IT) department builds a new quality dashboard for the unit's computers. The quality dashboard designed specifically for 2E provides up to date quality data on patient falls, MAE rates, HAI rates, and the most recent safety culture survey results. Some hospital units choose to have their quality dashboard appear as a banner in the bottom of their unit computer screens.
- 2E healthcare team members have other ideas for a visual campaign on 2E to promote improvement in safety culture and specific patient safety outcomes. Other ideas include a Red, Yellow, Green Performance Indicator Board for the four targeted quality outcomes. Red indicates project challenges that are being addressed, yellow indicates in-process work, and green indicates completed process steps with initial outcomes. Another visual tool for strengthening 2E's Safety Culture is an Idea Board where the 2E Team, patients, and families can post 2E Safety Culture successes and ideas to grow 2E's safety culture.
- Physicians and Advanced Practice Practitioners approach Amy asking for improved communication among all team members. Communication is not standardized, and providers realize they are missing key insights from the other members of the healthcare team. Daily safety huddles are implemented to improve group communication, team collaboration, and increase psychological safety for all team members.
- Amy works with interested team members in specific interventions for patient falls, medication administration, and HAIs. Amy empowers Champion team members with evidence-based tools and successful initiatives to guide improvement work targeting these three patient outcomes.

Data to track over time: As 2E continues to address patient falls, medication administration, HAIs, and safety culture, data will be transparently shared to guide and reward 2E's healthcare team. Data collection will focus on:

- Repeated results from the Manchester Patient Safety Framework and Safety Attitude Questionnaire to track the emerging strength of safety culture on 2E.
  - Relevant subscale data specific to Just Culture, leadership, teamwork, communication, and commitment to quality will be reviewed as training in these areas occur.

- Monthly data on patient falls, medication errors, and HAIs will populate the unit's quality dashboard.
- Amy will also track nurse turnover on 2E. Some evidence suggests that stronger safety culture is correlated with improved teamwork and increased nurse satisfaction.

6 Summary

Culture can be an elusive phenomenon to assess and improve because it is variable and composed of a group's attitudes, beliefs, assumptions, and values. Safety culture is built over time and is built on trust. Through growing safety culture, healthcare team members learn to trust each other, leadership, and the system. And with stronger safety culture, patients and families are able to fully trust the healthcare team.

There are practices that contribute to safety culture, but no one practice can ensure safety culture. Many practices reinforce the priority of safety and contribute to the growth of trust. Practices that contribute to safety culture include standards that support psychological safety, Just Culture, safety huddles, reporting of errors and near misses, sharing of data to facilitate transparency, and open disclosure about errors and near misses with patients and families. Measurement of safety culture using valid and reliable tools can assist healthcare teams in tracking their success or decrease in developing safety culture. Many safety culture tools include subscales that will assist healthcare teams in targeting which elements of their safety culture need reinforcement.

Key Points

- Safety culture is the product of individual and group values, attitudes, perceptions, competencies, and patterns of behavior that determine the commitment to, and the style and proficiency of an organization's safety management.
- Safety culture is the foundation for effective, sustainable patient safety improvements.
- Addressing key components of safety culture provides the necessary context for the success of improvement work.
- Psychological safety is necessary, so all healthcare team members feel free to speak up to address safety concerns.
- Just Culture shifts traditionally blame-oriented responses to error to an emphasis on curiosity about why an error occurred.
- Reporting systems are often cumbersome for healthcare workers. Streamlining reporting systems can facilitate higher reporting rates for errors and near misses.
- Incentivizing reporting near misses through a Good Catch Program can counterbalance healthcare team members' fear about the liability of reporting an error or near miss.

- Making quality data more transparent in quality dashboards can provide positive feedback to frontline works as patient safety outcome data improves.
- Safety huddles can support transparency of sharing safety concerns in real time.
- There are several reliable and valid tools to measure safety culture so a team can track its progress over time.

References

1. Donaldson MS, Corrigan JM, Kohn LT, editors. To err is human: building a safer health system. 2000.
2. Eldridge N, Wang Y, Metersky M, et al. Trends in adverse event rates in hospitalized patients, 2010-2019. JAMA. 2022;328(2):173–83. https://doi.org/10.1001/jama.2022.9600.
3. Casey T, Griffin MA, Flatau Harrison H, Neal A. Safety climate and culture: integrating psychological and systems perspectives. J Occup Health Psychol. 2017;22(3):341–53. https://doi.org/10.1037/ocp0000072.
4. Rodziewicz TL, Houseman B, Hipskind JE. Medical error reduction and prevention. In: StatPearls. Treasure Island, FL: StatPearls Publishing; 2022.
5. INSAG. Basic safety principles for nuclear power plants (Safety Series No 75-INSAG-3). Vienna: International Nuclear Safety Advisory Group, International Atomic Energy Agency; 1988.
6. Cullen WD. The public inquiry into the piper alpha disaster. London: His Majesty's Stationary Office (HMSO); 1990.
7. Kohn KT, Corrigan JM, Donaldson MS, editors. Committee on quality health care in America. Washington, DC: Institute of Medicine, National Academy Press; 1999.
8. Sammer CE, Lykens K, Singh KP, Mains DA, Lackan NA. What is patient safety culture? A review of the literature. J Nurs Scholarsh. 2010;42(2):156–65. https://doi.org/10.1111/j.1547-5069.2009.01330.x.
9. Halligan M, Zecevic A. Safety culture in healthcare: a review of concepts, dimensions, measures and progress. BMJ Qual Saf. 2011;20(4):338–43. https://doi.org/10.1136/bmjqs.2010.040964.
10. Lee SE, Scott LD, Dahinten VS, Vincent C, Lopez KD, Park CG. Safety culture, patient safety, and quality of care outcomes: a literature review. West J Nurs Res. 2019;41(2):279–304. https://doi.org/10.1177/0193945917747416.
11. Agency for Healthcare Research and Quality. Culture of safety. https://psnet.ahrq.gov/primer/culture-safety. Accessed 22 Apr 2023.
12. Bisbey TM, Kilcullen MP, Thomas EJ, Ottosen MJ, Tsao K, Salas E. Safety culture: an integration of existing models and a framework for understanding its development. Hum Factors. 2021;63(1):88–110. https://doi.org/10.1177/0018720819868878.
13. Kilcullen MP, Bisbey TM, Ottosen MJ, Tsao K, Salas E, Thomas EJ. The safer culture framework: an application to healthcare based on a multi-industry review of safety culture literature. Hum Factors. 2022;64(1):207–27. https://doi.org/10.1177/00187208211060891.
14. Dombrádi V, Bíró K, Jonitz G, Gray M, Jani A. Broadening the concept of patient safety culture through value-based healthcare. J Health Organ Manag. 2021;35:541. https://doi.org/10.1108/JHOM-07-2020-0287.
15. Alshyyab MA, FitzGerald G, Dingle K, et al. Developing a conceptual framework for patient safety culture in emergency department: a review of the literature. Int J Health Plann Manag. 2019;34(1):42–55. https://doi.org/10.1002/hpm.2640.
16. Noh J, Lee S, Cho HC. The impact of corporate culture on industrial accidents in high-risk industries: a cross-sectional survey. Ind Health. 2023;61(2):102–11. https://doi.org/10.2486/indhealth.2021-0252.

17. Naji GMA, Isha ASN, Mohyaldinn ME, et al. Impact of safety culture on safety performance; mediating role of psychosocial Hazard: an integrated modelling approach. Int J Environ Res Public Health. 2021;18(16):8568. https://doi.org/10.3390/ijerph18168568.
18. Hessels AJ, Paliwal M, Weaver SH, Siddiqui D, Wurmser TA. Impact of patient safety culture on missed nursing care and adverse patient events. J Nurs Care Qual. 2019;34(4):287–94. https://doi.org/10.1097/NCQ.0000000000000378.
19. Millson T, Hackbarth D, Bernard HL. A demonstration project on the impact of safety culture on infection control practices in hemodialysis. Am J Infect Control. 2019;47(9):1122–9. https://doi.org/10.1016/j.ajic.2019.02.026.
20. Moghimian M, Farzi S, Farzi K, et al. Patient safety culture in burn care units from the perspectives of healthcare providers: a cross-sectional study [Published correction appears in J Burn Care Res. 2022 May 17;43(3):757]. J Burn Care Res. 2022;43(4):841–5. https://doi.org/10.1093/jbcr/irab208.
21. Skoogh A, Bååth C, Hall-Lord ML. Healthcare professionals' perceptions of patient safety culture and teamwork in intrapartum care: a cross-sectional study. BMC Health Serv Res. 2022;22(1):820. https://doi.org/10.1186/s12913-022-08145-5.
22. Pimentel MPT, Choi S, Fiumara K, Kachalia A, Urman RD. Safety culture in the operating room: variability among perioperative healthcare workers. J Patient Saf. 2021;17(6):412–6. https://doi.org/10.1097/PTS.0000000000000385.
23. Verbakel NJ, Langelaan M, Verheij TJ, Wagner C, Zwart DL. Improving patient safety culture in primary care: a systematic review. J Patient Saf. 2016;12(3):152–8. https://doi.org/10.1097/PTS.0000000000000075.
24. Pimenta Lopes Ribeiro OM, de Lima Trindade L, Silva Fassarella C, et al. Impact of COVID-19 on professional nursing practice environments and patient safety culture. J Nurs Manag. 2022;30(5):1105–14. https://doi.org/10.1111/jonm.13617.
25. Newman A, Donohue R, Eva N. Psychological safety: a systematic review of the literature. Hum Resour Manag Rev. 2017;27(3):521–35.
26. Greene MT, Gilmartin HM, Saint S. Psychological safety and infection prevention practices: results from a national survey. Am J Infect Control. 2020;48(1):2–6. https://doi.org/10.1016/j.ajic.2019.09.027.
27. Reason J. Managing the risks of organizational accidents. Aldershot, Hants, England: Ashgate; 1997. p. 25.
28. Edmondson AC. Teaming: how organizations learn, innovate, and compete in the knowledge economy. San Francisco, CA: Jossey-Bass Publishers; 2012. p. 26.
29. Edmondson AC, Lei Z. Psychological safety: the history, renaissance, and future of an interpersonal construct. Ann Rev Organ Psychol Organ Behav. 2014;1:23–43.
30. Aranzamendez G, James D, Toms R. Finding antecedents of psychological safety: a step toward quality improvement. Nurs Forum. 2015;50(3):171–8. https://doi.org/10.1111/nuf.12084.
31. Ridley CH, Al-Hammadi N, Maniar HS, et al. Building a collaborative culture: focus on psychological safety and error reporting. Ann Thorac Surg. 2021;111(2):683–9. https://doi.org/10.1016/j.athoracsur.2020.05.152.
32. Bradley V, Liddle S, Shaw R, et al. Sticks and stones: investigating rude, dismissive and aggressive communication between doctors. Clin Med (Lond). 2015;15(6):541–5. https://doi.org/10.7861/clinmedicine.15-6-541.
33. Wright C. The disruptive physician and impact on the culture of safety. Curr Opin Anaesthesiol. 2021;34(3):387–91. https://doi.org/10.1097/ACO.0000000000000968.
34. Dekker S. Just culture: restoring trust and accountability in your organization. CRC Press; 2018.
35. Marx D. Patient safety and the just culture. Obstet Gynecol Clin North Am. 2019;46(2):239–45. https://doi.org/10.1016/j.ogc.2019.01.003.
36. Petschonek S, Burlison J, Cross C, Martin K, Laver J, et al. Development of the just culture assessment tool: measuring the perceptions of health-care professionals in hospitals. J Patient Saf. 2013;9(4):190–7. https://doi.org/10.1097/PTS.0b013e31828fff34.
37. Ulrich B. Just culture and its impact on a culture of safety. Nephrol Nurs J. 2017;44(3):207–59.

38. O'Donovan R, Ward M, De Brún A, McAuliffe E. Safety culture in health care teams: a narrative review of the literature. J Nurs Manag. 2019;27(5):871–83. https://doi.org/10.1111/jonm.12740.
39. Fencl JL, Willoughby C, Jackson K. Just culture: the Foundation of Staff Safety in the perioperative environment. AORN J. 2021;113(4):329–36. https://doi.org/10.1002/aorn.13352.
40. Small D, Small RM, Green A. Improving safety by developing trust with a just culture. Nurs Manage (Harrow). 2022;29(2):32–41. https://doi.org/10.7748/nm.2021.e2030.
41. Howell AM, Burns EM, Hull L, Mayer E, Sevdalis N, Darzi A. International recommendations for national patient safety incident reporting systems: an expert Delphi consensus-building process. BMJ Qual Saf. 2017;26(2):150–63. https://doi.org/10.1136/bmjqs-2015-004456.
42. Shojania KG. Incident reporting systems: what will it take to make them less frustrating and achieve anything useful? Jt Comm J Qual Patient Saf. 2021;47(12):755–8. https://doi.org/10.1016/j.jcjq.2021.10.001.
43. Adamson L, Beldham-Collins R, Sykes J, Thwaites D. Safety culture and incident learning systems in radiation oncology: staff perceptions across Australia and New Zealand. J Med Imaging Radiat Oncol. 2022;66(2):299–309. https://doi.org/10.1111/1754-9485.13335.
44. Fox MD, Bump GM, Butler GA, Chen LW, Buchert AR. Making residents part of the safety culture: improving error reporting and reducing harms. J Patient Saf. 2021;17(5):e373–8. https://doi.org/10.1097/PTS.0000000000000344.
45. Afaya A, Konlan KD, Kim DH. Improving patient safety through identifying barriers to reporting medication administration errors among nurses: an integrative review. BMC Health Serv Res. 2021;21(1):1156. https://doi.org/10.1186/s12913-021-07187-5.
46. Rocco C, Rodríguez AM, Noya B. Elimination of punitive outcomes and criminalization of medical errors. Curr Opin Anaesthesiol. 2022;35(6):728–32. https://doi.org/10.1097/ACO.0000000000001197.
47. He H, Yu P, Li L, et al. Patient safety culture and obstacles to adverse event reporting in nursing homes. J Nurs Manag. 2020;28(7):1536–44. https://doi.org/10.1111/jonm.13098.
48. Armstrong G. Commentary: the effect of patient safety culture on nurses' near-miss reporting intention: the moderating role of perceived severity of near misses. J Res Nurs. 2021;26(1–2):17–8. https://doi.org/10.1177/1744987120979756.
49. Wallace SC, Mamrol C, Finley E. Promote a culture of safety with good catch reports. PA Patient Saf Advisory. 2017;14(3).
50. Simmons D, Mick J, Graves K, Martin SK. 26,000 close call reports: lessons from the University of Texas Close Call Reporting System. In: Henriksen K, Battles JB, Keyes MA, Grady ML, editors. Advances in patient safety: new directions and alternative approaches, Assessment, vol. 1. Rockville, MD: Agency for Healthcare Research and Quality; 2008.
51. Herzer KR, Mirrer M, Xie Y, et al. Patient safety reporting systems: sustained quality improvement using a multidisciplinary team and "good catch" awards. Jt Comm J Qual Patient Saf. 2012;38(8):339–47. https://doi.org/10.1016/s1553-7250(12)38044-6.
52. Putnam LR, Anderson KT, Diffley MB, et al. Meaningful use and good catches: more appropriate metrics for checklist effectiveness. Surgery. 2016;160(6):1675–81. https://doi.org/10.1016/j.surg.2016.04.038.
53. Tanz M. Improving safety knowledge, skills, and attitudes with a good catch program and student-designed simulation. J Nurs Educ. 2018;57(6):379–84. https://doi.org/10.3928/01484834-20180522-11.
54. Crandall KM, Almuhanna A, Cady R, et al. 10,000 good catches: increasing safety event reporting in a pediatric health care system. Pediatr Qual Saf. 2018;3(2):e072. https://doi.org/10.1097/pq9.0000000000000072.
55. Ibrahim M, Szeto WY, Gutsche J, et al. Transparency, public reporting, and a culture of change to quality and safety in cardiac surgery. Ann Thorac Surg. 2022;114(3):626–35. https://doi.org/10.1016/j.athoracsur.2021.08.085.
56. Mazor KM, Simon SR, Yood RA, et al. Health plan members' views about disclosure of medical errors. Ann Intern Med. 2004;140(6):409–18. https://doi.org/10.7326/0003-4819-140-6-200403160-00006.

57. Gleason JL, Swisher E, Weiss PM. Transparency and disclosure. Obstet Gynecol Clin N Am. 2019;46(2):247–55. https://doi.org/10.1016/j.ogc.2019.01.007.
58. Eaves-Leanos A, Dunn EJ. Open disclosure of adverse events: transparency and safety in health care. Surg Clin N Am. 2012;92(1):163–77. https://doi.org/10.1016/j.suc.2011.11.001.
59. Lamming L, Montague J, Crosswaite K, et al. Fidelity and the impact of patient safety huddles on teamwork and safety culture: an evaluation of the huddle up for safer healthcare (HUSH) project. BMC Health Serv Res. 2021;21(1):1038. https://doi.org/10.1186/s12913-021-07080-1.
60. McCain N, Ferguson T, Barry Hultquist T, Wahl C, Struwe L. Influencing a culture of quality and safety through huddles. J Nurs Care Qual. 2023;38(1):26–32. https://doi.org/10.1097/NCQ.0000000000000642.
61. Franklin BJ, Gandhi TK, Bates DW, et al. Impact of multidisciplinary team huddles on patient safety: a systematic review and proposed taxonomy. BMJ Qual Saf. 2020;29(10):1–2. https://doi.org/10.1136/bmjqs-2019-009911.
62. Nieva VF, Sorra J. Safety culture assessment: a tool for improving patient safety in healthcare organizations. Qual Saf Health Care. 2003;12 Suppl 2(Suppl 2):ii17–23. https://doi.org/10.1136/qhc.12.suppl_2.ii17.
63. Pronovost P, Sexton B. Assessing safety culture: guidelines and recommendations. Qual Saf Health Care. 2005;14(4):231–3. https://doi.org/10.1136/qshc.2005.015180.
64. Ellis LA, Pomare C, Churruca K, Carrigan A, Meulenbroeks I, Saba M, Braithwaite J. Predictors of response rates of safety culture questionnaires in healthcare: a systematic review and analysis. BMJ Open. 2022;12(9):e065320. https://doi.org/10.1136/bmjopen-2022-065320.
65. Azyabi A, Karwowski W, Davahli MR. Assessing patient safety culture in hospital settings. Int J Environ Res Public Health. 2021;18(5):2466. https://doi.org/10.3390/ijerph18052466.
66. Sorra JS, Nieva VF. Hospital survey on patient safety culture. (Prepared by Westat, under Contract No. 290-96-0004). AHRQ Publication No. 04-0041. Rockville, MD: Agency for Healthcare Research and Quality; 2004.
67. Waterson P, Carman EM, Manser T, Hammer A. Hospital survey on patient safety culture (HSPSC): a systematic review of the psychometric properties of 62 international studies. BMJ Open. 2019;9(9):e026896. https://doi.org/10.1136/bmjopen-2018-026896.
68. Kirk S, Parker D, Claridge T, Esmail A, Marshall M. Patient safety culture in primary care: developing a theoretical framework for practical use. Qual Saf Health Care. 2007;16(4):313–20. https://doi.org/10.1136/qshc.2006.018366.
69. Mohr DC, Chen C, Sullivan J, Gunnar W, Damschroder L. Development and validation of the veterans health administration patient safety culture survey. J Patient Saf. 2022;18(6):539–45. https://doi.org/10.1097/PTS.0000000000001027.
70. Sexton JB, Helmreich RL, Neilands TB, Rowan K, Vella K, Boyden J, Roberts PR, Thomas EJ. The safety attitudes questionnaire: psychometric properties, benchmarking data, and emerging research. BMC Health Serv Res. 2006;6:44.
71. Tocco Tussardi I, Moretti F, Capasso M, et al. Improving the culture of safety among healthcare workers: integration of different instruments to gain major insights and drive effective changes. Int J Health Plan Manage. 2022;37(1):429–51. https://doi.org/10.1002/hpm.3348.
72. Kho ME, Carbone JM, Lucas J, Cook DJ. Safety climate survey: reliability of results from a multicenter ICU survey. BMJ Qual Saf. 2005;14(4):273–8.

Safety in Sight: Illuminating Hidden Barriers to Zero Harm

Jane S. Braaten and Kelly Wild

A strong program of achieving zero harm to patients lies within the ability of individuals to identify safety issues, speak up to prevent issues from causing harm, participate in mitigation strategies and learnings, and to adapt when faced with safety problems in the moment [1, 2]. Although all these areas are important, the key to protecting patients from preventable harm is early identification of error producing conditions and mitigating effectively prior to patient harm [3]. There are still many obstacles within the healthcare culture that constrain those elements of patient safety that are hidden within a well-established program.

Nurses are at the frontline of healthcare and have a responsibility to speak up and stop harm from reaching a patient when they identify it in progress. Although we have come a long way in improving teamwork, promoting speaking up behavior, and encouraging reporting, we still have major obstacles to effectively prevent an error from causing patient harm. These obstacles are not always outwardly apparent and exist within a culture that has developed and been accepted over time. Key areas covered in this chapter include the following cultural aspects that undermine safety:

- Power distance: Barriers to speaking up in the moment due to hierarchy
- Normalization of deviance and the toleration of lowered safety standards
- Error reporting: Barriers to reporting errors, near misses, and close calls
- Failure of a just culture program to effectively prevent future errors and further harm

J. S. Braaten (✉) · K. Wild
AdventHealth Parker, Parker, CO, USA
e-mail: jane.braaten@adventhealth.com; Kelly.Wild@adventhealth.com

C. A. Oster, J. S. Braaten (eds.), *The Nexus between Nursing and Patient Safety*,
https://doi.org/10.1007/978-3-031-53158-3_3

43

1   Power Distance in Healthcare: Barriers to Speaking Up and Communication

"Speaking up for safety" has been a mantra to patient safety since the Institute of Medicine report, "To Err is Human" [4] was published. This push has been supported unanimously with ample research and reviews on the subject [5]. It seems that speaking up is the answer, however, it still has not been fully realized. Strong individual and organizational factors are required to facilitate and support speaking up behavior. There is evidence that healthcare providers in many different disciplines and contexts do not always speak up [6–8] even though the call to do so is clear. Simply asking healthcare providers, specifically nurses, to speak up is not as easy as it sounds.

1.1   What Is Power Distance?

Power distance is a complex cultural concept that greatly influences the decision to speak up that was developed in the late 1950s by Mauk Mulder [9]. Mulder described power distance as the inequality of power and influence between lower and higher powered individuals within the same society. Geert Hofstede [10] further developed the concept as it applies to systems such as organizations, workplaces, schools, and countries. Hofstede described power distance as the acceptance of inequality in society. That means that individuals accept their standing and the expectations of who they should defer to, who is in control and who is not. Power distance is a factor in daily interaction within workplace environments that affects employee relationships, management styles, and effective communication.

For many safety issues in which preventable harm occurred, we frequently find that there is someone on the team who had identified an issue and did not bring it forward. Many factors lead to speaking up or choosing not to speak up. Top reasons that nurses cite for not speaking up about a safety concern can be personal as well as those reflective of leadership response including:

- Concern that no change will occur
- Fear of retaliation
- Fear of disregard of opinion
- Fear of negative feedback
- Fear of being wrong [8]

The decision to speak up about a patient safety concern is impacted by balancing the perceived benefit to a perceived negative outcome. Moreover, speaking up and the fears noted above are heavily influenced by power dynamics and hierarchy. An example of this hierarchical influence is evident in nursing students and the prevalence of not speaking up while on clinical rotations [6]. This study, conducted in

Austria, measured speaking up behavior in a group of nursing students by using the "Speaking Up for Patient Safety Questionnaire" (SUPS-Q) as well as asking for feedback on a scenario which involved observing a senior physician not complying with hand hygiene prior to entering a patient room. The results revealed that although nursing students are given extensive training and education on patient safety and speaking up, it is difficult for them to apply it in their clinical rotations due to hospital hierarchy. Overall, during their 4-week clinical rotation, up to 84% of the students noticed a harm producing event, a rule violation, or had specific concerns. More troubling is that up to 74% of these students did not feel that they would bring up errors, share ideas for improvement, or address a colleague not following a safety specific rule.

Furthermore, few students felt that they would address a senior physician who did not follow hand hygiene protocol. The main factors cited by the students included fear of negative response, fear of ineffectiveness, and fear of unpredictable reactions. Also, students more senior in the program were even more hesitant to bring up concerns [6]. This reinforces the knowledge that inhibition of speaking up behaviors is rooted in fear, possibly due to prior experience. This is embedded deeply in our culture due to a persistent hierarchical system and the effect of power distance.

1.2   Examples of Power Distance in Healthcare

Speaking up for safety is an essential practice to ensure that risks, issues, and concerns identified by members of the healthcare team are brought forward, listened to and acted upon. The absence of this practice is a major cause of safety issues that go undetected and cause patient harm. Although there has been much work on teamwork and communication, power differentials that affect communication still exist within modern healthcare.

One reason for this is that training on speaking up exists but does not address the main barriers: positional hierarchy and the emotional skills and psychological safety required to voice concerns [11]. Kim and colleagues [11] performed a scoping review of studies that focused on the training of interventions targeted to speaking up. They found that most interventions:

- Trained just one discipline rather than interdisciplinary
- Were conducted as a one-time training
- Only focused on verbal skills and not emotional ones

Health care organizations have historically been hierarchical between disciplines, and this imbalance continues to exist within medicine and nursing [12]. Hierarchy also exists within disciplines based on experience and within the management structure of the organization leading to power differentials within nursing itself [13].

Examples of power distance behaviors and circumstances in healthcare and nursing include but are not limited to:

- A nurse not questioning a physician's decision even though they have concerns
- Agreeing with a questionable decision made by a nurse manager to avoid conflict
- Acceptance that nurse aides do not escalate issues above the primary staff nurse
- Holding back suggestions in an emergent situation due to fear of being wrong
- Higher power individuals such as executives not allowing frontline decisions to be made without their input
- Special considerations for those in power such as free parking or free lunches

Consider these examples:

Safety situation: A new surgeon is finishing up a case. The surgeon closes the incision before the instrument/sponge count is completed. Staff do not speak up to stop the surgeon before protocol is violated. The count is missing one sponge which later is found inside the patient. The patient requires another operation to remove.
Power differential: Nurse to physician.
Possible reason for not speaking up: New surgeon with possible unpredictable reaction; easier not to speak up.
Solution: Interdisciplinary acknowledgment of perceived power distance. Surgeon could introduce self and say "I know we don't know each other well but please, I depend on you to call out issues if you see them and I will always appreciate the input"

Safety situation: A nurse practitioner feels that a physician is prescribing too many narcotic pain relievers to patients. She discussed this with the physician, the physician disagreed and reported her to her supervisor as insubordinate. The nurse practitioner does not bring up the situation again. One of the patients is given too much narcotic and is later found unresponsive.
Power differential: Nurse practitioner to physician.
Possible reason for not speaking up: Fear of retaliation.
Solution: Leadership acknowledgment of perceived power distance. The nurse practitioner's supervisor could say "I understand that you were concerned about patient safety, and you did not get an acceptable response. Please keep reporting this issue if it occurs and I can assist in discussion to assure the concerns are heard."

Safety situation: A medical surgical nurse is caring for a transferred patient from the critical care unit. She was told she could call the critical care unit at any time if she had questions or needed help. She calls for assistance about a possible arrythmia and is asked "Didn't you take the class?" She says "never mind; I'll figure it out." The patient was discovered to have a heart block and emergently needed a pacemaker.

Power differential: Medical surgical nurse to critical care nurse (perceived inexperience to experience).

Possible reasons for not speaking up: Fear of looking incompetent, fear of unpredictable reaction.

Solution: intradisciplinary acknowledgment of perceived power distance and communication.

The critical care nurse could recognize the perceived power distance and inexperience and say "This is a complicated rhythm, let me look at it and we can discuss."

As the previous examples show, power differentials that affect patient safety and speaking up behavior occur frequently, often are based on individual decision-making within the specific context and are deeply rooted in an unspoken fear. The key to creating a safer culture for speaking up and teaching its importance is not solely the responsibility of the individual. Instead, it lies within the whole system to recognize who is seen to have the power in situations and includes training to assess how those in power encourage speaking up behavior.

1.3 The Way Forward: Decreasing the Power Distance

As noted earlier, training to effectively decrease power distance and encourage speaking up behavior is fairly limited by education provided to only one discipline during a one-time educational session. This might help but keeps the hierarchy in control. This is not adequate. Four main areas of focus to equalize the playing field in a hierarchical system include the following:

1. Recognizing the imbalance of power and its effect on communication

    Power distance is prevalent in all areas of healthcare but does not just focus on one discipline or one clinical area. As a system of healthcare dedicated to support safe patient care, it is imperative to recognize that imbalances of power exist within all contexts and disciplines. When safety events occur, it is important to ask if all voices in the room were heard, and if not, to ask "why"? When all voices are heard, it is equally important to ask about the factors that made speaking up possible.

2. Interdisciplinary training

One educational session and teaching skills to those in so-called subordinate positions is not the full answer to decrease the safety challenge of power distance. There is a shortage of information on the best way to improve speaking up behavior as outcomes and interventions are not clear [14]. However, improvement is not contained within just the individual. It is contained within teams and dyads within an interdisciplinary context. Patient safety is enabled when speaking up behavior is practiced and encouraged as a team effort within the contexts in which it occurs [15].

3. Reflecting on approachability as the team leader

Approachability of a person in power is a key factor in speaking up behavior. Pack and colleagues [15] used interdisciplinary simulation to allow team leaders to reflect on how their behavior encourages or discourages others voicing concerns in an obstetrical setting. The team leaders were surprised to learn that some were not seen as approachable even though they believe they are civil and do not have disruptive behaviors. This is a key finding to begin the journey to lessen power distance. Approachability is something that is created actively by team leaders and the perception of the team leader may be different than what the team perceives. Effective actions include actively seeking other opinions, thinking out loud and facilitating a debriefing so all can ask questions and learn. Moreover, it is constantly reinforced by the actions and behavior of the leader. It is imperative for the positional leader to actively commit to creating a safe space for questions.

4. Actively promoting psychological safety

Amy Edmondson [16] defined the term "psychological safety" as the ability to take interpersonal risks without fear of repercussions. Psychological safety is the foundation to speaking up behavior and as we have noted, it can be fostered more from the group level than at the individual level. Those with positional power have the most responsibility to assure that they create a culture where everyone can share ideas, disagree, and question. Practices to consider include:

- Sharing vulnerability: "I am unsure about this decision, does anyone have other suggestions?"
- Asking for assistance: "I am depending on you to stop me if you have questions"
- Inviting response: "I really value your opinion, please tell me what you think"
- Positive response: "Thank you for pointing that out. I might have made an error without your help"

In summary, power distance is a pervasive cultural issue that can be present in all teams and interactions within healthcare with a huge impact to patient safety when the power distance is large. The problems with power distance are that it is easily accepted in our hierarchical system, not recognized by those in power, and it has few interventions that have been shown to be successful. The way forward to encourage speaking up behavior is to actively identify when power differentials could exist and place more emphasis on how the team, and especially the team leader, actively promotes leveling this power distance to assure safe care that is truly a collaborative team process.

2 Normalization of Deviance: Underlying Threat to a Safety Culture

Normalization of deviance is a term that was coined by Dianne Vaughn [17] to describe the culture at NASA that led to the Space Shuttle Challenger exploding and killing all astronauts on board. Vaughn described a culture at NASA, driven by production and prior success, as one that took risks, tolerated defects because they hadn't failed yet, and did not create a space for individuals to question risky decisions and have their concerns acknowledged. In other words, the organization did not ever imagine that an identified risk that had not failed, ever would. This led to disaster.

A concept analysis defined normalization of deviance as the gradual acceptance of lower standards due to periods of time in which the lower standard is performed with no negative consequences and perhaps perceived positive benefits. This leads to reinforcement that the standard is acceptable [18]. Normalization of deviance does not occur overnight. It becomes a part of an organization's or work unit's culture that develops with experience over time. It is a gradual acceptance of nonstandard practices because they do not appear to cause negative consequences. Normalization of deviance does not stand out until an issue occurs or there is a deliberate focus on recognition because it becomes embedded into culture and appears as "the way we do things around here." Furthermore, as deviance is the accepted way of operations, it is difficult for members of the team to speak up without risking non-acceptance by the group.

For Example
A new graduate nurse is hired onto a medical surgical unit and is very excited. He is taught in orientation to never take verbal orders from providers as this is an opportunity for error. One physician on the unit continues to give staff verbal orders and staff continue to place these orders for the physician. The new nurse asked why this occurs. Coworkers say the physician is very important to the organization and gets angry when asked to enter her own orders. Furthermore, it takes less time to enter the verbal orders than ask and wait for the physician to do it herself. It is easier to not challenge the physician and to instead, work around the policy for her. The new nurse does not want to cause trouble for his coworkers and the unit, so he does what everyone else on the unit does to keep the status quo and to save time.

This example illustrates the need to conform to the norm of the work unit but also makes visible the main reasons that normalization of deviance occurs; production pressure and the perceived advantage of non-compliance.

Production pressure or the pressure to complete tasks and move on to the next is ever present in healthcare and has been found to be a driving factor that encourages staff to find workarounds to meet the production metric [18]. The Cambridge Dictionary defines a workaround as "a way of dealing with a problem or making something work despite the problem, without completely solving it" [19]. There is an uneven balance between the processes needed to create safety in a situation and the time constraints of completing the task to a productivity metric. This balance between safety and productivity in task completion leads to workarounds to complete the task in the allotted time.

Operating or procedural suites where the turnover of patients is most often one of the highest indicators of a successful program is a prime area for normalization of deviance. Surgical services are one of the most lucrative areas in the hospital, and the pressure to do more cases is immense. This type of pressure, where success of the service and the day-to-day operations depend not only on outcome but on the amount that can be completed in a day, sets up a situation for workarounds to occur. For example, completing a thorough time out checklist prior to surgery and then a post-procedure debriefing can be difficult when the team is pressed to complete a surgery and move on to the next in an allotted amount of time. This predicament then causes safety workarounds to get the job done quickly which can mean sacrificing safety for productivity. Ultimately, the productivity metric appears to hold more value than an absence of safety events that day. Most often, safety events do not occur, so the workaround is accepted.

Another common area for workarounds is in medication administration in hospitals. van der Veen and colleagues [20] found that workarounds by nurses to bar code administration were frequent. This is a common problem with multiple causes including technology issues, such as computer or barcode scanners not working, difficulties with reading or scanning a label, or simply being in a high-pressure situation. Again, this reemphasizes the perceived need for workarounds in a high-risk process with safety critical steps that might be outweighed by the desire for productivity.

Example: Workaround in Medication Safety

Safety process and task to be accomplished: Nurses in hospitals need to administer medications safely. "Smart pumps" have programmed safeguards for many medications that prompt a hard stop when an unsafe dosage is entered.

Issue: A particular medication is not programmed into the pump, so no hard stop is provided. There is no real time fix, and the nurse needs to give the medication urgently.

Workaround: The nurse administers the medication without utilizing the safety programming.

Normalization of deviance: The issue is not escalated, and no adverse event occurs, so the practice continues shift after shift until a mistake causes harm.

The example above illustrates how normalization of deviance develops from a safety process that is not complete or effective for the task at hand. There is a need to expedite the task quickly (production pressure), thus a workaround is performed

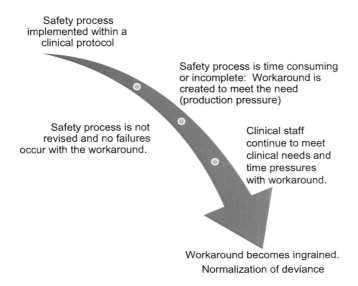

Safety process implemented within a clinical protocol

Safety process is time consuming or incomplete: Workaround is created to meet the need (production pressure)

Safety process is not revised and no failures occur with the workaround.

Clinical staff continue to meet clinical needs and time pressures with workaround.

Workaround becomes ingrained. Normalization of deviance

Fig. 1 The development of normalization of deviance in healthcare

to complete the task. The workaround continues because the problem is not corrected so the workaround becomes "how we do the work" or normalized. Figure 1 illustrates the development of normalization of deviance.

2.1   The Way Forward: Identify High-Risk Areas and the Signs of Normalization of Deviance

Normalization of deviance does not occur overnight as it develops and becomes accepted over time. Recognizing this practice can be difficult. However, the key to recognition is to seek out the contexts where the conditions for normalization of deviance exist. Sedlar et al. [21] analyzed the literature on normalization of deviance and found that it occurs in situations of risk normalization, production pressure, and a lack of negative consequences. McGaffigan [22] summarizes the cause of normalization of deviance as "Rules that don't make sense and impede productivity, particularly when under time pressure and heavy loads." The first step then is to go to the areas where those conditions exist and include these areas as a focus for safety rounds. Consider asking the following questions to locate normalization of deviance:

- What are the most time critical and high-risk processes that occur on a daily basis?
- Where and in what context exists the most pressure for production?
- What do frontline staff list as the most difficult safety protocols to follow?

The answers to these questions will reveal pressure points and workarounds.

The healthcare system is continually becoming more complex, not only from decade to decade, but from year to year and sometimes day to day. The struggles of frontline staff to keep up with the need to provide effective, safe, and timely care to the many who need it are real and only getting more troublesome. Frontline clinicians will always strive to meet the demands placed upon them. Thus, the development of workarounds and normalization of deviance. In these cases, "deviance" is really about clinicians trying to do the best they can to give care. Amalberti and Vincent [23] suggest that we examine strategies that look at managing risk through a new lens:

1. Accept the fact that conditions in healthcare will not return to the days of old. We will continue to be placed in conditions that are unsafe due to production pressure and we must realize that deviations will develop from that pressure.
2. We cannot reduce all hazards. We can mitigate hazard with safety strategies that are targeted to the risks.
3. Focus not always on the unexpected but deal with the expected. We have risk when we have the regular staffing shortages, pressure on throughput and pressure to treat patients quickly. This is expected and occurs daily.
4. All levels of the organization need to be involved in this management of risk when stress affects all work units. This involvement demands changing cumbersome protocols and investigation into what can work safely at the frontline.

As deviations develop insidiously over time at the frontline of care, it is imperative that we encourage caregivers at the frontline to identify and recognize the issues. Below are some tips to recognize issues:

Ask staff at the frontline:

• What equipment failures have you experienced lately? How does that impact the work you need to do?
• How does this safety process work for you when it is busy, and you have limited time? What do you do to meet the demand?
• What kind of pressure are you under to complete tasks such as medication management, discharging patients, turnover in procedural areas? What happens to safety processes when the pressure is high?
• What workarounds do you use when you experience a barrier in these processes?

Look for the statements that indicate a normalization of deviance might be occurring:

• "This piece of equipment is always breaking down."
• "It takes so long to discharge patients safely with this new process."
• "I can't properly sterilize instruments when they are needed within an hour."
• "We can't adequately clean the room when we have to get the next patient up within 15 min."
• "The surgical team won't slow down to complete a proper time out."

In summary, normalization of deviance has become part of the way we do work within a high-pressure environment. This phenomenon can be completely invisible because it becomes a part of our practice and is accepted to cope with pressure. However, ignoring the deviation will not protect patients. Identification and recognition of the pressures that are encountered in daily healthcare work coupled with identification of workarounds implemented by frontline staff are a start to a higher level of patient safety.

3   Barriers to Error Reporting

Improving patient safety requires learning from previous mistakes. Analyzing the circumstances of an incident and identifying how the error occurred, enable patient safety professionals to develop strategies to prevent similar incidents in the future. Transparency of this process and open communication of learnings are essential to guiding healthcare workers toward a culture of zero harm. Reporting an event or a near miss is critical to provide data to understand the circumstances surrounding the event [24]. Voluntary incident reporting is a cornerstone of error prevention and has been shown to improve the safety of patients when used effectively [25]. A strong incident reporting system that workers feel safe to use is key to identifying underlying vulnerabilities.

Healthcare organizations are heavily reliant on voluntary reporting to improve patient safety. However, there are many drawbacks to this method and under-reporting remains a critical issue, particularly for near-miss events in which the error is identified and mitigated prior to reaching the patient. These near-miss events are especially important because they provide an opportunity to recognize and address safety concerns before there is any patient harm.

There is no way to learn from events that are not reported, or to prevent that error from reaching the patient next time. It is estimated that nearly half of serious incidents are not reported, and that events with moderate or minimal patient harm are reported less than 30% of the time [26]. Next, we will discuss the common barriers to reporting patient safety events listed below and in Fig. 2:

- Fear
- Lack of leadership support
- Lack of time and resources
- Low motivation or lack of knowledge

3.1   Fear

The single most cited barrier to incident reporting is the fear of negative repercussions. Most adverse events occur as part of a system or process failure that leads to

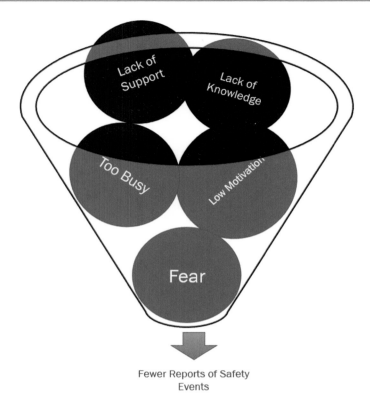

Fewer Reports of Safety
Events

Fig. 2 Barriers to reporting safety events

a mistake that is made by a single person. This person may feel concerned about being blamed for the resulting adverse outcome. This fear can be related to many factors [27]:

- Fear of being blamed
- Fear of punishment or retaliation
- Fear of disciplinary action, legal action, or liability
- Fear of stigmatization
- Fear of looking incompetent and humiliation
- Fear of conflict
- Fear of being wrong

Even in organizations with a strong non-punitive patient safety culture, fear is prevalent and a difficult barrier to overcome. Only 45% of nurses feel that the management of errors is non-punitive in nature [28]. Consistency in transparently demonstrating a fair and just culture is imperative to gain the trust of healthcare workers to feel safe when reporting patient safety incidents.

3.2   Lack of Leadership Support

The behavior of management in responding to errors and the perceived lack of support from leadership is another common barrier to reporting [8]. These are dynamic with varied reasons which include:

- Blame culture
- Dismissiveness
- Lack of investigation into the issue
- No perceived change or benefit from reporting
- Lack of feedback
- Lack of accountability
- Attitude of leadership toward reporting practices
- Lack of positive feedback for "good catches"

A positive organizational attitude toward reporting and management of patient safety concerns can assist in encouraging reporting. Healthcare workers need to know that every incident is reviewed and taken seriously. Managers must work to provide feedback on events and share any learnings that may have been identified and acknowledge when events are reported. Consistent messaging is important in all levels of leadership as well as in multidisciplinary roles, as frontline support has the most positive impact on patient safety outcomes. Often, unit culture has a stronger influence than that of the organization [29].

3.3   Time and Resources

A frequently cited barrier to reporting is the lack of time and resources to do so [25]. Documentation often takes a backseat to hands on patient care and is often not considered a priority. Other factors include:

- Too busy to report
- Time consuming reporting process
- Reporting system confusing or difficult to use
- Concerns for lack of confidentiality using the reporting system

The reporting system must be easily accessible, and every healthcare worker should have training on how to use the system. Having more than one way to report, for example, an electronic system and a call-in line, with the ability to remain anonymous, are helpful features to encourage use. A simpler and easier platform will increase the likelihood of use, whereas a complex reporting platform can be a significant barrier [30].

3.4   Motivation and Knowledge

Attitudes and perceptions of reporting errors are mixed among healthcare workers. There is a prevailing belief that the responsibility to report patient safety events is not a priority when compared to patient care and management, which can lead to unintentional omissions of reporting. Education on patient safety and the importance of reporting should be mandatory. Motivation and knowledge-related reasons for lack of reporting include [30]:

- Lack of knowledge of reporting system and responsibility to report
- Lack of knowledge that an error occurred
- Ambiguity on what consists of an error
- Error considered "not serious enough" to be reported
- Thinking situation is already well known or reported
- Belief that incident was unpreventable
- Negative association with reporting
- Insufficient training in patient safety concepts

The following examples illustrate these barriers:

Jamie was taking care of a high acuity ICU patient who decompensated and has a cardiac arrest. The resuscitation ended up being very time consuming with many complications. There was difficulty and delay in setting up suction, nobody knew where the equipment was in the code cart, and there were crowd control issues. Jamie knows that reporting these issues is the right thing to do but his patient is very sick, and he is already going to be staying late this shift to finish charting. He isn't even sure how he would start making the report. Jamie decides to let it go and thinks that maybe somebody else will report it instead.

Chris receives a patient transfer from another unit and realizes that many of the orders have not been completed. The patient never received their blood pressure medication, and their blood pressure was extremely elevated. Chris looks back into the record and notices the blood pressure had been elevated all shift. When assessing her patient, she notices the patient has had neurological changes and notifies the doctor. The doctor orders a stat CT scan which reveals that the patient has developed an intracranial hemorrhage. The patient ends up transferring to the ICU. Chris knows the elevated blood pressure probably contributed to the intracranial hemorrhage, but doesn't report this situation, not realizing that patient care issues like these should be reported.

3.5   The Way Forward: Organizational Transparency and Supportive Work Environment

Unfortunately, under-reporting remains one of the largest challenges to overcome. In the US, it is estimated that 50–90% of errors are not reported [30]. There are many opportunities to encourage and normalize the practice of reporting.

Organizational transparency and providing "loop closure" is a major facilitator to encourage reporting. This includes providing information on learnings that have occurred from an error back to the frontline staff, following up directly with reporting individuals when possible, during an investigation, and celebrating the reporting of near misses and good catches. When an incident is reported and it is perceived by staff that nothing has been done with the report, staff feel discouraged to keep reporting which undermines the culture of safety. The loop closure assists in demonstrating to staff that reporting is expected, with a focus on learning and improving system processes instead of punitive reactions.

The reporting system itself is also a significant factor in error reporting. The system must be readily available, easy to use, and provide option for anonymity. Staff must be educated on not only how to enter a report, but also what happens to the information after it is reported. Visible presence of the quality and safety team on patient units can provide reassurance and comfort that a reporting culture is an expectation [25]. To summarize, strategies to overcome barriers to reporting include:

- Providing loop closure
- Transparency in discussing medical errors
- Sharing learnings from investigations
- Maintaining a positive attitude toward reporting
- Providing education on the criteria for error reporting and use of the reporting system

4   Barriers to a Just Culture: More Than Just an Algorithm!

It is imperative to cultivate a strong patient safety culture to ensure reporting of events. A safety culture with a non-punitive response to errors who acknowledges that most errors are induced by a system or process failure is commonly referred to as a "just culture." A just culture recognizes that mistakes will happen in the complexity of a healthcare system and seeks to address the root cause of an event rather than blaming an individual. This requires interdisciplinary commitment and collaboration from all members of the healthcare team, from front line staff to administration [31].

Most healthcare facilities are familiar with the philosophy of just culture and may have an algorithm that they use when faced with safety events that are attributed to individuals. However, the presence of an algorithm alone does not create a true just culture. The examples below demonstrate that even in organizations that proclaim to have a fair and just culture, the application of the concept at the frontline is not consistent. Unit culture and influence can have a huge effect on behavior.

Annie is an experienced medical nurse working at a new facility for the last 3 months. She has noticed that the charge nurses on her unit tend to make fun of the other nurses when they have questions or ask for help. Annie has been trying hard to work independently even when she is very busy to avoid being teased. On a busy shift with several high acuity patients, she is rushing to give medications to a patient while on the phone with the lab regarding another patient. She scans her medications into the electronic health record and automatically clicks through all the "pop-ups". After finishing giving a medication intravenously, she realizes the medication was supposed to be given subcutaneously. Annie isn't sure what to do. She doesn't think the patient will be harmed from this mistake, but she is worried about getting in trouble and doesn't feel comfortable talking to the charge nurse about the situation, thinking they will humiliate her. Annie decides not to say anything, as she feels the repercussions for disclosing the error will be more harmful to her than to the patient, since there was no patient harm. She has heard that the facility has a just culture algorithm, but she has not seen it used.

Aaron has been a nurse on the oncology unit for 5 years. He has noticed an issue in which there can be a delay in obtaining medications for patients experiencing oncologic emergencies and has reported this concern several times. He has even come up with some other ideas to help. However, Aaron has never received a response to his concerns and is starting to feel like no one is listening. He decides that he will work around the problem by gathering medications at the patient bedside, so they are available quickly. Recently a patient of his had an emergency that he was able to quickly manage with the medications that were readily available, and he started telling his co-workers about his idea. Soon, many nurses on the unit are keeping medications at bedside. One day Aaron goes to use the medications and finds out they are missing, causing a delay in treatment, and the patient ends up transferring to the ICU with complications. He realizes the medications, which include controlled substances, may have been stolen from the patient room. He discusses the situation with his manager who advises him against reporting. Aaron is conflicted as he knows this could be a major patient safety concern, but also doesn't want to upset his manager and get blamed for the situation.

In the above situations, visible leadership support of a just culture may promote learning and communication instead of avoidance and fear. Active participation in patient safety activities and promoting the values of a just culture leads staff to trust that they will be supported in case of an adverse safety event. Healthcare workers must trust that reporting an error is safe, makes a difference, and is reliable.

Developing this trust requires consistent behavior toward a fair and just culture, open communication regarding the handling of errors, and providing constructive feedback and shared learnings that were gathered from an event [31].

Open communication, transparency, acknowledging that an error occurred, and sharing the learnings to all staff create and influence a positive patient safety culture [32]. Discussions on patient safety initiatives and providing the opportunity to voice concerns and suggestions should be a regular part of ongoing engagement with staff. Providing all staff with awareness of safety incidents and what is being done to address them encourages collaboration and improves teamwork.

All healthcare workers should be provided with basic patient safety training, including how to report events and near misses. Participation in activities such as root cause analysis or critical event reviews should be encouraged by leadership. Ongoing education is critical, as patient safety culture builds on evidence-based practices and continuous improvement of processes in the constant analysis of events and near-miss opportunities to prevent future events.

Reporting patient safety incidents should be considered a duty of every healthcare worker. All healthcare workers must be aware of their role in providing a safe patient environment and in preventing medical errors [33]. Creating a strong patient safety culture requires a sustained effort from the entire healthcare team. When this does not occur, the impact is significant to the patient, the hospital, and the individual involved.

Key aspects of a strong patient safety culture include [32]:

- Transparency and open communication
- Role modeling by leaders
- Support system for second victims
- Organizational commitment to just culture
- Timely feedback on shared learnings
- Non-punitive, investigative approach to errors
- Empowerment and expectation at all levels to report
- Clear definitions of errors and near misses
- Emphasis on learning from mistakes

5   The Second Victim

The psychological impact of making an error can be significant to the clinician. The second victim refers to a healthcare worker involved in an unintentional adverse patient event who becomes a victim from the trauma of guilt and blame over the event [34].

When an adverse event occurs, the immediate focus is on the impact to the patient and prevention of secondary injury. The patient is the first victim. However, evidence shows that the long-term emotional and psychological effects of the second victim can be just as devastating. Feelings of guilt, embarrassment, and shame can lead to self-doubt and a loss of confidence that can last for years. Lasting emotional distress can cause effects like that of post-traumatic stress disorder, such as depression, anxiety, pervasive thoughts of the event, insomnia, and emotional outbursts [35].

The second victim phenomena is thought to be widely prevalent, with some studies estimating 43% of healthcare workers having experienced it at some point in their career [36]. Those who experience symptoms as the second victim are more likely to worry about job performance, report burnout, and consider leaving the profession [37]. These effects are only compounded in an organization that blames and punishes rather than investigates and identifies what other factors may have led to the error.

Support for the second victim is vital to help with the potential long-term effects, though organizational interventions for support are not yet common as research on the second victim phenomena remains relatively new [37]. There are a number of institution-based second victim support resource programs and toolkits available [34]. Unfortunately, without a strong patient safety culture, many healthcare workers continue to experience blame or punishment, which not only worsens the trauma but also makes that person less likely to report an error if it occurs again [35].

Establishing a strong patient safety culture is the first step to providing a support structure for second victims with a non-punitive environment to reduce the emotional impact of adverse events. Organizations can assist in reducing the stigma of adverse events and encourage self-reporting of errors by taking measures to support the second victim:

- Create a confidential support network of peer counselors, chaplains, or mental health professionals that are specially trained to provide emotional support to second victims [34].
- Encourage management support by ensuring leaders are trained on recognizing the impact of adverse events on staff and how to approach situations in a non-judgmental manner immediately after an event.
- Recognize the second victim in the review process. Everyone who is involved in an event should have the opportunity to debrief in an event review, provide feedback, and contribute to learning from the experience [36].

6   Summary

Barriers to patient safety can be present even in well-established safety programs. These barriers usually involve unit culture, are not always easily identified, and are sometimes tolerated as the status quo. Power distance, normalization of deviance, poor culture of error reporting, and nonadherence to a true just culture are barriers that are not as easily corrected with a standard practice, algorithm, or behavioral intervention. These barriers are difficult to overcome if not intentionally uncovered and identified and may lead to patient or caregiver harm. In overcoming these formidable barriers to patient safety, we embark on a journey toward a healthcare system that truly prioritizes the well-being and trust of every patient, ultimately ensuring a brighter, safer future for all.

Key Points

- Although safety processes are often thought of as well established, barriers to patient safety can lie hidden in all of our programs of safety including speaking up behavior, drifting to normalization of deviance, error reporting, and within the application of just culture.
- Power differentials contribute to lack of speaking up behavior and can contribute to errors in all contexts of healthcare.
- Normalization of deviance is a gradual drift to tolerate a lowered safety standard in order to get the job done within a tight time constraint or high-pressure situation.
- Error reporting is the most important tool available to identifying patient safety concerns and is the duty of every healthcare worker.
- Failures of just culture exist even within an established system with a perceived strong safety culture. Work unit culture is an important influence in patient safety behavior.
- Second victim syndrome can lead to long-term emotional and psychological distress that can affect job performance and lead to leaving healthcare as a career.
- These barriers are not overtly obvious, but detrimental to safety, unless they are acknowledged and mitigated.

References

1. ECRI. Culture of safety: an overview. Health syst risk manage. 2019. https://www.ecri.org/components/HRC/Pages/RiskQual21.aspx
2. Frankel A, Haraden C, Federico F, Lenoci-Edwards J. A framework for safe, reliable, and effective care. White Paper. Cambridge, MA: Institute for Healthcare Improvement and Safe & Reliable Healthcare; 2017. ihi.org.
3. Weick KE, Sutcliffe KM. Managing the unexpected. 3rd ed. Wiley; 2015.
4. Institute of Medicine (US). Committee on quality of health care in America. In: Kohn LT, Corrigan JM, Donaldson MS, editors. To err is human: building a safer health system. National Academies Press (US); 2000.
5. Violato E. A state-of-the-art review of speaking up in healthcare. Adv in Health Sci Educ. 2022;27:1177–94. https://doi.org/10.1007/s10459-022-10124-8.
6. Hoffmann M, Schwarz CM, Schwappach D, et al. Speaking up about patient safety concerns: view of nursing students. BMC Health Serv Res. 2022;22:1547. https://doi.org/10.1186/s12913-022-08935-x.
7. Peadon R, Hurley J, Hutchinsin M. Hierarchy and medical error: speaking up when witnessing an error. Saf Sci. 2020;125:104648.
8. Etchegaray JM, Ottosen MJ, Dancsak T, Thomas EJ. Barriers to speaking up about patient safety concerns. J Patient Saf. 2020;16(4):e230–4. https://doi.org/10.1097/PTS.0000000000000334.

9. Mulder M. The daily power game. Leiden, Netherlands: Martinus Nijhoff; 1977.
10. Hofstede G. Cultures and organizations. Software of the mind. London: Harper Collins Publishers; 1994. p. 273.
11. Kim S, Appelbaum NP, Baker N, Bajwa NM, Chu F, Pal JD, Cochran NE, Bochatay N. Patient safety over power hierarchy: a scoping review of healthcare professionals' speaking-up skills training. J Healthc Qual. 2020;42(5):249–63. https://doi.org/10.1097/JHQ.0000000000000257.
12. Faisal A. Nurse-physician conflict and power dynamic. JOJ Nurse Health Care. 2017;5(3):555665. https://doi.org/10.19080/JOJNHC.2017.05.555665.
13. Bochatay N, Kuna Á, Csupor É, Pintér JN, Muller-Juge V, et al. The role of power in health care conflict: recommendations for shifting toward constructive approaches. Acad Med. 2021;96(1):134–41. https://doi.org/10.1097/ACM.0000000000003604.
14. O'Donovan R, McAuliffe E. A systematic review exploring the content and outcomes of interventions to improve psychological safety, speaking up and voice behavior. BMC Health Serv Res. 2020;20:101. https://doi.org/10.1186/s12913-020-4931-2.
15. Pack R, Columbus L, Duncliffe TH, et al. "May be I'm not that approachable": using simulation to elicit team leaders' perceptions of their role in facilitating speaking up behaviors. Adv Simul. 2022;7:31. https://doi.org/10.1186/s41077-022-00227-y.
16. Edmondson A. Psychological safety and learning behavior in work teams. Adm Sci Q. 1999;44(2):350–83. 16.
17. Vaughan D. The challenger launch decision. U of Chicago Press; 1986.
18. Wright MI, Polivka B, Odom-Forren J, Christian BJ. Normalization of deviance: concept analysis. ANS Adv Nurs Sci. 2021;44(2):171–80. https://doi.org/10.1097/ANS.0000000000000356.
19. WORKAROUND | definition in the Cambridge English Dictionary.
20. van der Veen W, Taxis K, Wouters H, Vermeulen H, Bates DW, van den Bemt PMLA, the BCMA Study Group. Factors associated with workarounds in barcode-assisted medication administration in hospitals. J Clin Nurs. 2020;29:2239–50. https://doi.org/10.1111/jocn.15217.
21. Sedlar N, Irwin A, Martin D, Roberts R. A qualitative systematic review on the application of the normalization of deviance phenomenon within high-risk industries. J Saf Res. 2023;84:290–305. https://doi.org/10.1016/j.jsr.2022.11.005.
22. McGaffigan_AvoidingDriftIntoHarm_HCExec_Sep2022.pdf. ihi.org.
23. Amalberti R, Vincent C. Managing risk in hazardous conditions: improvisation is not enough. BMJ Qual Saf. 2019;0:1–4.
24. Rutledge DN, Retrosi T, Ostrowski G. Barriers to medication error reporting among hospital nurses. J Clin Nurs. 2018;27(9–10):1941–9. https://doi.org/10.1111/jocn.14335.
25. Hamed MMM, Konstantinidis S. Barriers to incident reporting among nurses: a qualitative systematic review. West J Nurs Res. 2022;44(5):506–23. https://doi.org/10.1177/0193945921999449.
26. Fung WM, Koh SS, Chow YL. Attitudes and perceived barriers influencing incident reporting by nurses and their correlation with reported incidents: a systematic review. JBI Lib Syst Rev. 2012;10(1):1–65. https://doi.org/10.11124/jbisrir-2012-44.
27. Aljabari S, Kadhim Z. Common barriers to reporting medical errors. Sci World J. 2021;2021:6494889. https://doi.org/10.1155/2021/6494889.
28. Agency for Healthcare Research and Quality. Hospital survey on patient safety culture: 2019 User Database Report; 2019. https://www.ahrq.gov/sites/default/files/wysiwyg/professionals/quality-patient-safety/patientsafetyculture/hospital/2019/hosp19db.pdf.
29. Vrbnjak D, Denieffe S, O'Gorman C, Pajnkihar M. Barriers to reporting medication errors and near misses among nurses: a systematic review. Int J Nurs Stud. 2016;63:162–78. https://doi.org/10.1016/j.ijnurstu.2016.08.019.
30. Archer S, Hull L, Soukup T, Mayer E, Athanasiou T, Sevdalis N, Darzi A. Development of a theoretical framework of factors affecting patient safety incident reporting: a theoretical review of the literature. BMJ Open. 2017;7(12):e017155. https://doi.org/10.1136/bmjopen-2017-017155.
31. van Marum S, Verhoeven D, de Rooy D. The barriers and enhancers to Trust in a Just Culture in hospital settings: a systematic review. J Patient Saf. 2022;18(7):e1067–75. https://doi.org/10.1097/PTS.0000000000001012.

32. Wawersik D, Palaganas J. Organizational factors that promote error reporting in healthcare: a scoping review. J Healthc Manage. 2022;67(4):283–301. https://doi.org/10.1097/JHM-D-21-00166.

33. Rodziewicz TL, Houseman B, Hipskind JE. Medical error reduction and prevention. In: StatPearls. StatPearls Publishing; 2022.

34. Busch IM, Moretti F, Campagna I, Benoni R, Tardivo S, Wu AW, Rimondini M. Promoting the psychological well-being of healthcare providers facing the burden of adverse events: a systematic review of second victim support resources. Int J Environ Res Public Health. 2021;18(10):5080. https://doi.org/10.3390/ijerph18105080.

35. Cabilan CJ, Kynoch K. Experiences of and support for nurses as second victims of adverse nursing errors: a qualitative systematic review. JBI Database System Rev Implement Rep. 2017;15(9):2333–64. https://doi.org/10.11124/JBISRIR-2016-003254.

36. Seys D, Wu AW, Van Gerven E, Vleugels A, Euwema M, Panella M, Scott SD, Conway J, Sermeus W, Vanhaecht K. Health care professionals as second victims after adverse events: a systematic review. Eval Health Prof. 2013;36(2):135–62. https://doi.org/10.1177/0163278712458918.

37. Wade L, Fitzpatrick E, Williams N, Parker R, Hurley KF. Organizational interventions to support second victims in acute care settings: a scoping study. J Patient Saf. 2022;18(1):e61–72. https://doi.org/10.1097/PTS.0000000000000704.

When Accidents Happen: Investigations That Create Future Safety

Aurora Davis and Kristen A. Oster

1 Introduction

Ever since the publication of the landmark report *To Err is Human* [1], the healthcare industry has been well aware of the harm that medical errors can cause in our patients. Although improvements in safety have been made in the two decades since, there is still a high frequency of preventable harm in the healthcare industry [2] and a continued need for a focus on quality improvement [3]. Nurse leaders must be prepared to identify and respond to safety events. This chapter will describe effective and practical methods, informed by safety science, for investigation and mitigation of safety events.

2 Background

If the goal of healthcare as an industry is to do no harm, then it is important to have a standard by which harm can be identified [4]. The Joint Commission's Sentinel Event Policy [5] is careful to specify that safety events are events not primarily related to the patient's underlying medical conditions or illness. The policy recognizes the fact that, even when care is provided exactly as intended the outcome is not always what the care team would have wished for the patient. This interpretation also allows safety improvements to be focused specifically on areas where the care

A. Davis (✉)
University of Colorado Hospital, UCHealth, Aurora, CO, USA
e-mail: aurora.davis@uchealth.org

K. A. Oster
Mountain Region, CommonSpirit Health, Centennial, CO, USA
e-mail: kristen.oster@gmail.com

provided deviated from the ideal and can be improved, regardless of the ultimate outcome. Even near misses can provide a significant opportunity to improve the care for future patients and subsequently avoid a sentinel event before it can occur. Tools to identify these opportunities, such as a Safety Assessment Code (SAC) Matrix [6], can assist with determining if a near miss represents a significant enough risk that a higher level investigation (such as a root cause analysis) is warranted.

Once a safety event has been identified, standardized tools for categorizing the event and the level of harm to the patient are recommended for aggregating, classifying, analyzing, and reporting data [4]. The ability to review this data at a macro level provides a lens into the least reliable—and therefore riskiest—processes and outcomes. High functioning organizations will utilize formalized harm scoring systems conducive to interrater reliability, such as Healthcare Performance Improvement's Safety Event Classification [4] or the Agency for Healthcare Research and Quality's Common Format Harm Scale [7].

Once the event has been categorized and harm assessed, leaders will be better able to identify if it meets the Joint Commission's criteria to be considered a sentinel event [5] or is on the National Quality Forum's list of serious reportable events (aka a "never event") [8]. Most events will meet these criteria due to their high level of harm to the patient, such as death, permanent injury, or life-threatening harm. Therefore, most of the safety work occurs in response to these serious safety events and is reactive in nature.

However, it is important to note that there are also specific types of events considered critical indicators of flaws in a system and will therefore require a higher level of review regardless of their impact on the patient. In addition, highly reliable organizations will also invest time and resources in more proactive safety work, such as FMEA or other process improvement work [9]. A well-integrated safety program with both proactive and reactive aspects will result in better identification of risks [10] and a streamlined approach to any identified improvement work [11].

3 Tools for Success

3.1 Nursing Peer Review

Peer review is an important tool to ensure quality and safety in healthcare systems for nursing care [12].Peer review is defined as an organized effort where professionals review the quality and appropriateness of services performed by their peers. This definition's application to nursing is the process of nurses to systematically assess, monitor, and make judgments regarding the quality of nursing care provided by professional peers in comparison to professional standards of care [13, 14].

Nursing peer review focuses on:

- Evaluating the quality and quantity of care provided.
- Strengths and weaknesses of nursing care provided in comparison to standards of care.
- Provision of evidence to support recommended practice changes (if applicable).
- Identification of practice patterns where more knowledge is needed.

For peer review to be successful, six practice guidelines have been developed by the American Nurses Association (ANA) to provide a consistent, evidence-based approach [13]:

1. Peer is someone who has the same job role rank.
2. Peer review is focused on practice.
3. Feedback is timely, routine, and continuous.
4. Peer review fosters a culture of safety and best practice.
5. Feedback is not anonymous.
6. Feedback incorporates nurses' developmental stage.

The intention of peer review is not to be punitive. Peer review nurtures an environment focused on continuous learning culture of safety, best practice, and the provision of feedback to foster maintenance and development of standards of care [13, 14].

3.2   Just Culture

Humans are imperfect and at times may make unintentional mistakes in their daily life and work. Within the healthcare field, unintentional mistakes may have large consequences including patient harm and death. A just culture environment is an organizational framework utilized by leadership where staff members are empowered to share concerns, near misses, or errors freely without fear of punishment while still held to the responsibility of their choices. Just culture requires a shift from focus on errors to focusing on strengthening processes to decrease events from occurring and management of the choices of employees [15]. To create and sustain a just culture organizations need to provide understanding of errors, psychological safety, leader responsibility, and employee responsibility in the process [16].

Within a just culture, leaders focus not only on the why of an error occurring but also the individual's intent of the decision leading up to the error and then holding the individual accountable to the decision. Based on the intent leading to the error, the leader is then able to apply the appropriate interventions to the employee. Errors can be categorized into three types: human, at-risk, and reckless. Human errors occur due to human nature and are usually unintentional. At-risk errors occur when individuals either do not clearly understand the risk associated with the activity or believe the risk to be justified. Reckless errors occur when an individual knowingly makes a decision that can cause harm and disregards risks associated with the choice [15].

Psychological safety is a key component to a just culture where employees feel empowered to speak up when an error occurs without fear of punitive consequences. A psychologically safe environment ultimately leads to safer patient outcomes due to better communication, increased accountability, greater safety awareness, and improved reporting of safety events. Organization leaders play a key role in creating psychological safety and just culture in the workplace [17]. Leaders who are accessible and approachable provide a space where issues and problems can be brought with the focus on improvement and not consequence. For a just culture to thrive leaders need to establish clear expectations through direct communication, boundaries, and accountability of employees in a consistent manner [15]. Employees' role in a just culture is the commitment to reporting near miss and adverse events. When events are reported, employees are actively involved in the review process with leadership support to identify gaps and solutions to be implemented.

Creation of a just culture demonstrates to employees the organization and its leaders are committed to the provision of a safe environment focused on patient outcomes. A just culture values employees speaking up and accountability in their decision-making related to patient care events and outcomes. When organizations and leaders empower employees to speak up, this provides a strong foundation where employees and leaders work together to keep patients safe [17].

3.3   Root Cause Analysis

A root cause analysis (RCA) is a collective patient safety multidisciplinary team approach to review and analyze healthcare-related adverse events and near misses. The goal of an RCA is to determine what happened, why it happened, and how to prevent it from happening again. It is important to note an RCA is not meant to focus on the "who" involved in the event but the "how" and the "why" to identify action items to prevent an adverse event or near miss from occurring again [18, 19]. An RCA is conducted when an adverse event or near miss occurs resulting in actual or potential harm. Events can be identified through hospital safety reporting programs. Preliminary information is gathered through investigation, research of best practices, review of policies and procedures, and interviewing of individuals involved in the event. Through the initial investigation of the event, individuals to be included in the review can be identified [20].

At the RCA meeting, a timeline of the event is created and reviewed. All preliminary information is shared with the team to ensure all pertinent information is included to create the event timeline with focus just on the facts. From the timeline, the facilitator will lead the team to look deeper into the event by asking why, how, and what factors contributed to the event occurrence. Next the team reviews each contributing factor to work to identify the root cause. This can be done by digging deeper and utilizing tools such as the Five Whys and a Fishbone diagram. This process is done until all root causes are found [21].

Each root cause is evaluated to identify action items with the goal to prevent the event from occurring again. Action items should be categorized as high, intermediate, and weak using the action hierarchy to ensure that intermediate and high action items are selected [22]. Action items should be clearly written outlining when, how, and who will complete each item. Each action item should be measurable and continuously evaluated to determine the risk for future occurrence. Action items are successful when the goal was attained, and change is permanent.

3.4   RCA²

An issue with the RCA process is lack of standardization. The root cause analysis process has been evaluated to improve its effectiveness by the National Patient

Safety Foundation (NPSF) to examine best practices within RCAs with the goal being to prevent harm and improve patient outcomes [23]. Through this review, the RCA process has been renamed root cause analysis and action or RCA^2 with focus on efforts resulting in the implementation of sustainable, system-based improvements [24]. The aim of the RCA^2 process is to identify system vulnerabilities with the goal to eliminate or mitigate the vulnerabilities. RCA^2 process does not focus or address individual performance as this has been identified as a symptom of larger system-based issues [24].

To be effective, healthcare systems need to have a robust incident reporting structure in place allowing staff to be able to report events and near misses without fear. A robust reporting structure provides adverse events and near miss events to be reviewed with focus on mitigation and prevention [25]. For an RCA^2 to be successful, a risk-prioritization system needs to be in place as this system prioritizes hazards and vulnerabilities that may not have caused harm with the aim to mitigate or eliminate harm before it occurs. A risk-prioritization system provides credibility and objectivity to the process and decreases the chance of misconception.

A system should be in place to trigger an RCA^2 to ensure events, and near misses are reviewed. Immediate actions include taking care of the patient, disclosure, ensuring patient and staff safety, evidence preservation, and information gathering related to the event. Within 72 hours, the event should be scored using the risk-prioritization system implemented by the facility to determine if an RCA^2 meeting is required. If an RCA^2 meeting is required, the review is scheduled as soon as possible to ensure that details of the event are fresh to those involved, and resources are available for event review. A recommendation is to have standing RCA^2 meetings allowing for pre-scheduled time to review events as events occur. Depending on the severity of the event reviewed, multiple RCA^2 meetings may need to occur to complete the work.

Team size and membership for RCA^2 are recommended to range from four to six people including subject matter experts and an appointed RCA^2 team leader. All team members should be familiar with contributing factors and the RCA^2 process to increase effectiveness. It is key to point out that individuals involved in the event are not involved in the RCA^2 process as there may be feelings of guilt, defensiveness, and provide an environment where difficult questions may not arise as to not hurt those involved. Expertise and knowledge not represented or known by one of the RCA^2 team members can be obtained through interviewing. This includes the staff, patients, and family members who may have been involved in the event. Each will provide a different perspective assisting the team in identifying action items to move forward with.

During RCA^2 meetings, the team reviews information gathered during interviews, chart reviews, and evaluates process flow diagrams to look at what happened and why it happened. From this discussion, a causal statement is defined to describe the cause, effect, and event by using the five rules of causation [24]. Next the team should strive to identify multiple solutions and corrective actions to be implemented focusing on system issues. Using the action hierarchy, at least one intermediate and one strong corrective action should be identified for implementation [22]. Each action item should have either a process or outcome measure associated with an identified timeline. Process measures confirm an action is implemented while an outcome measure determines the action's effectiveness. For action items to be successful, each should be reviewed and approved by executive leadership for support. Organizations often recommend RCA[2] activities be completed no longer than 30–45 days post event.

Finally, feedback is essential. Staff, patients, and families involved in the event should be told the findings and next steps related to an RCA[2] meeting. Provision of feedback creates a culture of safety and shows there is action when events are reported. The RCA[2] process should be reviewed annually by executive leadership on its effectiveness and for continuous improvement [24]. Overall, RCA[2] is an essential tool utilized by healthcare systems to improve patient safety and reduce future adverse events. Visit https://www.ihi.org/resources/Pages/Tools/RCA2-Improving-Root-Cause-Analyses-and-Actions-to-Prevent-Harm.aspx for additional information on performing RCA[2], as well as templates and other resources.

3.5   Action Hierarchy

Use of the action hierarchy is recommended to identify high level corrective action items during investigation of patient harm events [22]. Action hierarchy was developed by the Institute for Healthcare Improvement and assists teams in identifying whether actions will have a strong, intermediate, or weak effect for successful and sustained improvement (see Table 1).

3.6   Apparent Cause Analysis

Patient safety events will occur which do not meet sentinel event criteria, but still represent an opportunity to improve the care of future patients by making systems more highly reliable. In these cases, an Apparent Cause Analysis (ACA) is a more appropriate tool than a Root Causes Analysis (RCA). Unlike RCA—which is discussed extensively in the literature—there is less consensus regarding the definition

Table 1 Action hierarchy [24]

Action	Description	Example
Strong	Less reliant on humans	Standardization of equipment or process Process simplification Physical environmental change
Intermediate	Moderately reliant on humans	Standardization of communication IT enhancements Changes in workload
Weak	More reliant on humans	Education Double checks Policies Training

Source: National Patient Safety Foundation (NPSF). (2015). *RCA[2]: Improving Root Cause Analyses and Actions to Prevent Harm.* Boston, MA: National Patient Safety Foundation

of an ACA [26, 27]. The term ACA is used for a more limited investigation performed in response to an event that caused little or no harm or did not reach the patient [28]. These investigations require less time and resources to complete than an RCA, but like RCAs, ACAs are also focused on identifying and addressing issues with the process of care rather than blaming individuals [24].

Because of the lower level of severity of the outcome, these investigations are less heavily regulated by both external (the Joint Commission, governmental agencies) and internal (hospital, departmental) policies, allowing a certain amount of freedom on the part of the investigating entity to tailor their tools for efficiency [28]. However, although ease and efficiency of use should be considered when building a tool for ACA (see Table 2), these goals should not sacrifice the thoroughness of the

Table 2 Example of an apparent cause analysis (ACA)

Question	Response			Explanations
1. Were policies, procedures, and/or protocols followed?		Yes	No	
	If "No" explain ➜			
2. List the relevant policies, procedures, and/or protocols governing actions before, during, and after the event.				
3. Was the expected level of care met?		Yes	No	
	If "No" explain ➜			
4. Were the policies, procedures, and protocols in place, and was the care delivered at the time of the event adequate to have prevented the event from happening?		Yes	No	
	If "No" explain ➜			
5. Related to policies, procedures, protocols and/or expected level of care, did staff have appropriate:				
• Training/education?		Yes	No	
• Competency?		Yes	No	
• Orientation?		Yes	No	
	If "No" explain ➜			
6. Did the capability and number of staff match the acuity and number of patients?		Yes	No	
	If "No" explain ➜			
7. Were non-facility staff involved in the event?		Yes	No	
	If "Yes" explain ➜			
8. Did equipment performance contribute to this event?		Yes	No	
	If "Yes" explain ➜			
9. What other external/environmental factors contributed to this event?				
10. What role did communication play in this event? For example, shift-to-shift handoffs, MD-to-RN communication, MD-to-MD communication, inter-departmental, etc.)				
11. Could this event happen in another department?	Yes	No		
	If "Yes" explain ➜			
12. Additional comments:				
13. Conclusion based on analysis:	• Human error • Systems error • No error identified Explanation of conclusion ➜			

analysis [26]. A simple template covering a broad variety of system issues at a high level can be reviewed quickly yet will maintain a level of insight allowing teams to identify areas requiring a deeper investigation.

3.7   Common Cause Analysis

At times, leaders may identify trends of events with similar outcomes but the common factors leading to those outcomes may not be immediately evident. Consider the following scenario:

> *An active birth center has noticed an increase in their volume of Code White calls. In this facility, a Code White is called in response to an uncontrolled maternal hemorrhage after the patient has given birth. Although the outcomes of these Code Whites were all positive— the mothers were successfully resuscitated with no loss of life—the facility is concerned by the overall volume of these occurrences. Facility leaders would like to investigate what is leading to this increase. Is it maternal factors? Errors in diagnosis or treatment? Faulty medications or equipment? The facility has decided to perform a common cause analysis to determine what these events have in common and may be leading to the need to call a Code White.*

As with an ACA, a Common Cause Analysis (CCA) is discussed less frequently in the literature than RCA [28]. CCA may be used to examine events with similarities to determine if those events have causative factors in common [29], but it may also be used to examine similarities between ACAs or RCAs findings to form a comprehensive needs assessment. If a facility is categorizing the types of root causes identified via RCA—such as the Press Ganey Healthcare Performance Improvement Failure Modes Taxonomy (HPI-FMT) [4, 30]—then leaders will already have a pool of data that can be readily examined by leveraging a common cause format.

The best way to begin a CCA is by gathering a team of subject matter experts to brainstorm the types of causes that might be leading to the trend of events. This group should be as multidisciplinary as possible, as well as consisting of both clinical and operational experts. A patient safety leader can act as the facilitator or can partner with a team member with performance improvement expertise (such as lean or other methodologies) to co-facilitate. The team should consider all possible patient, environmental, clinical, human, or other factors which may have influenced the occurrences, then decide which are relevant to the investigation. The team can then begin building the framework of their analysis.

Templates can be created for CCA frameworks but given the changing nature of root causes, it is important not to limit the team to the items chosen for the CCA form. For example, if CCAs are frequently performed based on patient outcomes, then a template listing basic demographic information for patients would be a great starting place. A simple spreadsheet format can be used for the framework, with factors listed in the rows and events (or patient cases) listed in the columns. Once the framework is built, the team can assign owners to complete the investigation required to fill in the cells where the rows and columns meet. When finished, every cell in the form will contain information for each chosen factor for each individual case. In terms of data management, it is helpful to stick to yes/no answers or short,

Table 3 Example of a common cause analysis

	Factor	Patient #1	Patient #2	Patient #3
Patient factors	Age	28	32	41
	Race	Caucasian	African-American	Asian
	Co-morbidities	Gest. diabetes	Gest. diabetes	Gest. diabetes
	Gestational age	38w2d	37w1d	40w1d
Treatment factors	Epidural?	Yes	No	Yes
	Induction?	No	No	Yes
	Physician	Dr. Smith	Dr. Jones	Dr. White
	Provider team	OBGyn	Family medicine	OBGyn
Fetal factors	Newborn weight	8 lb. 6 oz	7 lb. 11 oz	9 lb. 8 oz

standardized names—most spreadsheet applications include the ability to create flexible charts and graphs and can count the number of times various answers appear in the cells.

Part of the common cause analysis form for the previous scenario might look something like Table 3.

A team of clinical experts would quickly notice the one thing these patients have in common is a co-morbidity of gestational diabetes. This information can then be used to delve further into the cause of the events, likely by completing a second CCA focused on the team's management of gestational diabetes in their patients.

3.8   Failure Mode and Effects Analysis (FMEA)

Failure mode and effects analysis (FMEA) is a systematic proactive method to identify and address potential failures within a process or system before an adverse event may occur. Failure modes mean the way or how a process or system might fail [31]. Effects analysis refers to analyzing the consequences of the identified failures. FMEA was originally developed in 1949 by the United States military and later adopted by the National Aeronautics and Space Administration (NASA) in the 1960s [32]. This methodology has continued to be used in aviation, aerospace, nuclear power, and automotive industries before being adopted into the healthcare field [32]. FMEA has now been extensively adopted into healthcare after the Joint Commission on Accreditation of Healthcare Organizations expedited its use in hospitals to complete proactive safety reviews.

3.8.1   When to Use an FMEA
In healthcare, FMEA can be utilized to evaluate new and existing processes and systems. For new processes, FMEA identifies potential or unintended consequences and should be completed prior to implementation. For existing processes, FMEA is helpful in identifying how proposed changes will impact the system [18]. Overall, an FMEA can be used in various scenarios including:

- Setting up a new process.
- Improving an existing process.

- Changing an existing process.
- Periodically throughout the life of an existing process for quality control.

3.8.2 Steps of an FMEA [18]
An FMEA consists of seven primary steps to proactively identify and address potential failures within a system.

Step 1: Identify the process to review
- Determine which process or system is going to be the focus of the FMEA.
- Define the scope of the project and be as narrow as possible.

Step 2: Create a team
- Develop a diverse group of subject matter experts (SMEs) to gain insight into the potential failure modes of the identified process or system to be reviewed [33].
- This team is led by a project team leader who can organize the SMEs to work together utilizing their various expertise and knowledge to identify failures.
- Number of team members is based on scope of the problem being reviewed.

Step 3: Map the process
- Map out all steps and substeps of the process or system in a visual manner using the collective knowledge and expertise of the SMEs.
- Clearly defining each step of the process assists all team members understand what is being analyzed.

Step 4: Analyze each step of process and identify failures
- Create a safe environment where all SMEs can participate freely.
- Review of each step and substep is completed by the SMEs to identify potential failure modes of each.
- For each failure, identify all consequences to the process and the associated root cause of the failure.

Step 5: Prioritize identified failures
- For each failure ask [18]
- What is the outcome of this failure?
  - How serious would the outcome be?
  - How often can this outcome occur?
- Assign a numeric value to each identified failure using a scale of 0–10 quantifying the likelihood of occurrence, detection, and severity of impact [34].
- The assigned values will be multiplied together to calculate the Risk Priority Number (RPN), which is an overall numeric assessment of the risk of the failure [34]. The higher the RPN, the higher the risk associated with the potential failure.
- Based on RPN score, select the top priority failure to work on.

Step 6: Identify and implement solutions
- As a team, evaluate each identified failure to determine a solution to implement with the goal to reduce or eliminate the failure.
- Do not choose too many failures to work on at once.
- Aim for solutions that are stronger or intermediate actions such as implementation of technology or a checklist/cognitive aid versus a low action such as education [18].
- Design of the action plan timeline for a solution includes what will be done, by whom, and when.

Step 7: Monitor and measure effectiveness of solutions
- Monitor and measure success of implemented solutions to determine if making an impact on selected failure.
- Monitoring and measuring occur starting at implementation of the solution and are the responsibility of the team leader.
- Successful completion of an FMEA includes
  - Success was monitored and measures illustrating effectiveness
  - Identified goal was attained
  - Change will become permanent

Visit https://www.ihi.org/resources/Pages/Measures/RiskPriorityNumberfrom FailureModesandEffectsAnalysis.aspx for additional tools and templates for performing FMEAs.

3.9   Interviewing Techniques

Interviewing teams in response to safety events is a necessary—indeed, crucial—part of any investigation [24]. However, as important as the information obtained will be to the event review, it is key to remember these interviews are often seen as frightening to those who were involved in the occurrence. The phrase second victim is used to describe staff and providers who either witnessed or were directly involved in the event and may have been left feeling sad, scared, guilty, or otherwise emotionally traumatized [35, 36]. The interview may be the first time these individuals have ever interacted with a patient safety team member, and participants often do not know what to expect.

It may be helpful to get feedback from those familiar with standard workflows for the involved department before talking to the individual who actually participated in the event. This allows the interviewer to gain a better understanding of the process prior to conducting interviews, which may be emotionally charged or challenging. For individuals who are involved in clinical care, speak with their leader to ensure interviewee availability and clinical coverage. It is important to coach the leader, so the purpose of the interview is communicated appropriately. Leaders should be encouraged to explain the goal of the interview is to gain accurate knowledge of the details of the event without blaming the individual. It is essential that employees should feel comfortable sharing openly, as their candor will lead to a more accurate assessment of what caused the event.

Start things off on the right foot by not using the term "interview" to describe the meeting with these individuals. Rather, call it a discussion, a debrief, a conversation—something less intimidating and with less connotation of wrong-doing. View this discussion as an opportunity to build trust with the individual on behalf of the patient safety team and the event review process. Use it as a way to reinforce just culture principles and systems thinking [37]. Meet in person whenever possible; if a remote meeting is required, try to schedule a virtual meeting rather than a phone conversation. Limit the number of people in the conversation to only one to two interviewers. Although some literature does recommend leaders not be present [24] if a staff member requests their direct leader be present to support them, be open to the idea.

During the meeting, express gratitude for the individual's participation in the conversation. Let the individual know you appreciate how difficult it can be to discuss an event with a poor outcome. Tell the person you are sorry the event occurred, and the intention of the review is to find and address any systems issues so that similar events will not happen again. Assure the individual the review will not be focused on assigning blame in response to individual actions. Perhaps most important—offer the person access to the peer support resources available at your organization, early and often! [38]

Begin by introducing yourself and your role, then proceed by asking the interviewee for their version of the event. Keep questions in the beginning of the conversation as open-ended as possible. Promote psychological safety by using active listening skills [37]. Avoid interrupting or preparing your next question while the interviewee is speaking. Repeating back or asking for clarification about what the individual has said helps people engage in this type of listening. Once the interviewee has finished their narrative of events, ask for clarification or expansion as needed. A list of systems-based questions [24, 25] can be helpful to ensure the interviewer doesn't forget to ask about potential factors that may have influenced the outcome of events. See Table 4 for some examples of systems focused interview questions. For a more comprehensive list of questions, visit https://www.ihi.org/resources/Pages/Tools/RCA2-Improving-Root-Cause-Analyses-and-Actions-to-Prevent-Harm.aspx.

During the final moments of the interview, ask the interviewee *if he/she could go back and do anything differently, what would he/she do?* This simple question is often quite effective at identifying what staff view as the root cause of the event. Pay close attention to the answer given here, as it will also often point to potential solutions (although that's getting ahead of ourselves). Place these proposed solutions in a virtual "parking lot" for future consideration during the event review. Give the interviewee an opportunity to ask questions about next steps or what will happen during the event review meeting. Tell the interviewee your discussion is confidential and remember to thank him/her for their time and again offer support resources. A follow-up email with your contact information is also a good idea.

Table 4 Examples of systems focused interview questions [24]

Systems category	Question
Human factors	• How often do staff perform this task? Were staff adequately trained? Can staff demonstrate competency? • Were the results of training monitored over time? • Consider whether the outcome was impacted by the individual's level of experience or by the presence of distractions/interruptions, slips/lapses, or cognitive biases. • Were fatigue, hunger, illness, or other physiological conditions a factor?
Task factors	• Were there any deviations from normal processes? • Were the policies and procedures related to this event current, clear, understandable, and readily available to all staff? • If policies and procedures were not followed, what positive and negative incentives may have influenced this? Is there a culture of normalized deviance? • Are the processes involved efficient and effective? What are the barriers to completion of the process or task?
Team factors	• Can you describe the teamwork during the event? Do you have thoughts about strengths or weaknesses of this team? • Were there barriers to communication? • Was there a handoff involved in the event? • Did existing documentation provide a clear picture of the work-up, the treatment plan, and the patient's response to treatment? • Was the correct technical information adequately communicated to the people who needed it?
Organizational factors	• Did the overall culture of the department encourage or welcome observations, suggestions, or "early warnings" from staff about risky situations and risk reduction? Are staff safe to speak up? • Was leadership or management involvement and/or oversight adequate? • Did leadership have an audit or quality control system to provide feedback on how key processes related to the adverse event were functioning? • Was communication between management/supervisors and frontline staff adequate?
Information technology	• Were there any issues with information technology? • Consider usability issues, downtime, and individual knowledge gaps.
Equipment	• Was equipment misuse (including user error) or malfunction a factor in the event? • Was routine preventative maintenance performed? • Are there any manufacturer recalls for this device? • Did staff receive the appropriate training for safe use? • Were backup systems available in case of equipment failure?
Physical work environment	• Did the physical environment have a negative impact? • Consider how the environment may be impacted by the time of day, day of week, temperature, lighting, room layout, and noise or other distractions.

(continued)

Table 4 (continued)

Systems category	Question
Resources	• Were there appropriate resources to complete the required work? • Was there sufficient staff on hand for the workload at the time? Were there contingency plans in place if this was not the case? • Was there adequate equipment to perform the work processes?
Closing	• Were there any unusual aspects of the patient such as unexpected patient complications or conditions? • How would you describe your interaction with the patient? • Is there anything else you think I should know? • If you could go back and do anything differently, what would you do?

3.10 Meeting Facilitation

Choosing the correct group to participate in a review meeting will make the facilitator's job much simpler. Gathering a multidisciplinary group including not only experienced clinicians, but also operational leaders, safety specialists, and process improvement experts will ensure all points of view are represented and the skills needed to identify root causes and develop strong action items are present [39]. Opinions are mixed regarding whether frontline staff and providers who were involved in the event should be present at the meeting [24, 37, 40]. Individuals who work on the frontline of patient care are subject matter experts when it comes to how policies and procedures are being put into practice [40]. Staff and providers are also the end user of any new processes being developed by the review team. However, frontline workers' presence can also lead to a "blame and shame" environment or can lead to heightened emotions as they relate their experiences [24]. Safety leaders should assess whether the individuals involved have a strong desire to attend, as well as whether their organization's safety and just culture are advanced enough to support the presence of frontline staff at a review meeting [41].

The meeting facilitator should always open by describing the review team's guiding principles of just culture and psychological safety. This can also be performed by the highest leader in the meeting, as it demonstrates the importance of the review and just culture ideals to the organization's executive leadership team [42]. The meeting should also include reminders of confidentiality per your organizational needs [37] and any meeting etiquette suitable for the venue (for example, in-person attendees may be asked to sign an attendance sheet, while virtual attendees may be asked to turn on their cameras and raise their hand if he/she would like to speak).

There are many challenges a facilitator may face, including difficulty engaging participants, blaming language, emotional sensitivities, and premature problem-solving. Many of these challenges can be addressed using active listening techniques like those used during interviewing [21, 24, 37]. Always acknowledge the emotions and ideas of participants, and avoid shutting down open dialogue. Keep the group focused on systems issues and learning opportunities, rather than the decisions of an individual. Place premature solutions in a "parking lot" and reassure the team you will bring these ideas back up after root causes are identified. When appropriate, leverage excitement about problem-solving to assign owners to action items.

3.11 Avoiding Cognitive Bias

Facilitators should also be alert for potential biases that may influence the review team. Implicit bias is unintentional discriminatory behavior caused or influenced by unconscious attitudes and feelings [43], even when the individual or group is driven by the best of intentions [44]. These biases may keep the team from establishing an environment of psychological safety for participants, identifying the true root cause of an occurrence, or developing strong action items. Facilitators should be mindful of cognitive shortcuts leading to causes or solutions shaped by implicit bias and ask the team questions to guide the discussion toward more introspective solutions. Facilitators may also wish to take a self-assessment to help identify their own internal biases, allowing facilitators to be more mindful about their own assumptions, as well as those of others. An example assessment can be found at https://implicit. harvard.edu/implicit.

Hindsight bias is another risk a review team faces when analyzing a safety event. Fischhoff describes hindsight bias as believing the outcomes of events could or should have been seen in advance [45]. This is commonly seen in occurrence reviews as believing decisions or actions should have failed the substitution test [46]; in other words, a similar individual with similar knowledge, training, and experience would not have made the same choice in the same circumstances [47]. This bias often results in an oversimplification of circumstances surrounding decisions and ignores the influence of systems issues upon these decisions [48]. RCA tools such as the "5 Whys" [49, 50] are designed to counteract hindsight bias by prompting the group to continually ask "but why...?" until a nuanced root cause is reached, rather than surface rationales.

3.12 Fishbone Analysis and Process Mapping

The Ishikawa diagram, commonly known as the cause-and-effect diagram or fishbone diagram, is a tool utilized during event reviews where the team evaluates different categories of contributing factors related to the event occurrence [51]. It is a structured approach providing a systematic review, through a visual graph digging deep into root causes of contributing factor categories. Examples of categories include manpower, machinery, measurement, material, and method [52] (see Fig. 1).

A process map is another planning tool that visually describes the flow of work. Other names include a flowchart, process chart, or workflow diagram. This method visually shows the who and what is involved in a process being reviewed, the relationships between steps, and can be used to reveal where the process can be improved [53].

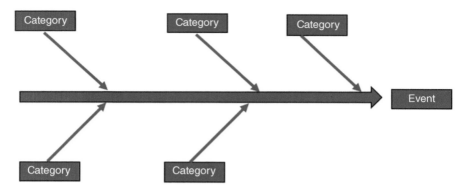

Fig. 1 A fishbone or Ishikawa diagram

3.13   Causal Trees

A causal factor tree diagram is another visual analysis tool displaying a logical hierarchy of causes leading to an occurrence. When gaps are encountered, the tree exposes the gaps but does not provide a means to resolve. The basic principle of the diagram is the occurrence as the result of changes or variations in a process. The diagram is constructed from the main occurrence as the tree's "trunk" with causal effects deductively categorized into "branches," thus explaining both causal factors and their relationship to the original occurrence [54].

3.14   The 5 Whys

The Five Whys is a simple technique to assist an investigator to determine the cause of a problem and understand contributing factors or causes to where a system fails. The strategy involves asking why to the original problem statement with the answer prompting a second why and so on [55]. The group completing the five whys should include a primary facilitator and a team of subject matter experts related to the problem statement being evaluated. To start the Five Whys the group facilitator should clearly identify the initial problem statement and asks "why?" If the answer provided is a contributing factor or cause to where the system failed, this will prompt the facilitator to ask why again. The five whys process is complete once the group comes to consensus—the root cause of the problem statement [49] (see Fig. 2). The Five Whys process can be used in conjunction with the fishbone diagram to determine contributing factors and causes for failure in different categories [21].

3.15   Gemba Walk

The word Gemba can be translated to "actual place" and was developed in the automotive industry [56]. A Gemba walk is an opportunity for leaders to complete a walkthrough of the actual workplace to gain knowledge and insight through

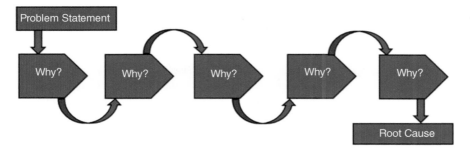

Fig. 2 A visual depiction of the 5 Whys

observation and inquiry with those actively involved in the work and can be used in conjunction with interviews to better understand what happened when responding to safety events. During this process, leaders are able to observe and directly speak with those completing the work to determine where value is focused and where opportunities can be implemented to eliminate waste [57, 58]. This is a simple but powerful method utilized to promote continuous improvement in the workplace. Using techniques like Gemba walk to improve the reliability of healthcare delivery is a strategy to develop a safer environment for both patients and providers [59].

3.16   Improvement Sustainability

It is helpful to begin thinking about the sustainability of identified improvements as early as the review meeting itself. The entire goal of an action item should be to improve the system and thereby **prevent recurrence** of the initial event. This cannot happen if the solution is unworkable over a long period of time, is too impractical, or proves overly complex. The development of strong action items that are less dependent on humans are generally more successful and sustainable over time [60]. The meeting facilitator should discuss the need for long-term solution success during action item development, and a process should be in place to design the sustainability plan in partnership with action item owners.

A simple audit performed at appropriate intervals can often be effective on many levels: it allows for an immediate assessment of the solution's success at addressing identified root causes, provides an opportunity for education and reinforcement with participants, identifies implementation barriers, and shows leadership's commitment to the success of the solution. FMEA can also be used for the proactive risk assessment of new processes [61]. Determining where a process may fail in advance allows for targeted changes and will help ensure the solution's success.

Process improvement (PI) tools are used in implementation science and are designed to measure and monitor workflow changes. PI tools can also be leveraged to ensure the success and sustainability of RCA action items [37, 62]. Lean Six Sigma uses the DMAIC (define, measure, analyze, improve, control) model [63] for structured process improvement work; this model integrates with many other RCA tools, and can provide a more detailed framework if a clearly defined PI workflow is needed. Visit https://www.dmaictools.com/ for templates.

4   Selecting the Right Methodology

It is important to select the correct tool for the job when investigating and responding to safety events. Organizers should consider multiple factors when selecting which methodology to use, including event severity, team skill set, institutional policies and culture, and regulatory requirements. If the incorrect tool is selected, it may hinder the team in identifying and implementing process changes to prevent harm to future patients. See Table 5 for an overview of the criteria used to select the appropriate tool for investigation or response.

5   Case Study

Let's review a case study. Imagine the following scenario:

> *It's late in the afternoon on a Friday and you're working in the Quality Department of a large urban medical center. You receive a phone call from a charge nurse who tells you she's calling about a code blue called for a patient on her surgical unit about an hour ago. A medication was ordered and administered incorrectly and caused the patient to experience a cardiac arrest. The patient was resuscitated and transferred to the critical care unit.*

Event response can be divided into three primary phases: immediate response, investigation, and analysis/action.

5.1   Immediate Response

Begin by considering if there is anything to be done immediately to prevent another patient from experiencing a similar adverse event. Ask the caller about anything already done to mitigate risk, as well as who has been notified of the occurrence. Sequester any evidence or equipment needed for the investigation, including taking photos of the scene. Remember to offer peer and other support resources early and often. Then, think about communication. Who in the facility will need to be notified of this event immediately? Are there standard communication channels for sharing this kind of information, such as a phone/email tree?

> *You thank the caller for taking the time to notify you of the event and ask who else has been told about the occurrence. She has already notified the unit's Manager and the Hospital's Manager, who notified the Administrator on call. There are no other patients on the unit who are receiving the medication involved, so she doesn't think it will impact any other patients. The Manager is already working to organize peer support for those involved. You ask her to sequester the IV pump involved in the error, as well as the medication bag and the IV tubing, and you arrange a time to pick this evidence up. After you hang up, you immediately activate your department's notification tree. You also notify Risk Management and your Pharmacy Safety team.*

Table 5 Tools and methodologies for safety event investigation and response

Tool/method	Description	Indication for use
RCA (root cause analysis)	A structured tool used in response to a serious safety event to identify and address the event's root causes, thereby preventing future harm [24]. https://www.ihi.org/resources/Pages/Tools/RCA2-Improving-Root-Cause-Analyses-and-Actions-to-Prevent-Harm.aspx	Sentinel events (events resulting in serious patient harm, including death, life-threatening harm, or severe permanent harm) or a near miss of these events [5].
Peer review	A process by which health care professionals evaluate each other's clinical performance to ensure consistent, high-quality care [64].	Care concerns such as perceived substandard care or perceived deviations from standard of care [5]. Cases may also be referred from RCA for an examination of clinical decision-making.
Collaborative case review	An interprofessional group retrospectively reviews individual patient encounters to improve future patient outcomes [60].	Indications may include adverse events (not meeting RCA criteria) that the team deems appropriate for review based on outcomes of interest or identified trends; these are not necessarily based on harm or poor outcomes.
FMEA (failure modes and effects analysis)	A process analysis tool used to identify all the ways a new design, process, product, or service could fail to perform as intended [31]. https://asq.org/quality-resources/fmea	Proactive risk assessment prior to the implementation of a new process or product.
Risk review/ assessment	An assessment that examines an existing process in detail and prioritizes areas for improvement based on the actual or potential impact (i.e., harm) [65]. There are a variety of tools depending upon the type of process involved, such as human reliability analysis to review human factors or probabilistic risk assessment for a review of complex systems.	Identified problematic processes, potential process vulnerabilities, or high-risk procedures that could result in a poor outcome.
Debrief	A relatively brief meeting, typically held immediately post-event, with the intention of identifying what went well and what did not go well during event response [66].	An adverse event requiring immediate response from multiple people and/or teams, such as a code blue or rapid response.
Audit	A quality management tool designed to review actual processes against defined criteria to identify adherence and gaps [67].	Identified gaps between best practice and actual practice. Frequently used to gauge adherence to process changes after an improvement event or root cause analysis [24].

5.2   Investigation

Determine if the event meets sentinel event criteria. In this case, the patient experienced life-threatening harm as a result of a medication error, which would meet the definition of a sentinel event [5]. Per the Joint Commission's Sentinel Event Policy (2023), sentinel events require "a thorough comprehensive systematic analysis (most commonly a root cause analysis) to determine why the event occurred. The organization must then create a corrective action plan to prevent similar events from happening again, implement the plan, and monitor its effectiveness." The team would follow the guidelines for an RCA to investigate the event. These may be supplemented by additional tools as indicated, such as a process map if there is a complex process to analyze or a Gemba walk if observational data will be helpful for the team's understanding.

During your call with your manager, you confirm you will be performing an RCA to review the event. You discuss who should attend, executive ownership, and the physician teams involved. You review the patient's chart and start a list of staff, providers, and pharmacists to interview. You contact leadership teams to discuss staff support and the timeline of the investigation. You interview those involved and organize the information you learn into an organized summary to share during the RCA meeting. You decide to use a fishbone diagram to map out what you have learned during your investigation. You also perform a literature search to identify best practices to help the RCA team during action item development.

5.3   Analysis and Action

The team will continue to use the RCA guidelines during the meeting to analyze the findings. The team can use a visual tool, such as a fishbone or causal tree, to organize the findings and assist with the identification of root causes. The 5 Whys are a simple and highly effective way to validate the analysis has gone deeply enough to identify a root cause, rather than a contributing factor. Finally, action items are developed and assigned to owners who have sufficient ownership of the processes involved to drive change. Executives should be prepared to remove barriers when owners escalate issues.

During the RCA meeting you are able to facilitate the team to identification of two root causes by utilizing both your fishbone diagram and the 5 Whys. Together the team identifies several action items, but you're concerned these actions may not be strong enough to provide sustained success over time. When you point this out and share the definition of a strong action item, the team is able to come up with an additional solution that will take longer to implement but will be more highly reliable in the long run. With your guidance, the team also comes up with a plan for auditing the success of the action items to ensure the changes are hardwired. After the meeting is over, you share the action plan with the RCA team, as well as any other stakeholders who weren't present at the meeting. You also schedule regular check-in meetings at 30, 60, and 90 days to review audit findings and ensure the action items have been successful in driving improvements.

6   Summary

Leaders who are investigating and responding to safety events must be able to identify which of many different tools are most suited to the work at hand. While an RCA can be effective at preventing future harm if it leads to strong, sustainable action items [24], RCA should not be considered a "one size fits all" solution. Instead, safety leaders need to select the right tool for the right event review to ensure the needed results. In addition, successful review and abatement of safety events are supported through the use of a just culture environment and peer support resources. Finally, leaders can leverage high reliability principles and process improvement tools to supplement safety investigations and increase the success of identified solutions [37, 59, 62].

Key Points

- There remains a high frequency of preventable harm in the healthcare industry and a continued need for a focus on quality improvement.
- The successful review and abatement of safety events are supported through the use of just culture and peer support resources.
- Critical tools for the investigation of and response to safety events include Root Cause Analysis (RCA), Apparent Cause Analysis (ACA), Common Cause Analysis (CCA), and Failure Mode and Effects Analysis (FMEA).
- Safety leaders should select the right tool for the right event review to ensure their work produces the needed results.
- Ensuring the sustainability of interventions is crucial to prevent recurrence and to improve care for future patients.

References

1. Institute of Medicine. To err is human: building a safer health system. The National Academies Press; 2000. https://doi.org/10.17226/9728.
2. Bates DW, Singh H. Two decades since to err is human: an assessment of progress and emerging priorities in patient safety. Health Aff. 2018;37(11):1736–43. https://doi.org/10.1377/hlthaff.2018.0738.
3. Dzau VJ, Shine KI. Two decades since to err is human: progress, but still a "chasm". JAMA. 2020;324(24):2489–90. https://doi.org/10.1001/jama.2020.23151.
4. Throop C, Stockmeier C. SEC & SSER patient safety measurement system for healthcare, rev. 2. Virginia Beach VA. Healthcare Performance Improvement (HPI) white paper series. 2011.
5. Joint Commission Resources. Comprehensive accreditation manual: CAMH for hospitals. Oakbrook Terrace, IL: Joint Commission Resources, Inc.; 2023.
6. Switaj TL, Cummings BM, Logan MS, Mort EA. Adopting RCA2: the interrater reliability of safety assessment codes. Am J Med Qual. 2019;34(2):152–7. https://doi.org/10.1177/1062860618793945.

7. Williams T, Szekendi M, Pavkovic S, Clevenger W, Cerese J. The reliability of AHRQ common format harm scales in rating patient safety events. J Patient Saf. 2015;11(1):52–9. https://www.jstor.org/stable/26633078
8. National Quality Forum (NQF). Serious reportable events in healthcare—2011 update: a consensus report. Washington, DC; 2011.
9. Noor Arzahan IS, Ismail Z, Yasin SM. Safety culture, safety climate, and safety performance in healthcare facilities: a systematic review. Saf Sci. 2022;147:105624. https://doi.org/10.1016/j.ssci.2021.105624.
10. Bender JA, Kulju S, Soncrant C. Combined proactive risk assessment: unifying proactive and reactive risk assessment techniques in health care. Jt Comm J Qual Patient Saf. 2022;48(6):326–34. https://doi.org/10.1016/j.jcjq.2022.02.010.
11. Simsekler MCE, Gurses AP, Smith BE, Ozonoff A. Integration of multiple methods in identifying patient safety risks. Saf Sci. 2019;118:530–7. https://doi.org/10.1016/j.ssci.2019.05.057.
12. Kaehne, A., Simcock, T., Onochie, D. (2019). A literature review of peer review models in healthcare.
13. American Nurses Association (ANA). Peer Review Guidelines. Kansas City, MO: ANA; 1998.
14. Haag-Heitman B, George V. Peer review in nursing. Principles for successful practice. Boston, MA: Jones and Bartlett Publishers; 2011.
15. Fencl JL, Willoughby C, Jackson K. Just culture: the foundation of staff safety in the perioperative environment. AORN J. 2021;113(4):329–36.
16. Kim BB, Yu S. Effects of just culture and empowerment on patient safety activities of hospital nurses. Healthcare. 2021;9:1324. https://doi.org/10.3390/healthcare9101324.
17. Paradiso L, Sweeney N. Just culture: it's more than policy. Nurs Manag. 2019;50:38–45.
18. CMS. Guidance of performing failure mode and effects analysis with performance improvement project. 2023. https://www.cms.gov/medicare/provider-enrollment-and-certification/qapi/downloads/guidanceforfmea.pdf. Accessed 2 Sept 2023.
19. Tang J, Liu Y, Lin K, Li L. Process bottlenecks identification and its root cause analysis using fusion-based clustering and knowledge graph. Adv Eng Inf. 2023:55.
20. Bogen SA. A root cause analysis into the high error rate in clinical immunohistochemistry. Appl Immunohistochem Mol Morphol. 2019;27(5):329–38. https://doi.org/10.1097/PAI.0000000000000750.
21. Latino MA, Latino RJ, Latino KC. Root cause analysis: improving performance for bottomline results. 5th ed. CRC Press; 2019. https://doi.org/10.1201/9780429446573.
22. Wood L, Wiegmann D. Beyond corrective action hierarchy: a systems approach to organizational change. Int J Qual Health Care. 2020;32(7):438–44. https://doi.org/10.1093/intqhc/mzaa068.
23. Hussain al Mardawi G, Rajendram R. Investigation of medication safety incidents using root cause analysis and action. Glob J Qual Saf Healthc. 2021;4:50–2. https://doi.org/10.36401/JQSH-20-X9.
24. National Patient Safety Foundation (NPSF). RCA²: improving root cause analyses and actions to prevent harm. Boston, MA: National Patient Safety Foundation; 2015.
25. Balakrishnan K, Brenner MJ, Gosbee JW, Schmalbach CE. Patient safety/quality improvement primer, part II: prevention of harm through root cause analysis and action (RCA²). Otolaryngol Head Neck Surg. 2019;161(6):911–21. https://doi.org/10.1177/0194599819878683.
26. Crandall KM, Sten M-B, Almuhanna A, Fahey L, Shah RK. Improving apparent cause analysis reliability: a quality improvement initiative. Pediatric Quality & Safety. 2017;2(3):e025. https://doi.org/10.1097/pq9.0000000000000025.
27. Parikh K, Hochberg E, Cheng JJ, Lavette LB, Merkeley K, Fahey L, Shah RK. Apparent cause analysis: a safety tool. Pediatrics. 2020;145(5):e20191819. https://doi.org/10.1542/peds.2019-1819.
28. Toncray KA. Cause analysis. In: Rampersad SE, Katz CB, editors. Patient safety and quality improvement in anesthesiology and perioperative medicine. Cambridge Core: Cambridge University Press; 2023. p. 40–9. https://doi.org/10.1017/9781108125758.

29. Buitrago I, Seidl KL, Gingold DB, Marcozzi D. Analysis of readmissions in a mobile integrated health transitional care program using root cause analysis and common cause analysis. J Healthc Qual. 2022;44(3) https://journals.lww.com/jhqonline/fulltext/2022/06000/analysis_of_readmissions_in_a_mobile_integrated.5.aspx:169.
30. Congenie K, Bartjen L, Gutierrez D, Knepper L, McPartlin K, Pack A, Sava K, Smith L, Watts H. Learning from latent safety threats identified during simulation to improve patient safety. Jt Comm J Qual Patient Saf. 2023;49:716. https://doi.org/10.1016/j.jcjq.2023.08.003.
31. American Society for Quality. Failure mode and effects analysis (FMEA). 2023. https://asq.org/quality-resources/fmea. Accessed 29 Aug 2023.
32. Anjalee JA, Rutter V, Samaranayake NR. Application of failure mode and effect analysis (FMEA) to improve medication safety: a systematic review. Postgrad Med J. 2021;97:168–74. https://doi.org/10.1136/postgradmedj-2019-137484.
33. Ullah E, Mansoor Baig M, GholamHosseini H, et al. Failure mode and effect analysis (FMEA) to identify and mitigate failures in a hospital rapid response system. Heliyon. 2022;8:e08944. https://doi.org/10.1016/j.heliyon.2022.e08944.
34. IHI. Risk priority number (from failure modes and effects analysis). 2023. https://www.ihi.org/resources/Pages/Measures/RiskPriorityNumberfromFailureModesandEffectsAnalysis.aspx. Accessed 29 Aug 2023.
35. Nydoo P, Pillay BJ, Naicker T, Moodley J. The second victim phenomenon in health care: a literature review. Scand J Public Health. 2020;48(6):629–37. https://doi.org/10.1177/1403494819855506.
36. White RM, Delacroix R. Second victim phenomenon: is 'just culture' a reality? An integrative review. Appl Nurs Res. 2020;56:151319. https://doi.org/10.1016/j.apnr.2020.151319.
37. Allison D, Peters H. Root cause analysis (RCA) for the improvement of healthcare systems and patient safety. 1st ed. CRC Press; 2021. https://doi.org/10.1201/9781003188162.
38. Heiss K, Clifton M. The unmeasured quality metric: burn out and the second victim syndrome in healthcare. Error Traps Cult Saf. 2019;28(3):189–94. https://doi.org/10.1053/j.sempedsurg.2019.04.011.
39. Hayden C, Kazi RR, Bylund J, Rasper A, Strup S, Harris A. MP20-11 UTILIZING a MULTIDISCIPLINARY APPROACH TO NEAR MISS EVENT ANALYSIS LEADS TO SUCCESSFUL IMPLEMENTATION OF ACTION ITEMS. J Urol. 2021;206(Supplement 3):e340–1. https://doi.org/10.1097/JU.0000000000002005.11.
40. Swamy L, Worsham C, Bialas MJ, Wertz C, Thornton D, Breu A, Ronan M. The 60-minute root cause analysis: a workshop to engage interdisciplinary clinicians in Quality improvement. MedEdPORTAL. 2018;14:10685. https://doi.org/10.15766/mep_2374-8265.10685.
41. Murray JS, Clifford J, Larson S, Lee JK, Sculli GL. Implementing just culture to improve patient safety. Mil Med. 2023;188(7–8):1596–9. https://doi.org/10.1093/milmed/usac115.
42. Haskins HEM, Roets L. Nurse leadership: sustaining a culture of safety. Health SA Gesondheid. 2022;27:1–8.
43. Narayan MC. Addressing implicit bias in nursing: a review. Am J Nurs. 2019;119(7):36. https://doi.org/10.1097/01.NAJ.0000569340.27659.5a.
44. Edgoose JYC, Quiogue M, Sidhar K. How to identify, understand, and unlearn implicit bias in patient care. Fam Pract Manag. 2019;26(4):29–33.
45. Fischhoff B. Hindsight ≠ foresight: the effect of outcome knowledge on judgment under uncertainty. Qual Saf Health Care. 2003;12(4):304. https://doi.org/10.1136/qhc.12.4.304.
46. Groß J, Kreis BK, Blank H, Pachur T. Knowledge updating in real-world estimation: connecting hindsight bias and seeding effects. J Exp Psychol. 2023. https://doi.org/10.1037/xge0001452.
47. Reason J. Managing the risks of organizational accidents. 1st ed. Routledge; 1997. https://doi.org/10.4324/9781315543543.
48. Cohen JB, Patel SY. Getting to zero patient harm: from improving our existing tools to embracing a new paradigm. Anesth Analg. 2020;130(2) https://journals.lww.com/anesthesia-analgesia/fulltext/2020/02000/getting_to_zero_patient_harm__from_improving_our.39.aspx:547.

49. CMS. Five whys tool for root cause analysis. 2023. https://www.cms.gov/medicare/provider-enrollment-and-certification/qapi/downloads/fivewhys.pdf. Accessed 9 Sept 2023.
50. Soliman MHA. Jidoka: the Toyota principle of building Quality into the process. 2020.
51. Carvalho R, Lobo M, Oliveria A, Lopes F, et al. Analysis of root causes of problems affecting the quality of hospital administrative data: a systematic review and Ishikawa diagram. Int J Med Inform. 2021;156:104584.
52. Tufail MM, Shakeel M, Sheikh F, Anum N. Implementation of lean six-sigma project in enhancing health care service quality during COVID-19 pandemic. AIMS Publ Health. 2021;8(4):704–19. https://doi.org/10.3934/publichealth.2021056.
53. Whitaker J, Amoah AS, Dube A, Chirwa L, et al. Novel application of multi-facility process map analysis for rapid injury care health system assessment in northern Malawi. BMJ Open. 2023;13:e070900. https://doi.org/10.1136/bmjopen-2022-070900.
54. Ikwan F, Sanders D, Hassan M. Safety evaluation of leak in a storage tank using fault tree analysis and risk matrix analysis. J Loss Prev Process Ind. 2021;73:104597.
55. Gangidi P. A systematic approach to root cause analysis using 3 x 5 why's technique. Int J Six Sigma, vol. 10; 2019. p. 295.
56. Tortorella G, van Dun DH, de Almeida AG. Leadership behaviors during lean healthcare implementation: a review and longitudinal study. J Manuf Technol Manag. 2020;31(1):193–215. https://doi.org/10.1108/JMTM-02-2019-0070.
57. Dempsey A, Robinson C, Moffatt N, Hennessy T, et al. Lean six sigma redesign of a process for healthcare mandatory education in basic life support—a pilot study. Int J Environ Res Public Health. 2021;18(21):11653. https://doi.org/10.3390/ijerph182111653.
58. Quon C, Lopez I, Nill E, Miller R, et al. Using lean methodology to improve ophthalmology medication workflow processes. J Nurs Care Qual. 2023;38(3):199–202. https://doi.org/10.1097/NCQ.0000000000000687.
59. Thull-Freedman J, Mondoux S, Stang A, Chartier L. Going to the COVID-19 Gemba: using observation and high reliability strategies to achieve safety in a time of crisis. Can J Emerg Med. 2020;22(6):738–41. https://doi.org/10.1017/cem.2020.380.
60. Lacson R, Khorasani R, Fiumara K, Kapoor N, Curley P, Boland GW, Eappen S. Collaborative case review: a systems-based approach to patient safety event investigation and analysis. J Patient Saf. 2022;18(2):e522–7. https://doi.org/10.1097/PTS.0000000000000857.
61. Liu H-C. Improved FMEA methods for proactive healthcare risk analysis. Springer; 2019.
62. Braithwaite J, Ludlow K, Testa L, Herkes J, Augustsson H, Lamprell G, McPherson E, Zurynski Y. Built to last? The sustainability of healthcare system improvements, programmes and interventions: a systematic integrative review. BMJ Open. 2020;10(6):e036453. https://doi.org/10.1136/bmjopen-2019-036453.
63. Ahmed S. Integrating DMAIC approach of Lean Six Sigma and theory of constraints toward quality improvement in healthcare. Rev Environ Health. 2019;34(4):427–34. https://doi.org/10.1515/reveh-2019-0003.
64. Bader H, Abdulelah M, Maghnam R, Chin D. Clinical peer review; a mandatory process with potential inherent bias in desperate need of reform. J Community Hosp Intern Med Perspect. 2021;11(6):817–20. https://doi.org/10.1080/20009666.2021.1965704.
65. Ostrom LT, Wilhelmsen CA. Risk assessment: tools, techniques, and their applications. Wiley; 2019.
66. Twigg S. Clinical event debriefing: a review of approaches and objectives. Curr Opin Pediatr. 2020;32(3):337–42. https://journals.lww.com/co-pediatrics/fulltext/2020/06000/clinical_event_debriefing__a_review_of_approaches.2.aspx.
67. Abimanyi-Ochom J, Bohingamu Mudiyanselage S, Catchpool M, Firipis M, Wanni Arachchige Dona S, Watts JJ. Strategies to reduce diagnostic errors: a systematic review. BMC Med Inform Decis Mak. 2019;19(1):174. https://doi.org/10.1186/s12911-019-0901-1.

Part II

Nursing and Patient Safety

Role of Nursing in Patient Safety

Cynthia A. Oster and Kristen A. Oster

1 Introduction

The global nursing workforce is composed of 27.9 million men and women, of which 19.3 million are professional nurses [1]. A professional nurse is an individual licensed to practice who has completed a program of nursing education and is qualified and authorized in his/her country to practice nursing. "Professional nurses assume responsibility for the planning and management of the care of patients, including the supervision of other health care workers, working autonomously or in teams with medical doctors and others in the practical application of preventive and curative measures" [2]. Professional nurses include clinical nurses, public health nurses, nurse educators, advanced practice nurses, and nurse leaders.

In the United States (US), nursing is the largest healthcare profession and the largest component of the healthcare workforce with about 4.2 million registered nurses (RNs) nationwide [3]. Most healthcare services in the US involve some sort of care by nurses. With more than three times as many RNs as physicians, nurses are the primary providers of hospital patient care and deliver most of the nation's long-term care as well as provide care in settings such as private practices, health maintenance organizations, public health agencies, primary care clinics, home health care, outpatient surgical centers, mental health agencies, insurance and managed care companies, hospices, the military, industry and healthcare research [4]. Nursing

C. A. Oster (✉)
Nursing and Professional Development, CommonSpirit Health – Mountain Region,
Centennial, CO, USA
e-mail: oster.cynthia.a@gmail.com

K. A. Oster
Mountain Region, CommonSpirit Health, Centennial, CO, USA
e-mail: kristen.oster@gmail.com

© The Author(s), under exclusive license to Springer Nature
Switzerland AG 2024
C. A. Oster, J. S. Braaten (eds.), *The Nexus between Nursing and Patient Safety*,
https://doi.org/10.1007/978-3-031-53158-3_5

in the twenty-first century is the glue that holds the patient's health care journey together [5]. Nurses are indispensable in the work to improve patient safety and quality. Efforts to detect and remedy error-producing defects in the healthcare system are dependent on the eyes, ears, cognitive powers, and interventions of the professional nurse [6]. This chapter will discuss the historical background of nursing and patient safety, evolution of nursing in promoting patient safety, and the essentiality of nursing to patient safety.

2   Historical Background of Nursing and Patient Safety

Patient safety is considered one of the central issues in the healthcare environment. The nursing profession was founded to protect, promote, and improve health for all ages of patients. Florence Nightingale, often considered the founder of modern nursing, advocated for safe patient care. She proposed that nurses through their practice had to put the patient in the best condition possible for nature to act upon the patient. Today Nightingale's proposition is reflected in nursing practice as the provision of a caring relationship that facilitates health and healing. Nightingale viewed nursing quality as dependent on consistent reliable care and argued patient safety and restorative care to be dependent on effective leadership, standard procedures, and reliable processes [7]. The greatest threats to patient safety continue to be frailties of the human condition, complacent attitudes, and unconscious behaviors.

The Institute of Medicine (IOM) report *Keeping Patients Safe: Transforming the Work Environment of Nurses* made it explicit that nurses are the most likely member of the healthcare team to intercept errors and prevent harm to patients [6]. However, nursing was concerned with defining and measuring quality and safety long before the current national and state-level emphasis on quality improvement and patient safety. In 1854, Florence Nightingale oversaw nurses in Turkey during the Crimean War and was horrified by the unsanitary conditions and lack of medical supplies. She observed there was no clean linen; the clothes of the soldiers were dirty and infested with lice and fleas; and the walls, floors, and ceilings in the hospital building were filthy. Furthermore, she discovered the morbidity and mortality in the hospital far exceeded those on the battlefield. Nightingale gathered data to show it was typhus, typhoid, dysentery, and cholera rather than battle injuries that took the lives of more than 4000 British soldiers during her first year in service. She attributed these deaths to unsanitary conditions specifically overcrowding, poor hygiene, and lack of ventilation. Florence Nightingale analyzed mortality data among British troops and accomplished significant reduction in mortality through organizational and hygienic practices by implementing routine changing of bed linens, utilization of clean water, revision of patient diets, and cleaning up the hospital wards and kitchens [8, 9]. Nightingale used her passion for statistics and a "coxcomb," her innovative shaded color-coded data visualization strategy, to illustrate the number of unnecessary deaths during the Crimean War due to preventable infections [10]. Furthermore, she used data to illustrate that mortality dropped from 42% to less than 2% following her improvements in hospital sanitary conditions [11]. Nightingale showed the environment in which nursing care is provided is imperative to a patient's ability to heal as "what nursing has to do ... is to put the patient in the best condition for nature to act upon him" [12, p. 75].

Clearly Florence Nightingale was a pioneer of patient safety and quality improvement [13]. Since her priority was the well-being of the patient, she began to immediately uncover quality problems along with their root causes during her service in Crimea. For example, processes intended to serve patients were ineffective due to lack of supplies. The root cause being the British army supply chain function was not prepared to meet the demands and challenges during the Crimean War. Supply chain methodology or the purveying system was designed to prevent fraud rather than to promote low cost and high service to the soldier or customer. Furthermore, the supply inventory was unreliable. The system required duplicate paperwork to order supplies and lacked efficiency as often the system failed to deliver supplies. She improved safety and quality by reducing variation, improving efficiency, and using statistical expression of data as a tool for persuasion [14]. Nightingale envisioned a system in which the patient ceased to be a soldier and became a patient from the moment he crossed the hospital doors. He left his possessions in a storeroom and left supplies, or anything used in the hospital behind to become a soldier again. Customer focus or the well-being of the patient was the priority.

Nightingale is recognized as one of the first safety and quality leaders in healthcare [15]. Nightingale can be credited with creating the framework for quality management and safety as she understood and exposed cause and effects, promoted outcomes measurement based on credible data and understood that problems could be caused by not only individuals but also by systems as well [16]. She identified aims, changes to be made and measures to monitor changes made. This technique is timelessly relevant and is currently reflected in the science of improvement. Science of improvement is "an applied science that emphasizes innovation, rapid-cycle testing in the field, and spread in order to generate learning about what changes, in which contexts, produce improvements" [17]. It embodies a blend of expert subject knowledge and improvement methods and tools through a multidisciplinary lens that draws from clinical science, systems theory, psychology, statistics, and other disciplines.

A commonly used model in improvement science is the model for improvement created by Associates for Process Improvement [18]. This model is grounded in the work of W. Edwards Deming who is widely acknowledged as a leading thinker in the field of quality [19]. Deming created a method that allowed individuals and organizations to plan and continuously improve themselves, their relationships, processes, products, and services through a philosophy of cooperation and continual improvement that avoids blame and redefines mistakes as opportunities for improvement. The model for improvement is composed of two components: three fundamental questions followed by the Plan-Do-Study-Act (PDSA) cycle [18]. The three fundamental questions are: (1) What are we trying to accomplish? (Aims); (2) How will we know that a change is an improvement? (Measures); and (3) What changes can we make that will result in improvement? (Changes). The PDSA "uses repeated cycles of planning through problem identification, doing an active intervention to change processes associated with the problem, studying data associated with the process change, and acting on the data to address what was learned in the process

Table 1 Nightingale's focus on improvement science and lessons learned

Improvement on science focus	Lesson learned	Example
Total systems safety	Everyone in the healthcare system contributes to quality and safety.	Asserted the entire healthcare team should be held accountable for safe, high-quality care from those who deliver frontline care, to purveyors, educators, and hospital administrators.
Science of improvement tools/methods	Using the right improvement tools and methods matters.	Used diagrams to understand problems, set aims, assigned metrics for improvement, and translated evidence into practice that made handwashing, bathing, and other principles of asepsis and infection control mandatory and reduced hospital death rate by two-thirds during Crimean War.
Patient-centered	Improving quality means addressing what matters to patients.	Championed innovations designed to treat patients with dignity and respect such as creating a kitchen to make appetizing meals, establishing a library and classroom for entertainment and intellectual stimulation, and starting a laundry to provide clean sheets.
Culture of safety	Culture and outcomes are linked.	Showed courage in speaking up and challenging the traditional medical authority, which was instrumental in advancing collaborative, high-quality care, and defining components of safety culture.
Patient and workforce safety	Nurses are high-impact leaders.	Recognized the privilege of nurses to view, understand, and transform healthcare systems and believed hospital leaders must ensure patient and workforce safety as core values.
Data driven	Understanding data is essential for improvement.	Used data to understand current state, evaluate priorities, and assess progress in improving patient outcomes. Her version of root cause analysis revealed British soldiers were more likely to die because of typhoid, cholera, and dysentery spread through unsanitary conditions and practices than from injuries sustained in battle.

Adapted from: McGaffigan, P. (2019). Why Florence Nightingale's Improvement Lessons Still Matter Today. Accessed 06/16/23 at https://www.ihi.org/communities/blogs/why-florence-nightingales-improvement-lessons-still-matter-today [15]

change" [20, p. 209]. Nightingale was using these ideas most productively long ago as she linked causes with effects, used data to understand outcomes, and analyzed problems as flawed systems rather than as flawed individuals [16]. See Table 1 for a few highlights of Nightingale's focus on improvement science and lessons learned.

3   Evolution of Nursing in Promoting Patient Safety

Since the time of Florence Nightingale, the goal of nursing has remained unchanged, namely to provide a safe and caring environment that promotes patient health and well-being [21]. Nightingale analyzed mortality data among British troops in 1855 and accomplished significant reduction in mortality through organizational and hygienic practices [22]. She is also credited with creating the world's first performance measures of hospitals in 1859 [23]. In addition, she transformed army sanitation practices to improve the hospital barracks environment and thus decrease soldier mortality [9]. Nursing has been concerned with defining and measuring safety and quality long before the current national and state-level emphasis on safety and quality improvement.

The historical and contemporary role of the nurse in promoting patient safety is described in a content analysis of 1086 articles published in American Journal of Nursing from October 1900 through December 2015 [24]. From 1900 to 1919, safety in nursing focused on preventing post-operative complications such as pressure injuries and pneumonia and maintaining cleanliness through handwashing and asepsis in the time before antibiotic discovery. Physicians wrote many of the published papers centered on pathophysiology and symptomatology with little mention of nursing care. The 1920s continued to focus on knowledge and new technology with emphasis on the proper use and application of technology rather than on the associated nursing care and safety precautions or considerations. Patient safety was largely neglected in the 1930s, but nurses did increase attention to the importance of medication administration safety for medications such as insulin, digitalis, and sulfanilamide. In the 1940s, nurses were active inventors of safety equipment and protocols. Nurses recognized that patient survival required close observation and rapid intervention and helped create "shock wards," recovery rooms, and "shock carts." Nurses played a significant role in fire prevention, fire control, and patient evacuation as hospital fires were a frequent occurrence. Rapid intervention for high-risk patients based on their overall medical and nursing needs was a safety priority during the 1950s. Patients were assigned to intensive care, intermediate care, self-care, or home care based on medical and nursing needs. Specialized nursing education and in-service programs were identified as fundamental to patient safety. There was growing recognition that specialized care for premature infants could reduce mortality. The introduction of more complex medication regimens and hospital equipment prompted more discussion about potential dangers of equipment and medication errors. The risk of hospital acquired infection and the role of the nurse in prevention began to emerge in the 1960s. The 1970s saw the call for comprehensive reform in medication delivery practices using a team approach that involved a nurse, physician, and pharmacist in response to the increasing complexity of pharmacologic interventions. Patient care equipment was recognized as potentially hazardous, and nurses were encouraged to report equipment malfunction. In the 1980s, there was renewed focus on accident and medication error prevention, as well as equipment and procedural errors. The increased use of unlicensed assistive personnel arose as a factor in patient safety in the 1990s. In response, nursing developed staffing and delegation principles to promote patient safety. Institutions were encouraged to improve safety and quality by investigating causes of errors rather than blaming individuals. Reducing patient restraint became a top nursing priority. System factors with systemic solutions rather than individual performance factors with individual solutions emerged as the patient safety focus of the 2000s. System issues such as poor communication among healthcare team members, workforce and work environment issues, or disruptive behaviors became the emphasis rather than human performance. Care bundles were developed to mitigate development of hospital acquired conditions or "never" events in response to changes in Medicare reimbursement. See Table 2 for an overview of nursing's evolving role in patient safety from 1900 to 2015.

Table 2 Overview of nursing's evolving role in patient safety

Time period	Nursing's role in patient safety
1900–1919	• Focus on germ theory, importance of hand hygiene and preventing contagion • Frequent patient position change associated with decubitus ulcer and pneumonia prevention
1920–1929	• Safety precautions not associated with potentially harmful interventions (i.e., electrotherapy, IV warmers, hot surgical dressings) • Unit manuals ("ward standard books") recommended to increase efficiency and standardize patient care • Actions connected to insulin administration and hypoglycemia prevention
1930–1939	• Actions for medication administration safety and error prevention (i.e., no interruptions while medications are being prepared or administered; consistent use of either trade or generic medication names; identification of patients by name prior to medication administration; verification with prescriber; recognizing toxicity) • Insulin administration identified as high risk for error medication due to the availability of multiple concentrations • No safety precautions connected to analgesia for labor and delivery
1940–1949	• Active inventors of safety equipment, protocols, policies, and procedures to prevent accidents • Major role in fire prevention, fire control, and patient evacuation in response to numerous hospital fires • Recognized close observation and rapid intervention during World War II (shock wards, shock carts, and recovery rooms) improved survival of surgical and obstetric patients • Developed/implemented system to assure uniform and consistent use of card file system to reduce patient care errors
1950–1959	• Emphasis on positive patient identification before administering any treatment • Safety precautions for medications posing greatest risk to patients (barbiturates, opioids, sedatives) • Patients assigned to care at various levels of intensity based on acuity • Strategies to prevent suicide and self-harm • Specialized care for premature infants • Inservice educational programs to increase patient safety
1960–1969	• Initiated prevention programs for hospital acquired infections • Fall prevention received some attention • Common source of litigation was hot bottle burns • Increasing complexity of nursing care recognized as patient safety factor
1970–1979	• Call for comprehensive reform of medication delivery practices to include interdisciplinary team approach, nurse-oriented resource materials, and unit dose medication systems. • Developed procedures for reporting defective or malfunctioning equipment as recognized patient care equipment as potentially hazardous • Encouraged family member presence to avoid use of patient restraints • Recognized intermittent positive pressure breathing treatments as potential cause for pneumothorax • Continued focus on actions to mitigate hospital acquired infections and conditions

(continued)

Table 2   (continued)

Time period	Nursing's role in patient safety
1980– 1989	• Focus on accident awareness, more frequent patient rounds, fall prevention measures—bed alarms, nonskid footwear, bed brakes • Double-check systems to reduce medication errors and transcription errors, unit dose medication systems • Include patients in medication administration process to decrease errors • No reuse of single-use equipment and critical invasive devices
1990– 1999	• Focus on numerous reasons medication errors occur, using electronic medication administration records and refining policies and procedures through system theory • Developed staffing and delegation principles as increased use of unlicensed assistive personnel emerged as a patient safety factor • Reducing patient restraints became a priority as nurses required to try alternatives before restraining patients
2000– 2015	• Systemic factors recognized as contributing to errors • Rapid response teams established in hospitals • Care bundles (multi-intervention protocols) developed (i.e., VAP, CLABSI) to remedy problems • Medication reconciliation to reduce medication errors during patient transition periods • "Failure to rescue" used to evaluate nursing care

Adapted from: Kowalski, S. L., & Anthony, M. (2017). Nursing's evolving role in patient safety. *American Journal of Nursing*, *117*(2), 34–48 [24]

The past two decades have focused on the systemic factors that affect patient safety rather than the actions of individuals. The importance of nursing's role in the healthcare system has been and is vital to patient safety. In 2000, the IOM published *To Err is Human: Building a Safer Health System* that reported at least 44,000 people, and perhaps as many as 98,000 individuals, die in hospitals each year because of medical error that could have been prevented. The report discusses the toll associated with safety compromises and healthcare errors in terms of human lives, suffering, and financial burden to healthcare systems and services [25]. Major emphasis was placed on the essential role of leadership in addressing errors; the need for and structure of error reporting systems; the development of performance standards; and recommendations regarding elements key to safety design in healthcare systems.

The committee moved beyond a focus of perfection based on individual human performance to a system focus. Specifically, the report called for healthcare systems to be designed to make it easy for nurses to engage in safe practices and hard for nurses and others to make errors. The report outlined both internal and external drivers to improve the quality and safety of healthcare that included nursing care. External drivers influencing quality of nursing care identified in the report were regulation and legislation (state scope-of-practice laws), accrediting organizations (The Joint Commission Patient Safety Goals), efforts to link payment with performance (Centers for Medicare and Medicaid Services), the need for interdisciplinary guidelines (clinical practice guidelines), the commitment of professional organizations (safety content at conferences), and the level of public engagement (safety as part of public policy agenda). Internal drivers influencing quality and safety of nursing care included policies and management decisions. Nurse leaders were called upon to ensure highly visible patient safety programs, implement nonpunitive reporting processes, and incorporate safety principles into daily practice. Nurses were called upon to be more attuned to determining and addressing sources of potential error and utilize available protocols, checklists, and team training to improve team functioning and communication.

Crossing the Quality Chiasm: A New Health System for the Twenty-First Century described the work of healthcare as being "characterized by more to know, more to manage, more to watch, more to do, and more people involved in doing it at any time in the nation's history" [26, p. 25] and made the call for meaningful approaches to improve healthcare quality. Specifically, the report stated the purpose of the healthcare system as "All health care organizations, professional groups, and private and public purchasers should adopt as their explicit purpose to continually reduce the burden of illness, injury, and disability, and to improve the health and functioning of the people of the United States" [26, p. 39]. These statements reflect not only complexities of the healthcare system and the nature of nursing knowledge but also acknowledge the complexities of nursing practice. Six specific aims were articulated to provide focus for nurses and other clinicians to meet this purpose. The aims are safe care, effective care, patient-centered care, timely care, efficient care, and equitable care. See Table 3 for a definition of each aim and an example of nursing's ongoing contribution to achieving each aim. In addition, the report proposed a twenty-first century healthcare redesign to include care based on continuous healing relationships; customization based on patient needs and values; the patient as the source of control; shared knowledge and free flow of information; evidence-based decision-making; safety as a system property; the need for transparency; anticipation of needs; continuous decrease in waste; and cooperation among clinicians. Implementation of each of these redesign tenets has implications for nursing practice, education, and research.

The IOM reports *To Err is Human* and *Crossing the Quality Chasm* provide evidence on how the healthcare delivery system should be modified to keep patients safe from the complexities of a technologically driven, compartmentalized, US healthcare system and the fallibility of human care providers, managers, and leadership [25, 26]. These reports speak to "how the experiences of patients should be changed, how teams of health care workers should interact, how health care organizations can better design work and institute proactive error-reduction strategies, and how policy officials and health care purchasers can reshape health policy to create a safer health care system" [6, p. ix]. *Keeping Patients Safe: Transforming the Work Environment of Nurses* examined patient safety from a different lens—the perspective of the work environment of the nurse [6]. Evidence showed that the typical nurse work environment is characterized by several serious threats to patient safety such as frequent failure to follow management practices necessary for safety; unsafe workforce deployment; unsafe work and workspace design; and punitive cultures that hinder the reporting and prevention of errors. Each work environment characteristic poses a serious threat to patient safety. Page and colleagues argued the need for bundles of mutually reinforcing patient safety defenses in nurses' work environments as no one

Table 3 IOM's six aims for improving healthcare quality and example of nursing's ongoing contribution to achieving each aim

Aim	Definition	Example of nursing contribution to achieve
Safe care	Avoiding injuries to patients	Standardized patient handoff during inter- and intra-facility patient transfers; shift to shift and communication from one clinician to another clinician
Effective care	Providing care based on scientific knowledge	Evidence-based practice grounded in nursing science as well as other evidence produced by other disciplines relevant to nursing practice (i.e., medicine, psychology, sociology)
Patient-centered care	Providing respectful and responsive care that ensures that patient values guide clinical decisions	Respect for patients' values, preferences, and expressed needs; coordination and integration of care; information, communication, and education; physical comfort; emotional support; and involvement of family and friends
Timely care	Reducing waits for both recipients and providers of care	Application of technology such as use of call-a-nurse lines, telehealth sessions, and virtual nursing
Efficient care	Avoiding waste	Nursing practice models that mitigate high costs while sustaining or improving quality and safety, i.e., APRNs
Equitable care	Ensuring that the quality of care does not vary because of characteristics such as gender, ethnicity, socioeconomic status, or geographic location	Diversity, equity, and inclusion initiatives

Adapted from: Wakefield MK. The Quality Chasm Series: Implications for Nursing. In: Hughes RG, editor. Patient Safety and Quality: An Evidence-Based Handbook for Nurses. Rockville (MD): Agency for Healthcare Research and Quality (US); 2008 Apr. Chapter 4. Available from: https://www.ncbi.nlm.nih.gov/books/NBK2677/ [27]

single action can keep patients safe from errors. The report lays out guidelines for improving patient safety by changing nurses work environment conditions through transformational leadership and evidence-based management; maximizing workforce capability; designing work and workspace to prevent and mitigate errors; and creating and sustaining a culture of safety.

Following the passage of the Affordable Care Act in 2010 that provided insurance coverage for 32 million more Americans, Committee on the Robert Wood Johnson Foundation Initiative on the Future of Nursing, at the Institute of Medicine developed a vision for a transformed healthcare system that makes quality care accessible to the diverse populations of the US, intentionally promotes wellness and disease prevention, reliably improves health outcomes, and provides compassionate care across the lifespan. *The Future of Nursing: Leading Change, Advancing Health* [28] sought to explore what roles nursing could assume to address the increasing demand for safe, high-quality, and effective healthcare services. The committee examined the capacity of the nursing workforce to meet the demands of a redesigned healthcare system that delivers the right care—quality care that is patient-centered, accessible, evidence-based, safe, and sustainable—at the right time.

Achieving this reimagined care system requires transforming the work environment, scope of practice, education, and numbers of nurses in the US. Four key messages of the report are: (1) Nurses should practice to the full extent of their education and training; (2) Nurses should achieve higher levels of education and training through an improved education system that promotes seamless academic progression; (3) Nurses should be full partners, with physicians and other health professionals, in redesigning healthcare in the US; and (4) Effective workforce planning and policy making require better data collection and an improved information infrastructure.

For health professionals to function in redesigned and reimagined care systems, attention was directed on determining essential skills and knowledge needed to function and then disseminating those essential skills along with the knowledge across the healthcare workforce. *Health Professions Education: A Bridge to Quality* delineated the necessary change in skills and knowledge of various health professions [29]. The report described the shortcomings of health professions education programs and made a call for change that was clear, direct, and blunt—"Education for the health professions is in need of major overhaul" [29, p. 1]. The vison statement was "All health professionals should be educated to deliver patient-centered care as members of an interdisciplinary team, emphasizing evidence-based practice, quality improvement approaches, and informatics" [29, p. 8]. This vision stipulated five competencies applicable to all healthcare disciplines including nursing: patient-centered care, teamwork and collaboration, evidence-based practice, quality improvement and informatics, and safety.

The Quality and Safety Education for Nurses (QSEN) initiative commenced to address the challenge of preparing future nurses with the knowledge, skills, and attitudes (KSAs) necessary to continuously improve the quality and safety of the healthcare systems in which they work [30]. In Phase I (2005–2007), using the IOM competencies, the QSEN faculty and a National Advisory Board defined six competencies with associated pre-licensure KSAs: patient-centered care; teamwork and collaboration; evidence-based-practice (EBP); quality improvement (QI); safety and informatics [31]. Pilot schools integrated the six competencies into their nursing programs during Phase II (2007–2009). Phase III (2009–2012) QSEN faculty and the American Association of Colleges of Nursing (AACN) worked to develop the faculty expertise necessary for the nation's nursing schools to teach the competencies; focused on instilling the competencies in textbooks, licensing, accreditation, and certification standards; and promoted continued innovation in teaching the competencies. AACN hosted faculty development institutes across the US to better prepare nurse faculty in undergraduate programs to teach quality and safety content. The reach of the QSEN initiative has extended to graduate education programs with the help of AACN. This last phase of the project provides educational resources and training to enhance the ability of faculty in master's and doctoral nursing programs to teach quality and safety competencies. The overall goal through all phases of QSEN has been to address the challenge of preparing future nurses with the KSAs necessary to continuously improve the quality and safety of the healthcare systems in which they work. A comprehensive understanding of the QSEN competencies is available in the third edition of *Quality and Safety Education for Nurses: Core Competencies for Nursing Leadership and Care Management* [32].

In addition to developing faculty expertise necessary for the nation's nursing schools to teach the QSEN competencies, the AACN provides an entry-level and advanced-level educational framework for nursing faculty at colleges and universities to prepare nurses for professional nursing practice. *The Essentials: Core Competencies for Professional Nursing Education* represents the essence of professional nursing practice and serves to bridge the gap between education and practice [33]. The expert practice of professional nursing at entry and advanced levels requires integration and "employment of established and emerging principles of safety and improvement science. Quality and safety, as core values of nursing practice, enhance quality and minimize risk of harm to patients and providers through both system effectiveness and individual performance" [33, p. 11]. Nursing education programs in the twenty-first century are striving to prepare graduates who are "work ready" to apply quality improvement and safety principles in care delivery and contribute to a culture of patient safety and further a culture of provider and work environment safety.

4   Essentiality of Nursing to Patient Safety

What the discipline of nursing and individual professional nurse "brings to the future is a steadfast commitment to patient care, improved safety and quality, and better outcomes" [28, p. xi]. Nurses provide care in virtually all places in which healthcare is delivered. Thus, nurses are the providers that spend the greatest amount of time with patients and are most often likely to intercept errors and prevent patient harm. Nursing is essential in the delivery of person and family-centered care. Person-centered approaches to planning and providing care are a central element of quality and safety in nursing practice [34]. Nurses provide patient/family-centered care by recognizing the patient or their designee as the source of control and in full partnership provide compassionate and coordinated care based on respect for the patient's preferences, beliefs, and values with emphasis on collaborating with people of all ages [35, 36]. Nurses provide a vital blend of clinically competent care delivered with compassion through a positive nurse-patient relationship to facilitate patient empowerment and participation in their care [37]. The delivery of patient-centered care, care that supports patient participation positively influences patient safety perception among inpatients [38]. In addition, patient participation in patient safety activities in hospitals is positively related to nurses' competency in patient-centered care as well as teamwork and safety culture [39].

Building safe clinical practice environments is essential in minimizing adverse patient care events [6]. Leaders are essential to building a safe practice environment. A healthy work environment contributes to a culture of safety and is created and sustained by leaders [6, 40, 41]. Healthcare system executive and nursing leadership are pivotal to the provision of safer care because leaders direct and influence safety culture [42]. A culture of safety is an explicit top priority organizational goal driven by leadership and shown by strong direction and involvement of governance, management, and clinical leadership. Sammer and colleagues conducted a comprehensive review of the patient safety literature and identified leadership, teamwork, evidence-based, communication, learning, just and patient-centered as the important beliefs, attitudes, and behaviors that are integral to a culture of safety [43]. These culture of safety attitudes, beliefs, and behaviors are representative of the essence of professional nursing and nursing practice making nursing indispensable in the endeavor to improve patient safety. A culture of safety is a nursing leadership commitment to safety in the work environment that permeates all levels of the organization through acknowledgment of the high risk, error prone nature of healthcare activities, by supporting a blame-free environment where individuals can report errors without fear, the expectation of collaboration across ranks to seek solutions to vulnerabilities, and a willingness to direct resources to address safety concerns [44].

Leaders must foster psychological safety and be committed to nonpunitive event reporting that is transparent and monitored at all levels of the organization [45, 46]. Nursing leadership commitment to psychological safety in the work environment contributes to nurses speaking up, reporting mistakes and near misses quickly so that corrective actions can be made in a timely fashion. "Making the environment safe for open communication about challenges, concerns and opportunities is one of the most important leadership responsibilities of the twenty-first century" [47, p. 22]. Leadership styles, such as transformational leadership, transactional leadership, leader-member exchange, empowering leadership, and authentic leadership, do positively influence safety performance and outcomes; however, there is no clear agreement as to what leadership style or styles most influence a culture of safety [42, 48].

Nurses have kept watch over patients since the days of Nightingale and are the healthcare system's most reliable sentinels [12, 49, 50]. A sentinel is a lookout, a person employed to guard or keep watch over something or someone [51]. Nurses act as sentinels for safety to prevent errors from reaching patients and are expected to raise concerns when a harm or wrongdoing is committed against a patient or patients [52]. Nurses provide the broadest safety reporting from critical incidents to near misses and nurses are often the "whistle-blowers" regarding serious concerns about patient care safety and outcomes [53]. "Whistleblowing is an act which brings to relevant person(s) or the general public's attention information about something that has been done or is continuing to be done by an organization that is considered to be illegal and/or unethical and/or harmful" [52, p. 808–809]. Healthcare whistleblowing is the raising of concerns about unsafe, unethical, or poor-quality care to persons able to effect action [54]. According to Gagon and Perron, concerns that lead nurses to whistleblowing are related to working conditions (inadequate and unsafe staffing, work-related stress, and unsafe workload); nursing practice (inappropriate delegation, failure to follow policies and procedures, and failure to follow nursing standards); specific behaviors (unprofessional behavior, impairment at work, harassment, and behaviors indicative of a mental health issue); patient care and patient rights (poor quality of care, clinical incompetence, and changes in practice that put safety, health, and lives of patients at risk), and management or general governance of the organization (concealment of wrong doings and ineffective or harmful styles of management) [55]. Whistleblowing is often seen as a process that is gradual in nature, which starts by using the processes within an organization and gradually moves to a disclosure to an external body, should the internal process prove to be ineffective [56].

It is the professional duty of a nurse to report care that is harmful to patients [57]. The 2021 ICN Code of Ethics for Nurses states that nurses are active, not passive participants in the promotion of patient safety and are expected to take appropriate actions to safeguard individuals, families, communities, and populations when their health is endangered by a co-worker, any other person, policy, or misuse of technology [58]. Nurses promote ethical conduct by reporting errors or near misses when they occur, speak up when patient safety is threatened, advocate for transparency, and work with others to reduce the potential of errors. The 2015 ANA Code of Ethics for Nurses supports nurses as active participants in patient safety as Provision 3 of the code states "The nurse has authority, accountability, and responsibility for nursing practice; makes decisions; and takes action consistent with the obligation to provide optimal patient care" [59]. Nurses should report healthcare practices that put patients at risk for harm to leaders and should that practice that puts patients at risk for harm not be rectified, the nurse is ethically bound to voice their concerns to a regulatory agency or other external group. Nurses must actively intervene and voice their concerns should the delivery of care be not up to standard and put patients at risk for harm.

Nursing surveillance is a key intervention for early recognition of adverse events, preventing harm to patients and is central to patient health and safety [60, 61]. Nursing surveillance is described as a process to monitor and recognize early patient complications and deterioration [62]. Nursing Intervention Classification (NIC) defines surveillance as the purposeful and ongoing acquisition, interpretation, and synthesis of patient data for clinical decision-making [63]. NIC also defines the intervention of surveillance as safety, the purposeful and ongoing collection, and analysis of information about patients and the environment for use in promoting and maintaining patient safety [63]. Surveillance is a safety strategy that relies on nurses' ability to process and attend to a considerable number of cues or data during patient care. Nursing surveillance goes beyond monitoring and integrates assessment data to develop a dynamic plan of care for each patient. The goal is to detect subtle changes in the patient condition and to intervene using appropriate resources and tools to avoid a poor outcome.

Nurses report using surveillance as a safety strategy to identify and prevent medical errors. Studies of critical care nurses report surveillance is a strategy nurses use to interrupt medical errors and can bring about the nurse intervening on average of once a week to prevent potentially serious medical errors [64, 65]. Yang and colleagues report operating room (OR) nurses recovered an average of 11 errors per procedure [66]. "When built-in system defenses do not automatically avert potentially dangerous situations, nurses are uniquely poised and possess competencies to identify, interrupt, and correct medical errors. Such instances are referred to as a near miss, preventable error, or recovered medical error" [67, p. 1]. In addition, nurses use technology to enhance surveillance of patients to prevent adverse events. The use of remote, high-tech surveillance by critical care nurses in tele-ICUs helps bedside clinical nurses to identify patients whose condition may be worsening or provide disease surveillance for time-sensitive conditions such as sepsis [68]. Remote tele-ICU nursing surveillance can decrease adverse events such as cardiac and respiratory arrest, patient falls, and unplanned removal of tubes, lines, and airways [69, 70]. Furthermore, tele-ICU nurses conduct surveillance and serve as knowledge translators and mentors to prevent adverse events, provide safer and more timely care, while supporting fellow nurses practicing at the bedside [71].

The phenomenon of error recovery as a critical defense against medical errors is emerging [72]. Nurses work directly with patients and provide most of the inpatient care. Nurses represent the front line of patient defense and are well positioned to intercept and correct errors before patients are harmed. Error recovery is defined as the feature of the human factors or human system component to detect, localize, and correct system failures [73]. The recovery process consists of three sequential phases: detecting an error; intercepting and understanding the nature of the error; and correcting or counteracting the error. Error recovery proposes that errors can be prevented by adequate system defenses. However, when the system defenses are not able to control failures, it is the flexibility, experience, and intuition of the human who must stop the unintended chain of events before harm occurs. Thus, humans are the critical element in error recovery process [74].

Nurses are the human critical element in the medical error recovery process. Detection or identification of the error is the process of knowing if an error has occurred. Familiarity with all aspects of the plan of care allows nurses to anticipate and identify potential medical errors. Interception and understanding the nature of the error are when the nurse attempts to gather an explanation of how the error occurred to prevent it from happening again. Correcting or counteracting the error focuses in initiating corrective action to suppress the error by revising the plan or initiating a new plan. This is where nurses rely on creativity and flexibility to select the most appropriate strategy to interrupt and correct medical errors. "The recovery process is the unique difference between patient harm and a near miss and emphasizes the importance of professional decision-making and clinical reasoning as an expected behavior of nurses" [67, p. 2]. A study by Gaffney and colleagues illustrates the important role of nurses in the error recovery process and patient safety [67]. They report 184 medical-surgical nurses recovered a total of 3392 errors over the course of the 3-month study period, which could potentially equate to as many as 13,568 medical errors prevented each year. The team concluded "creating a safer healthcare system will depend on the ability of all nurses to fully use their education, expertise and role to identify, interrupt, and correct medical errors to prevent patient harm" [67, p. 10].

The essentiality of nurses and nursing to assess risks and take appropriate action to manage those risks is vital to patient safety [75]. Nurses are imperative to medication safety as nurses are often the last person to check that the medication is correctly prescribed and dispensed before administration [76]. They are well positioned to identify drug-related problems and minimize unnecessary drug-related patient harm that occur beyond the "five rights" (right patient, right drug, right route, right time, right dose) of medication administration to include checking medication orders with providers and follow up with the pharmacy on missing medications, assessing the patient, and preparing drugs to be administered [77, 78].

Nurses are crucial in the prevention of device-related healthcare associated infections. Device-related healthcare associated infections can be prevented by using evidence-based strategies as evidence-based guidelines, and prevention bundles are foundational to hospital acquired infection prevention efforts [79]. A prevention bundle is defined as a grouping of evidence-based practices that individually improve care and bundles have been used successfully to reduce CLABSI and CAUTI [80–82]. "Translating knowledge into practice requires an integrated approach to address both technical and adaptive work, including a deep understanding of the health care delivery system and human behavior, fostering engagement and ownership of the improvement process by local interdisciplinary teams, creating centralized support for the technical work, encouraging local adaptation of the intervention bundle, and ensuring a collaborative culture within the facility" [82, p. 2]. Nurses are ideally situated to collaborate, coordinate, and integrate the multiple aspects of hospital acquired infection prevention bundles as nurses are the lynch pin in encouraging adaptation of the prevention intervention bundle across care settings and fostering engagement of the interdisciplinary team.

The essentiality of nursing to patient safety cannot be ignored. Nurses are the end-users who often recognize an adverse event or near miss event and are implementers of safety initiatives. The nurse may be the first person to hear or observe an issue a patient is experiencing. The nurse may be the only person a patient tells that something happened or almost happened. The nurse is the patient's advocate and is accountable for each patient's safety. Nurses actively listen to seek to understand the patient's point of view and critically think about what could go wrong as the smallest decision could compromise the safety of a patient. As a patient advocate, nurses must report any errors, even their own error. Recognizing and reporting system failure, human error, drug reactions, and lack of adherence to infection control measures keep both current and future patients safe from adverse events and errors. Nurses must practice effective communication habits with other interdisciplinary members of the healthcare team to mitigate the opportunity for miscommunication to cause potential for harm. Nurses are optimally poised to collaborate, coordinate the teamwork, and integrate the multiple aspects of care across the care continuum to keep patients safe. Nurses are the healthcare team's most essential and reliable sentinels for safety to prevent errors from reaching patients in our healthcare systems.

5 Case Study: "How to" Application

A critical contribution of nursing to patient safety is the nurse's ability to collaborate, coordinate, and integrate the multiple aspects of care to mitigate the risk of error reaching the patient and thus prevent patient harm. The case study illustrates the role of the nurse in quality management and safety as she understood and exposed cause and effects, promoted outcomes measurement based on credible data, and understood that problems could be caused by not only individuals but by systems using science of improvement principles (aims, changes to be made and measures to monitor changes made). This case study is an example of how a perioperative clinical nurse specialist (CNS) at an urban hospital lessened the risk of pressure injury by piloting an alternating pressure overlay over a 12-month period to mitigate intra-operative pressure injury development in the head/neck surgical population.

5.1   Background

Pressure injuries are a painful, costly, and preventable complication. The presence or absence of a pressure injury is a nurse sensitive indicator and reflective of quality and safety in nursing care [83]. The operating room is a high-risk environment for pressure ulcer development related to patient intrinsic factors (advanced age, medications, presence of comorbid diseases) as well as extrinsic factors related to physical and environmental factors (shear, friction, moisture). Furthermore, the patient in the perioperative setting is at risk for the development of pressure injuries due to the inherent risk factors associated with surgery such as length and type of surgery, positioning, anesthetic agents, blood loss, low arterial pressure, and body temperature [84]. Positioning guidelines recommend a patient be repositioned every 2 hours intra-operatively; however, this recommendation can be difficult to accomplish [85].

The head and neck surgical population is at risk for development of pressure injuries because of surgery length and the inability to reposition the patient due to the type of procedure and necessary exposure of the surgical site. Duration of head and neck surgical procedures is frequently greater than four hours and is often longer than anticipated when unexpected pathology is revealed during a planned surgical procedure. Repositioning the patient during the procedure may not be possible because of necessary exposure of the surgical site. There are some techniques, supplies, and equipment that may prevent skin damage during surgical procedures [86].

5.2   Purpose

Three head and neck patients sustained pressure injuries following long surgical procedures with little ability for patient repositioning during the previous 2 years. The three pressure injuries developed within 2 days following a head and neck procedure were staged as suspected deep tissue injury–depth unknown and required extensive intervention and treatment for healing. Assessment of the head and neck surgical population identified the need for greater surveillance and targeted pressure injury prevention strategies. The purpose of the project was to pilot an alternating pressure overlay over a 12-month period to mitigate intra-operative pressure injury of head/neck patients when surgery was scheduled for four or more hours.

5.3 Materials/Methods

The CNS assembled an interdisciplinary team to investigate and evaluate additional measures to mitigate pressure injury development in the head/neck surgical population. The team was composed of two surgeons, a wound care nurse, the head and neck nurse program coordinator, three head and neck OR nurses, and the CNS. The CNS led team evaluated a variety of equipment and selected an alternating pressure overlay with power console for placement on the operating table to supplement the association of perioperative registered nurses (AORN) pressure prevention recommendations [84, 85, 87]. The intervention was to apply the alternating pressure overlay with power console to the operating table of head and neck patients when surgery was scheduled for four or more hours. The interdisciplinary team developed education materials including patient assessment, overlay indication, overlay application to operating table, console set-up, and medical record charting. Education was provided to 100% of the head and neck perioperative staff prior to intervention implementation. Patients included in the pilot were those with surgery scheduled for four or more hours with complete medical record charting. Excluded were head and neck patients with surgery scheduled for less than four hours, those with incomplete medical record charting or an error of the overlay power console occurred during the procedure. Measures were number of pressure injuries and average surgical time.

5.4 Results

One hundred and eighteen head/neck patients were assessed and assigned the alternating pressure overlay. One hundred and nine patients (92.4%) had complete overlay medical record charting and were included in the analysis. Average age of patients was 58.14 years with more males than females. Average surgical time was 5 hours and 37 minutes. Nine patients (7.6%) were excluded due to incomplete overlay medical record charting or error of overlay power console. One patient (0.9%) developed a pressure injury, and case review revealed indirect contact with the overlay where the pressure injury occurred.

5.5 Discussion/Conclusions/Implications for Practice/ Dissemination

Pressure injury occurrence was zero when the alternating pressure overlay was correctly applied to the operating table. Correct application and utilization of an alternating pressure overlay may be an effective supplementary measure to mitigate risk of pressure injury for surgical patients scheduled for procedures of 4 hours or greater in length. The overlay could be a useful addition to peri-operative nursing practice to pressure injury prevention beyond the head and neck patient population. Additional research is needed to identify best pressure injury prevention positioning and pressure relieve devices that may be applied to all types of surgical patients.

6   Summary

The occurrence of adverse events due to unsafe care is likely one of the ten leading causes of death and disability in the world, with an estimated one in ten patients harmed and more than three million deaths occurring annually [88]. More than 50% of this harm is avoidable and can be attributed to medication errors, unsafe surgical procedures, healthcare-associated infections, diagnostic errors, patient falls, pressure ulcers, patient misidentification, unsafe blood transfusion, and venous thromboembolism. Nurses have kept watch over patients since the days of Nightingale and are the reliable safety sentinels that often prevent errors from reaching patients in our healthcare systems. The most critical contribution of nursing to patient safety is the nurse's ability to collaborate, coordinate, and integrate the multiple aspects of care across care settings [89]. "It may seem a strange principle to enunciate as the very first requirement in a hospital that it should do the sick no harm" [11, p. 1].

Key Points

- Nurses have kept watch over patients since the days of Nightingale and are the healthcare system's most reliable sentinels.
- Nurses represent the front line of patient defense and are well positioned to intercept and correct errors before patients are harmed.
- Nursing surveillance is a key intervention for early recognition of adverse events, preventing harm to patients and is central to patient health and safety.
- A critical contribution of nursing to patient safety is the nurse's ability to collaborate, coordinate, and integrate the multiple aspects of care to mitigate risk of an error reaching a patient and thus preventing patient harm.
- Healthcare system leadership and nursing leadership commitment to psychological safety in the work environment contributes to nurses speaking up, reporting mistakes, and reporting near misses quickly so that corrective actions within the system can be made in a timely fashion.
- The essentiality of nursing to patient safety cannot be ignored. Nurses are the end-users who often recognize an adverse event or near miss event and are implementers of safety initiatives.

References

1. World Health Organization. State of the world's nursing 2020: investing in education, jobs and leadership. Executive Summary. 2020. https://apps.who.int/iris/bitstream/han dle/10665/331673/9789240003293-eng.pdf. Accessed 14 Mar 2023.
2. WHO European Region. European Health Information Gateway Data–Professional nurses, licensed to practice, total. 2016. https://gateway.euro.who.int/en/indicators/hlthres_220-professional-nurses-licensed-to-practice-total/. Accessed 14 Mar 2023.

3. Smiley RA, Ruttinger C, Oliveira CM, Hudson LR, Lauer, Allgeyer R, Reneau KA, Silvestre JH, Alexander M. The 2020 National Nursing Workforce Survey. J Nurs Regul. 2021;12(1):S1–S48.
4. American Association of Colleges of Nursing. Nursing Fact Sheet. 2022. https://www. aacnnursing.org/news-Information/fact-sheets/nursing-fact-sheet. Accessed 14 Mar 2023.
5. ANA. What is nursing? https://www.nursingworld.org/practice-policy/workforce/what-is-nursing/. Accessed 14 Mar 2023.
6. Page A, editor. Keeping patients safe: transforming the work environment of nurses. Washington, DC: The National Academies Press; 2004.
7. Reid J, Catchpole K. Patient safety: a core value of nursing-so why is achieving it so difficult? J Res Nurs. 2011;16(3):209–23.
8. Fee E, Garofalo ME. Florence nightingale and the Crimean war. Am J Public Health. 2010;100(9):1591–1.
9. Nightingale F. Army sanitary administration and its reform under the late Lord Herbert. McCorquodale; 1862.
10. Nightingale F. Notes on matters affecting the health, efficiency and Hospital Administration of the British Army: founded chiefly on the experience of the late war. Harrison and Sons; 1858.
11. Nightingale F. Notes on Hospitals: 1859. London: John W. Parker and Son, West Strand; 1863.
12. Nightingale F. Notes on nursing: what it is, and what it is not. London: Harrison and Sons; 1859.
13. Schmalbach CE. Patient safety/quality improvement (PS/QI) Florence Nightingale prevails. Otolaryngol Head Neck Surg. 2015;152(5):771–3.
14. Meyer BC, Bishop DS. Florence Nightingale: nineteenth century apostle of quality. J Manag Hist. 2007;13(3):240–54.
15. McGaffigan P. Why Florence Nightingale's Improvement Lessons Still Matter Today. 2019. https://www.ihi.org/communities/blogs/why-florence-nightingales-improvement-lessons-still-matter-today. Accessed 16 June 2023.
16. Dlugacz YD. Introduction to health care quality: theory, methods, and tools. Wiley; 2017.
17. Institute for Healthcare Improvement. Science of improvement. 2023. https://www.ihi.org/about/Pages/ScienceofImprovement.aspx. Accessed 16 June 2023.
18. Associates for Process Improvement. 2023. https://www.apiweb.org/. Accessed 16 June 2023.
19. The Deming Institute. About Dr. W. Edwards Deming Viewing the world through a different lens. 2023. https://deming.org/learn/about-dr-deming/. Accessed 16 June 2023.
20. Granger BB. Science of improvement versus science of implementation: integrating both into clinical inquiry. AACN Adv Crit Care. 2018;29(2):208–12.
21. Selanders L, Crane P. The voice of Florence Nightingale on advocacy. Online J Issues Nurs. 2012;17(1):Manuscript 1.
22. Hughes R, editor. Patient safety and quality: an evidence-based handbook for nurses. (Prepared with support from the Robert Wood Johnson Foundation.) AHRQ Publication No. 08–0043. Agency for Healthcare Research and Quality: Rockville, MD; 2008.
23. Nightingale F. Florence Nightingale: measuring hospital care outcomes: excerpts from the books notes on matters affecting the health, efficiency, and hospital administration of the British army founded chiefly on the experience of the late war, and notes on hospitals. Joint Commission Resources. 1999.
24. Kowalski SL, Anthony M. Nursing's evolving role in patient safety. Am J Nurs. 2017;117(2):34–48.
25. Institute of Medicine. To err is human: building a safer health system. Washington, DC: The National Academies Press; 2000. https://doi.org/10.17226/9728.
26. Institute of Medicine. Crossing the quality chasm: a new health system for the 21st century. Washington, DC: The National Academies Press; 2001. https://doi.org/10.17226/10027.
27. Wakefield MK. Chapter 4. The quality chasm series: implications for nursing. In: Hughes RG, editor. Patient safety and quality: an evidence-based handbook for nurses. Rockville, MD. Agency for Healthcare Research and Quality (US); 2008. https://www.ncbi.nlm.nih.gov/books/NBK2677/.

28. Institute of Medicine. The future of nursing: leading change, advancing health. Washington, DC: The National Academies Press; 2011. https://doi.org/10.17226/12956.
29. Institute of Medicine. Committee on the health professions education summit. In: Greiner AC, Knebel E, editors. Health professions education: a bridge to quality. Washington, DC: National Academies Press; 2003. https://www.ncbi.nlm.nih.gov/books/NBK221528/pdf/Bookshelf_NBK221528.pdf.
30. QSEN. Project overview. 2022. https://www.qsen.org/post/project-overview. Accessed 13 Sept 2023.
31. Cronenwett L, Sherwood G, Barnsteiner J, Disch J, Johnson J, Mitchell P, Sullivan DT, Warren J. Quality and safety education for nurses. Nurs Outlook. 2007;55(3):122–31.
32. Vana PK, Vottero BA, Altmiller, G. (Eds.). Quality and safety education for nurses: core competencies for nursing leadership and care management. 3rd ed. Springer Publishing Company; 2022.
33. American Association of Colleges of Nursing. The essentials: core competencies for professional nursing education. 2021. https://www.aacnnursing.org/Portals/0/PDFs/Publications/Essentials-2021.pdf. Accessed 11 Aug 2023.
34. Rossiter C, Levett-Jones T, Pich J. The impact of person-centred care on patient safety: an umbrella review of systematic reviews. Int J Nurs Stud. 2020;109:103658.
35. Halm MA, Barnsteiner J. Person/family-centered care. In: Sherwood G, Barnsteiner J, editors. Quality and safety in nursing A competency approach to improving outcomes. 3rd ed; 2022. p. 85–130.
36. Institute for Patient-and Family-Centered Care. Patient- and family-centered care. 2023. https://www.ipfcc.org/about/pfcc.html. Accessed 14 Aug 2023.
37. Sharp S, McAllister M, Broadbent M. The vital blend of clinical competence and compassion: how patients experience person-centred care. Contemp Nurse. 2016;52(2–3):300–12.
38. Choi N, Kim J, Kim H. The influence of patient-centeredness on patient safety perception among inpatients. PLoS One. 2021;16(2):e0246928. https://doi.org/10.1371/journal.pone.0246928.
39. Hwang JI, Kim SW, Chin HJ. Patient participation in patient safety and its relationships with nurses' patient-centered care competency, teamwork, and safety climate. Asian Nurs Res. 2019;13(2):130–6.
40. Huddleston P, Gray J. Measuring nurse leaders' and direct care nurses' perceptions of a healthy work environment in acute care settings. Part 1. J Nurs Adm. 2016a;46(7/8):373–8.
41. Huddleston P, Gray J. Describing nurse leaders' and direct care nurses' perceptions of a healthy work environment in acute care settings. Part 2. J Nurs Adm. 2016b;46(9):462–7.
42. Oster CA, Braaten JS. Safety leadership: commitment to high reliability organizing. In: Oster CA, Braaten JS, editors. High reliability organizations A healthcare handbook for patient safety & quality. 2nd ed. Indianapolis, IN: Sigma Theta Tau International, Honor Society for Nurses; 2020. p. 73–99.
43. Sammer CE, Lykens K, Singh KP, Mains DA, Lackan NA. What is patient safety culture? A review of the literature. J Nurs Scholarsh. 2010;42(2):156–65.
44. Wachter RM. Understanding patient safety. 2. New York, NY: McGraw-Hill Medical; 2012.
45. Appelbaum NP, Dow A, Mazmanian PE, Jundt DK, Appelbaum EN. The effects of power, leadership and psychological safety on resident event reporting. Med Educ. 2016;50(3):343–50.
46. Cawley PJ, Scheurer DB. Achieving high reliability through cultural mindfulness. Front Health Serv Manag. 2017;33(4):3–15.
47. Edmondson A. The fearless organization: creating psychological safety in the workplace for learning, innovation, and growth. Hoboken, NJ: Wiley; 2019.
48. Donovan SL, Salmon PM, Lenne MG. Leading with style: a literature review of the influence of safety leadership on performance and outcomes. Theor Issues Ergon Sci. 2016;17(4):423–42.
49. Ricci M, Goldman AP, De Leval MR, Cohen GA, Devaney F, Carthey J. Pitfalls of adverse event reporting in paediatric cardiac intensive care. Arch Dis Child. 2004;89(9):856–9.
50. Rowin EJ, Lucier D, Pauker SG, Kumar S, Chen J, Salem DN. Does error and adverse event reporting by physicians and nurses differ? Jt Comm J Qual Patient Safety. 2008;34(9):537–45.

51. Cambridge Dictionary. Sentinel. https://dictionary.cambridge.org/us/dictionary/english/sentinel. Accessed 24 June 2023.
52. Kearns AJ. The principle of double effect and external whistleblowing in nursing. Nurs Outlook. 2022;70(6):807–19.
53. Jackson D, Hickman L, Hutchinson M, Andrew S, Smith J, Potgieter I, Cleary M, Peters K. Whistleblowing: an integrative literature review of data-based studies involving nurses. Contemp Nurse. 2014;48:240–52.
54. Blenkinsopp J, Snowden N, Mannion R, Powell M, Davies H, Millar R, McHale J. Whistleblowing over patient safety and care quality: a review of the literature. J Health Organ Manag. 2019;33(6):737–56.
55. Gagnon M, Perron A. Whistleblowing: a concept analysis. Nurs Health Sci. 2020;22(2):381–9.
56. Mansbach A, Bachner YG. Internal or external whistleblowing: nurses' willingness to report wrongdoing. Nurs Ethics. 2010;17(4):483–90. https://doi.org/10.1177/0969733010364898.
57. Hodgson J. The legal dimension: legal system and method. In: Tingle J, Cribb A, editors. Nursing law and ethics. 4th ed. Chichester; Hoboken, NJ: Wiley; 2014. p. 321.
58. International Council of Nurses (ICN). The ICN code of ethics for nurses. Geneva; 2021. https://www.icn.ch/system/files/2021-10/ICN_Code-of-Ethics_EN_Web_0.pdf.
59. American Nurses Association. Code of ethics for nurses. American Nurses Publishing; 2015.
60. Halverson CC, Scott Tilley D. Nursing surveillance: a concept analysis. Nurs Forum. 2022, May;57(3):454–60.
61. Pfrimmer DM, Johnson MR, Guthmiller ML, Lehman JL, Ernste VK, Rhudy LM. Surveillance: a nursing intervention for improving patient safety in critical care environment. Dimens Crit Care Nurs. 2017;36(1):45–52. https://doi.org/10.1097/DCC.0000000000000217.
62. Kutney-Lee A, Lake ET, Aiken LH. Development of the hospital nurse surveillance capacity profile. Res Nurs Health. 2009;32:217–28.
63. Bulechek G, Butcher HK, Dochterman JM, Wagner CM, editors. Nursing interventions classification (NIC). 6th ed. St Louis, MO: Mosby; 2013.
64. Dykes PC, Rothschild JM, Hurley AC. Medical errors recovered by critical care nurses. J Nurs Adm. 2010;40:241–6.
65. Henneman EA, Gawlinksi A, Guiliano KK. Surveillance: a strategy for improving patient safety in acute and critical care units. Crit Care Nurse. 2012;32:e9–e18.
66. Yang YT, Henry L, Dellinger M, Yonish K, Emerson B, Seifert PC. The circulating nurse's role in error recovery in the cardiovascular OR. AORN J. 2012;95(6):755–62. https://doi.org/10.1016/j.aorn.2011.09.022.
67. Gaffney TA, Hatcher BJ, Milligan R, Trickey A. Enhancing patient safety: factors influencing medical error recovery among medical-surgical nurses. Online J Issues Nurs. 2016a;21(3):Manuscript 6. https://doi.org/10.3912/OJIN.Vol21No03Man06.
68. Rincon TA, Manos EL, Pierce JD. Telehealth intensive care unit nurse surveillance of sepsis. Comput Inform Nurs. 2017;35(9):459–64.
69. Olff C, Clark-Wadkins C. Tele-ICU partners enhance evidence-based practice: ventilator weaning initiative. AACN Adv Crit Care. 2012;23(3):312–22.
70. Williams LM, Hubbard KE, Daye O, Barden C. Telenursing in the intensive care unit: transforming nursing practice. Crit Care Nurse. 2012;32(6):62–9.
71. Rincon T, Henneman E. An introduction to nursing surveillance in the tele-ICU. Nurs 2020 Critical Care. 2018;13(2):42–6. https://doi.org/10.1097/01.CCN.0000527223.11558.8a.
72. Gaffney TA, Hatcher BJ, Milligan R. Nurses' role in medical error recovery: an integrative review. J Clin Nurs. 2016b;25(7/8):906–17. https://doi.org/10.1111/jocn.13126.
73. van der Schaaf TW, Kanse L. Errors and error recovery. In: Elzer PF, Kluwe RH, Boussoffara B, editors. Human error and system design and management, vol. 253. Godalming: Springer-Verlag London Ltd; 2000. p. 27–38.
74. Reason JT. The human contribution: unsafe acts, accidents and heroic recoveries. Farnham, England; Burlington, VT: Ashgate; 2008.
75. Choo J, Hutchinson A, Bucknall T. Nurses' role in medication safety. J Nurs Manag. 2010;18(7):853–61. https://doi.org/10.1111/j.1365-2834.2010.01164.x.

76. Elliott M, Liu Y. The nine rights of medication administration: an overview. Br J Nurs. 2010;19(5):300–5.
77. Macdonald M. Patient safety: examining the adequacy of the 5 rights of medication administration. Clin Nurse Spec. 2010;24(4):196–201.
78. Soerensen AL, Lisby M, Nielsen LP, Poulsen BK, Mainz J. Improving medication safety in psychiatry—a controlled intervention study of nurse involvement in avoidance of potentially inappropriate prescriptions. Basic Clin Pharmacol Toxicol. 2018;123(2):174–81. https://doi.org/10.1111/bcpt.12989.
79. Yokoe DS, Advani SD, Anderson DJ, Babcock HM, Bell M, Berenholtz SM, et al. Executive summary: a compendium of strategies to prevent healthcare-associated infections in acute-care hospitals: 2022 updates. Infect Control Hosp Epidemiol. 2023;44:1–15.
80. Pronovost P, Needham D, Berenholtz S, Sinopoli D, Chu H, Cosgrove S, Sexton B, Hyzy R, Welsh R, Roth G, Bander J, Kepros J, Goeschel C. An intervention to decrease catheter-related bloodstream infections in the ICU. N Engl J Med. 2006;355(26):2725–32.
81. Saint S, Olmsted RN, Fakih MG, Kowalski CP, Watson SR, Sales AE, Krein SL. Translating health care-associated urinary tract infection prevention research into practice via the bladder bundle. Jt Comm J Qual Patient Saf. 2009;35(9):449–55.
82. Septimus EJ, Moody J. Prevention of device-related healthcare-associated infections. F1000Res. 2016;5:F1000. https://doi.org/10.12688/f1000research.7493.1.
83. Elliott R, McKinley S, Fox V. Quality improvement program to reduce the prevalence of pressure ulcers in an intensive care unit. Am J Crit Care. 2008;17(4):328–34.
84. Engels D, Austin M, McNichols L, Fencl J. Pressure ulcers: factors contributing to their development in the OR. AORN J. 2016;103(3):271–81.
85. Association of perioperative Registered Nurses. Guideline for positioning the patient. In: Guidelines for perioperative practice. Denver, CO: AORN, Inc.; 2016. p. 649–74.
86. Allegretti AL, Malkiewicz A, Brienza DM. Measuring interface pressure and temperature in the operating room. Adv Skin Wound Care. 2012;25(5):226–30.
87. National Pressure Ulcer Advisory Panel, European Pressure Ulcer Advisory Panel and Pan Pacific Pressure Injury Alliance. Individuals in the operating room. In: Haesler E, editor. Prevention and treatment of pressure ulcers: clinical practice guideline. Osborne Park, Western Australia: Cambridge Media; 2014. p. 225–9.
88. World Health Organization. Patient safety. 2019. https://www.who.int/news-room/fact-sheets/detail/patient-safety. Accessed 26 Aug 2023.
89. Hughes RG, Clancy CM. Nurses' role in patient safety. J Nurs Care Qual. 2009;24(1):1–4.

Nursing Education: The Bridge to Patient Safety

Jennifer T. Alderman and Gwen Sherwood

1 Introduction

Education has been the bridge to creating safe quality healthcare delivery systems. Since the Institute of Medicine (now the National Academy of Medicine) reported the statistics of preventable harm in healthcare in the United States [1] and identified core quality and safety competencies for all health professionals [2], educators and clinicians have sought to transform health professions education in both what is taught and how that content is implemented in didactic and clinical learning environments.

Nurses are important members of the health care team in helping health care systems integrate ongoing improvement in quality and safety. Patient outcomes, quality, and safety are learned both at the systems level and at the individual level to advance professional development. When nurses understand those system improvements in the context of their individual patient, a transformation in mindset takes place, and quality and safety become an integral part of their daily work. The Institute of Medicine [2] issued a call for nurses and other health professionals to transform health care and to uphold and transmit core professional values for reducing risk while understanding and managing the full dimensions of interprofessional, safe, quality, evidence-based patient-centered care. Nurses and all health professionals must be able to deploy a complex array of competencies while maintaining a deep commitment to each patient's best interests. These competencies—patient-centered care, teamwork and collaboration, evidence-based practice, quality improvement, safety, and informatics—were identified by the 2003 IOM report on health professions education and operationalized through the Quality and Safety

J. T. Alderman · G. Sherwood (✉)
University of North Carolina at Chapel Hill, Chapel Hill, NC, USA
e-mail: jgtaylor@email.unc.edu; Gwen.sherwood@unc.edu

© The Author(s), under exclusive license to Springer Nature Switzerland AG 2024
C. A. Oster, J. S. Braaten (eds.), *The Nexus between Nursing and Patient Safety*,
https://doi.org/10.1007/978-3-031-53158-3_6

Education for Nurses (QSEN) project [3–5]. Reflective practice used for personal and professional development catalyzes transformative care through critical consciousness, critical reasoning, culturally based practice improvements.

The American Association of Colleges of Nursing (AACN) reimagined the essentials of nursing education in 2021, moving them toward a competency-based approach [6]. The 2021 Essentials provide a framework outlining the necessary curricular content for baccalaureate, master's, and Doctor of Nursing Practice programs [6]. There are ten domains in the 2021 Essentials. In each domain, competencies are provided for entry-level and advanced-level nursing practice. Domain 5 is entitled Quality and Safety. The 2021 AACN Essentials competencies can be found at https://www.aacnnursing.org/Portals/0/PDFs/Publications/Essentials-2021.pdf.

This chapter describes and explores the connection between nursing education and patient safety by describing the core mission of QSEN, the quality and safety domains of the AACN Essentials, the intersection of the interprofessional education and practice competencies, and the reimagining of nursing pedagogies for implementing the competencies. Interactive and narrative pedagogies include reflective practices that guide learner engagement and development also contribute to leadership development to prepare nurses for leading and working in systems grounded in cultures of safety. The chapter includes a cross walk between the QSEN competencies and the ten domains comprising the 2021 AACN Essentials.

2   Patient Safety: Driving Education Transformation

QSEN has been the core foundation for educating nurses about quality and safety. These separate but related terms are essential for changing outcomes first identified in the IOM 2000 report, and yet, patient safety continues as a global crisis. Education bridges to practice improvements, and culture shifts are required for changing outcomes. Transformative models for educating learners are driving changes in nursing education paradigms and hold the promise for patient safety as a part of every nurse's practice every day, every patient, and every time.

2.1   QSEN: Quality and Safety Education for Nurses

Since its launch in 2005, the national initiative Quality and Safety Education for Nurses (QSEN) has guided extensive curricula updates incorporating quality and safety competencies developed for pre-licensure [3] and graduate [5] learners. Developed as curricular guidelines, the knowledge, skills, and attitude (KSA) statements exemplifying each of the six quality and safety competencies are intended as practice guidelines as well. The competencies include patient-centered care, teamwork and collaboration, evidence-based practice, quality improvement, informatics, and safety. Detailed information on the competencies is found at www.QSEN.org.

The QSEN project team developed a set of knowledge, skills, and attitude (KSA) objective statements defining the six competences leveled for pre-licensure [3] and graduate education [5]: patient-centered care, teamwork and collaboration, evidence-based practice, quality improvement, informatics, and safety. The core definitions were integrated into nursing curricula and are explicitly defined in the 2021 American Association for Colleges of Nursing (AACN) Essentials for nursing pre-licensure and graduate education [6]. The QSEN project inspired transformation across nursing education and practice for integrating quality and safety into nurses' professional identity formation establishing quality and patient safety as integral to nurses' professional practice. Educators recognized that how we teach is as critical as what we teach, going beyond knowledge acquisition to create interactive pedagogies that include knowledge application. Redesigned academic-practice partnerships help bridge the gap between academic and workplace learning. Educators also recognized that each patient safety competency does not stand alone; each requires integration across the other five competencies [7].

As educators implemented the QSEN competencies across their curriculum, the need for education transformation became apparent. The 15 school Pilot Learning Collaborative [4] revealed an imperative for changing both content (what we teach) and education delivery (how we teach). It reached a ground swell as QSEN was referred to as a social movement [8]. Guidelines for using interactive pedagogies grounded in unfolding case studies incorporated reflective learning strategies in guiding learners to move from content acquisition to include content application [9]. The QSEN website has an open access compendium of dozens of teaching strategies for integrating the competencies at www.QSEN.org.

Reflective inquiry facilitates meaningful exploration of nurses' own roles and sense of professional responsibility [10]. New graduate nurses are increasingly exposed to foundational content in practice quality standards and national safety initiatives but lack focus on systems approaches [11]. Nursing education has historically focused more on tasks for providing individual patient care. Patient safety education requires curricula integrate exposure to systems thinking. Nursing students need to understand that safe systems of care and safe provision of care are different facets of the same phenomenon; now, systems thinking and design are included in the AACN Essentials [6]. Clinicians continually make important decisions at the individual practice level that influence quality and safety outcomes, but sustained change relies on systems applications.

Nursing is a high-stakes discipline. Nursing practice based on multiple types of knowledge is going beyond empirical evidence [12]. Nurses apply critical reasoning as they sift through available evidence, past experiences, and other ways of knowing (e.g., aesthetic, personal, ethical and legal, spiritual) for making choices in the context of a particular situation, developing a sense of salience (i.e., the ability to recognize what is urgent in a particular situation). Nurses build a multiplicity of knowledge by engaging in informational and transformational learning experiences through which they experientially apply what they know (knowledge), what they know how to do (skills), and how decisions fit within their ethical and moral framework (attitudes), thus develop competency. A spirit of inquiry that asks critical questions combine with engaging in the moment to create synergy through which nurses actively think and reason in dynamic situations, acting for the good of the patient, ever mindful of safety risks, person-centeredness, and interactions with the team.

A bibliometric analysis of QSEN penetration reported 221 articles published in peer reviewed journals between its first publication in 2007 and 2021: 165 focused on education with far less focused on practice (35) showing the gap between academic learning and practice application [13]. Cengiz and Yoder [14] reported nursing students' perceptions of how well they had achieved the QSEN competencies, finding patient-centered care rated highest and quality improvement rated lowest. Given the expectation that all learners would have been exposed to the QSEN competencies prior to completing their formal academic program, it is concerning that learners felt they had not mastered this essential learning, and that quality improvement was considered the least important when safety depends on continuous improvement. Furthermore, Altmiller and Armstrong [15] conducted a national survey of nurse faculty finding significant gaps in faculty members' readiness to integrate the QSEN competencies into their teaching continues. It is timely to reassess how we are providing safety education to explore transformative pedagogies for transforming practice.

3 Transforming Nursing Education: Pedagogies Integrating Quality and Safety

3.1 Transformational Education: Think like a Nurse

Transformational education engages learners in the deeper meaning and application of knowledge as they meld theory and content with real-world clinical application. Learners are challenged to "think like a nurse" [16]. Interactive learning that applies the pathophysiology underlying disease categories develops understanding of how signs and symptoms combine with evidence-informed interventions encourages critical reasoning and judgment leading to improved outcomes. Creating an interactive learning space holds the patient in the center of the learning experience. The purpose of nursing knowledge is caring for patients [17]; holding patients in the center of case study analysis that applies the taxonomies learners have worked on prior to coming together (i.e., flipped classroom style) emphasizes the QSEN competency of patient-centered care. Learners must apply what they know and know how to do with real people; someone's life will depend on their ability to sift through this array of knowledge to inform what and how they enact patient care [9, 18].

Transformational learning is a necessary component of practice development and speaks to the lifelong learning demanded of professional practice [19]. Developing safety practice derives from critical reflection that questions assumptions leading to critical thinking. Reflection helps to surface assumptions that limit an open perspective and full understanding of a situation or seeing a person as they are. Transformational learning promotes both personal and professional growth.

Who we are as a person is the person we bring to practice; the reflective foundation of transformational learning theory helps in developing emotional intelligence for improving self-awareness, relationships with others, empathy, and motivation [20]. Transformational learning based on learning from experience moves the learner or the nurse beyond acquisition of new knowledge and skills to increase capacity for asking questions about their work, challenging assumptions, values, and beliefs, and propels learners forward in their professional development.

Experiential education [21] incorporates adult learning theories for helping learners and nurses practice how they apply what they know, can do, and attitudes guiding their professional practice development. Experiential teaching is learner-centered focused on knowledge application. The educator is not trying to exert control nor simply deliver lecture content but co-create with the learner through narrative-based pedagogies [22].

Education transformation is a global challenge in combatting patient safety. Cheng [23] described the evolution of nursing education in Taiwan for preparing practice-ready graduates prepared to practice in safe quality systems. The goal was preparing nurses for engaging in knowledge transformation and skills demonstrations addressing current practice needs. New graduates often experience difficulties in transitioning into practice settings because of passive learning and lack of problem-solving skills and critical thinking [11]. Skills in reflective practice can enhance development of practice knowledge, self-assessment, and lifelong learning, develop future practice capability and professional identity, and critically appraise practice traditions rather than simply reproduce them. This mindset for questioning is a critical feature in safety education for monitoring risks of preventable harm and is developed through critical reflection in practice-based narratives. Various forms of interactive narrative learning are included in Table 1 with a brief summary for application. All apply narrative learning strategies [17].

Table 1 Experiential learning strategies adapted from [9]

Classroom strategy	Purpose
Narrative pedagogy	Learners and facilitators/educators use story or real patient situations to co-construct what is important, concerns, evaluate options, and determine an approach with patient shared decision-making
Unfolding case studies	Patient-based situations from practice are presented for analysis, discussion in small groups to discuss options, plan care, and share with all
Problem-based learning	Learners work with client cases to apply what they know to solve patient problems, either discipline specific or involving multiple disciplines
Simulation	Learners participate in mock client care scenarios with varying fidelity simulating the real world with reflection before and after the experience
Flipped classrooms	Focus on knowledge acquisition prior to coming to the session where the focus is on application of what they can apply to understand the situation and plan priorities and actions
Team-based learning	Learners are assigned to teams for working on a problem or scenario to discover and construct what they need to know to propose a solution

With careful planning, these strategies are effective for both in person and online delivery and can be used synchronously or asynchronously. The COVID-19 pandemic interrupted the usual pattern and processes of nursing education with a quick pivot to online delivery [24]. Educators developed innovative strategies to engage learners, yet, providing the same level or higher level of learner achievement of required competencies remains a challenge [25]. Transformative learning theory is a way to further develop experiential, interactive learning approaches such as in Table 1 to achieve the goals of education in changing behavior, attitudes, and skills to address patient safety. Each method or approach is grounded in experience and how nurses and learners reflect on the experience in developing knowledge and skills for practice and calls into their ethical and moral standards that guide decisions about practice.

3.2   Reflective Practices: Learning from Experience

Quality safe care is more than just applying knowledge and skills; it is how we approach our work with a spirit of inquiry. Asking questions about practice is fundamental to quality and safety to surface contradictions, gaps in care standards, and risks leading to preventable harm. Reflective practice builds from inquiry, from systematic questioning of what produces the outcomes we see. Reflection bridges theory and practice, helping make sense of practice [26]. The essence of learning through reflection is to surface contradiction between intention and actual practice. Reflection demands confrontation with factors and situations that limit achieving desirable work, both individually and at the organization or system level.

Reflection is a process of noticing, engaging, and thinking about what you are seeing and doing. Reflection is the art of asking questions that can result in new mental models. Reflective practices develop focused ways of thinking about practice for deeper awareness and understanding [22]. It is sometimes described as structured listening to your own voice to examine your own perspectives in relation to others. [27] mapped reflective tools and approaches used by nurses and learners in clinical settings. Both specific questions and open-ended questions sought to help learners and nurses in applying a reflective framework as a practice habit for improving quality and safety.

Reflective practice helps one see things from different perspectives by purposefully examining self and experiences [28]. We learn from experience through cycles of interpretation using our inner compass to search for truth and reconsider ways to improve. Reflective practices raise awareness about what we do to make better choices in the future by helping see the gap between actual actions alongside what was hoped, enabling one to monitor reactions for intentional, conscious, deliberate responses.

Reflective practice helps nurses and others ask the questions to identify current practice to compare with benchmarks for effective practice, a necessary aspect of quality improvement [29]. Reflective practice examines the theory-practice gap, development, and caring; in training, as learning, guided process, and development;

Fig. 1 Reflection model for monitoring patient safety risks

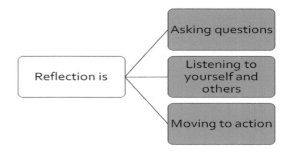

and in research, as knowledge, method, and social change [30]. By reliving experience through reflection, we can develop insights to take more appropriate action in the future guided by purpose to engage mindfully in our work by providing a mirror into one's own thinking and values, revealing what is beneath the surface of our actions and attitudes, uncovering initial assumptions and learning by looking inward to grow. We see what we did not see before. Reflection is looking at the same thing but seeing it differently, uncovering the layers. Figure 1 offers a three-prong reflection guide appropriate for developing safety awareness that leads to action: Asking questions (inquiry), listening to yourself and others (self-awareness), and moving to action (mitigating patient safety risks).

3.3   Learning from Story: Improving Patient Safety

Learning from story is one form of transformational education pedagogy that creates experiential, interactive learning [22]. Story builds from experiential learning theory [21] and reflecting on actions by story participants. Story-based learning is a type of narrative learning that examines a situation or experience from multiple perspectives; through reflection one can examine the same experience from the lens of the different participants, helping hone the skills of observation, cultural sensitivity, and seeing others for who they are. Stories represent experience. We learn as we reflect on experience to make sense of events, see other angles, and to consider what we can learn from the experience to change our responses in the future. Three questions can help in developing the habit of reflection on experience to increase awareness:

- What are you noticing?
- What concerns you?
- What are the important elements in the story so far?

Asking learners or nurses to view a photo or drawing is one way to practice seeing beyond the first glimpse, beyond surface assumptions of what something represents. It helps build awareness of previously unseen patient risks to prevent harm. Patient safety depends on recognizing patient risks, knowing what to do, and having the courage to act, therefore, apply knowledge, skills, and attitudes. Practice is a way to

Fig. 2 Examine the
picture from different
angles to discern the two
images [31]

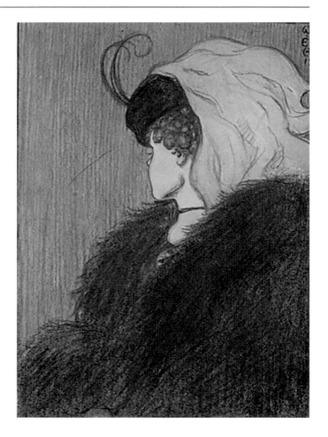

develop this type of situational awareness key to patient safety The picture below in
Fig. 2 depicts two different images. Discerning the images is an exercise in looking
past the first glimpse and seeing the whole picture.

Reflection provides an understanding of seeing the person behind the illness.
Reflection contributes to increased self-understanding and awareness of oneself as
a caring nurse [32]. A reflective model for developing a spirit of inquiry uses guided
questions to examine the story or experience to see from a new lens [18]:

- What stands out in this situation?
- What assumptions influence my thinking?
- What else could be going on?
- What previous experiences may help?
- What other perspectives could there be?
- Whose voice is missing in the story?

Textbox 1: Example of Learning from Story to Improve Patient Safety

Students in an undergraduate nursing leadership course use reflective practice and principles of quality and safety to perform a root cause analysis after reading the book, *Josie's Story* [33]. This book describes what happened to Josie King, an 18-month-old little girl who suffered from accidental burn injuries in 2001. Multiple healthcare errors contributed to the events that befell Josie. Students use the guiding questions below to complete this assignment. The root cause analysis allows students to analyze what happened and determine possible courses of action that would prevent a situation like this from happening again [34].

1. What happened in this case (case summary)?
2. What was your personal reaction to this case?
3. Why did it happen? List three active errors and three latent errors.
4. What are some evidence-based recommendations to keep it from happening again?

Textbox 1 provides another example of using a reflective model while learning from story.

3.3.1 Simulation-Based Learning

Nursing education relies heavily on workplace learning, yet clinical placements for students are in short supply. Simulation-based learning provides a safe space for learners to practice skills and apply what they know prior to real-world experience. Panda et al. [35] cited challenges encountered in clinical learning environments including experiencing an inadequate support structure, lack of a sense of belonging, fear of mistakes, staff shortages, and inconsistencies between theory and practice. Simulation provides learners with educator guided application interacting with other learners using a scenario that encourages critical thinking [36].

Simulation has provided alternatives to clinical practice and invites multiple strategies for working with learners. Sherwood and Day's [18] description of a reflective model to guide workplace learning that can be used both in analyzing scenarios in classrooms, simulation, or clinical debriefing as a safety focus. Developing a mindful engaged presence begins with reflection before taking action to identify the primary purpose of what you are undertaking. Helping nurses and learners develop the habit of purpose-based practice asks, what actions will achieve my goal? What do I need? What are the safety risks? Reflecting in action may require a pause to ask who can help me manage this situation or provide needed information? Am I on course to achieve the purpose or goal? Reflecting on action asks what went well? What could be improved? What will I do differently next time? What should be reported or measured to assure quality safe care?

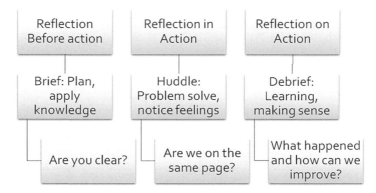

Fig. 3 Reflection framework for purpose-driven deliberate practice

Simulation has been shown to improve patient safety, although more rigorous research is needed in this field. Components of simulation that have linkages to patient safety include the ability to practice a skill or patient communication before taking care of an actual patient, interprofessional teambuilding, resilience building, and improving communication skills [37]. The specific skill of medication administration has been a frequent focus of simulations, emphasizing the critical safety issue of errors related to medication administration in healthcare [38]. Using simulation to teach medication administration has been shown to improve nursing students' medication administration safety competence so they are better prepared for real-world application [38]. Figure 3 provides a reflection framework that can be used in simulation-based learning.

4   Quality and Safety Education: Optimizing Transition to Practice

4.1   Key Components Driving Quality and Safety Education

Patient safety education is influenced by multiple components. We describe the intersection of the QSEN competencies with the ten domains from the AACN Essentials [6]. Interprofessional education is an essential competency for developing cultures of safety. Reimagining academic-practice partnerships has emerged as a strong driver for patient safety education by developing ways for learners to better integrate into the system and thus improved their understanding of safety culture.

4.1.1   Competency-Based Education
A chief driver in current education is the shift to competency-based education. The new paradigm stems from concern over content saturation that left too little emphasis on knowledge application. Competency-based education concentrates on learner

Table 2 AACN competency domains integrate with QSEN to improve patient safety education

Domain	Primary goal	Application to safety
1. Knowledge for nursing practice	Bridge theory and practice to develop clinical judgment	Each of the 6 QSEN competencies is described by knowledge statements for achieving the competency
2. Person-centered care	Develop and coordinate caring relationships, communication, assessment, and accountability for actions	Patient-centered care is an explicit QSEN competency that respects the patient as an active partner in their care
3. Population health	Develop partnerships, advocacy, and equitable approach to care delivery	In implementing the QSEN competencies, person-centered care considers patient and family unique cultures and beliefs
4. Scholarship for nursing practice	Develop and embrace multiple ways of knowing, using evidence-informed practices	Evidence-based practice is a QSEN competency at the core of care comparing actual care with benchmarks
5. Quality and safety	Cultivate culture of patient safety and quality improvement	Quality improvement and safety are two of the six competencies in the QSEN framework
6. Interprofessional partnerships	Create climate of mutual respect, working together with collaboration	Teamwork and collaboration are the QSEN competency
7. Systems-based practice	Recognize complexities in practice that interact across microsystems for patient safety	Systems thinking is as a core concept and strategy for achieving safe quality care
8. Information and healthcare technologies	Apply technologies and tools to enhance communication and care effectiveness	Informatics is a QSEN competency essential for communication and decision-support
9. Professionalism	Apply ethical comportment in practicing diversity, equity, and inclusion with participatory approach	Each QSEN competency describes attitude statements to formulate how one implements their practice, thus professional identity formation.
10. Personal, professional, and leadership development	Practice with inquiry, reflection grounded in caring for self and others in developing leadership and professional identity	Emotional intelligence supports personal development guiding how one applies their leadership skills in living the QSEN competencies

accountability of outcomes, easing the transition to practice for new graduates. The American Association for Colleges of Nursing published ten essentials domains, each with defined competencies leveled to guide baccalaureate and graduate nursing education. Each competency is leveled for baccalaureate, Master of Science in Nursing (MSN), and Doctor of Nursing Practice (DNP) programs [6]. The QSEN competencies are integrated throughout the ten domains but are intentionally defined in Domain 5, Quality and Safety. Table 2 demonstrates this integration of QSEN competencies and the AACN competencies.

4.2   Interprofessional Education and Practice: Working Together for Safety

Domain 6 of the AACN essentials is interprofessional partnerships. The goals for interprofessional partnerships begin with integration of the interprofessional education and practice frameworks guiding health professions education. The links between the QSEN competencies and the AACN essentials have already been established in this chapter and demonstrate how the Interprofessional Education Collaborative (IPEC) competencies can be leveraged in nursing education to impact quality and safety in healthcare.

The 2023 update of the Interprofessional Education Collaborative (IPEC) competencies can be found at https://www.ipecollaborative.org/assets/core-competencies/IPEC_Core_Competencies_Version_3_2023.pdf [39]. A 2023 update is currently under review. Many health professions' schools, including nursing, require IPE to be part of their respective curricula as required by accreditation standards. A key driver of this change was the need for health professions students to learn how to communicate and operate successfully in teams during their educational programs, thus resulting in practice-ready members of the health care workforce. Understanding roles and responsibilities, leading with effective teamwork, communication, and identifying personal values and ethics are the four IPEC competencies [39]. Noted in Domain 6 of the AACN essentials are competencies and sub-competencies that encompass the IPEC competencies, thus showing solid integration of the two frameworks.

Leadership development is a cornerstone in providing safe, quality care. One sub-competency in Domain 6 is to "apply principles of team leadership and management performance to improve quality and assure safety" (p. 47). Using teaching strategies endorsed by QSEN for ensuring safe and quality care is one path for addressing this sub-competency in the AACN essentials. Simulation-based learning, reflective practice, and problem-based learning are all effective strategies that can be used to improve safety and quality competencies [40]. Bleich [41] noted that quality and safety are core leadership competencies; academic programs need to integrate leadership throughout the curriculum rather than at the end of the academic program so that learners have opportunities to practice leadership skills. Leadership capacity helps when nurses understand the systems and processes in which they work and how they contribute to human safety behaviors [42].

Brewer et al. [43] conducted a scoping review to understand how leadership has been conceptualized through the lens of interprofessional education and practice. Results showed a trend approaching more collaborative models of leadership, focusing on interpersonal relationships and the idea that all members within interprofessional teams can serve as leaders at various times and in various ways. Improving leadership competence in pre-licensure nursing students may need to occur over successive courses in nursing school curricula [44]. Noting that leadership is more a process than a role, Hsieh et al. [44] reported that at the end of their academic study, nursing students viewed leadership as a team effort versus an individual one.

Multiple opportunities often exist in nursing school curricula for students to interact on interprofessional teams. Many nursing schools have intentionally embedded IPE encounters in their curricula to meet accreditation requirements. One goal of this intentionality is to improve teamwork and collaboration, thus leading to improved team communication and safety outcomes. For example, Banks et al. [45] found that interprofessional collaboration between nursing and social work students shifted the students' thinking from the silo effect and led to collaboration between the groups. Through interprofessional simulations, attaining a better understanding of roles and responsibilities enhances the students' abilities to work in teams and to come out of their siloed mindset [46]. Decreasing the silo effect in interprofessional teams improves patient safety and patient outcomes [45]. Textbox 2 provides an example of an active learning strategy that can be used as a case discussion in interprofessional education.

Textbox 2: Integrating Interprofessional Competencies for Improving Patient Safety

Lewis Blackman was a healthy 15-year-old who had elective surgery and died 4 days later due to a series of medical errors. His story is re-enacted in this video which embeds reflective questions to help viewers develop a mindset for patient safety and demonstrates the imperative of interprofessional education and practice for improving patient safety.

The film Transparent Health—Lewis Blackman Story is available at https://www.youtube.com/watch?v=Rp3fGp2fv88

- Identify elements of each QSEN competency in this story for their presence or absence.
- What were opportunities for any one clinician to speak up for patient safety?
- Describe how this story illustrates the imperative for including the patient and family as team members and patient safety allies.
- Rewrite the story using the QSEN competencies as guidelines.

---

5 Case Study: "How to" Application

5.1 Academic-Practice Partnership: Driving Quality and Safety

The benefits of academic-practice partnerships (APPs) provide essential linkages between nursing schools and practice organizations that supply needed avenues of learning and scholarship. All APPs have the core components of a nursing school (academic partner) and healthcare or community-based organization (practice partner) to provide nursing services to patient populations while furthering the school's teaching and scholarship missions [47]. Noting again that education has been the bridge to creating safe quality health care delivery systems, APPs serve in making this bridge possible.

Hahn et al. [48] reported on an APP that was created to give pre-licensure students additional valuable clinical experiences focused on providing quality care to patients with complex health needs. Managers, preceptors, nursing faculty, and students noted that this was a positive learning experience, with managers recruiting future hires and students improving in prioritization and communication skills. Named *Bridge to Professional Practice* and motivated by the need to produce a more practice-ready nursing workforce, this program is an example of an innovative solution to a workforce need. Aligning with Domain 7 in AACN's essentials, *Systems-Based Practice* [6], a partnership such as this shows how leaders within a group of health care organizations problem-solved a workforce issue. Knowing that nursing schools need to produce graduates who are ready to provide safe, quality care to patients with complex health needs lead to this successful partnership.

Reporting on the effect of the COVID-19 pandemic on APPs, Bejster et al. [49] noted that opportunities arose during the pandemic to be transformative with nursing education. Nursing faculty were able to pivot, identify curricular gaps, and provide education related to telehealth, health promotion, epidemiology, partnership-building, and resource navigation, thus allowing students to bring skills to clinical settings, meeting the demands of their future practice of providing quality, safe care. One example of creating a new APP during the pandemic was described by Gresh et al. [50]. There was a need to be pro-active in providing social connections to older adults in one community setting. One nursing program partnered with a community-based coalition to provide social support and assist with resource navigation by making phone calls to this population. This was one way to

---

Textbox 3: Example/Case Study of Academic-Practice Partnership

The intersection of nursing education and patient safety can be demonstrated through academic-practice partnerships. In one academic medical center and a partnering school of nursing, multiple initiatives have been developed and implemented with much success. Initiatives have included intraprofessional simulations, an experiential learning elective nursing course, a nursing faculty-new graduate residency program liaison, and a workload-share for practicing bedside clinical nurses.

Intraprofessional simulations: In a pre-licensure maternal/newborn nursing course, simulations occur at the end of the semester aimed at synthesizing student learning from the overall course [51]. Course leaders recruited bedside obstetric nurses to help facilitate the simulations. The nurses brought authenticity to the cases and in turn learned pedagogical strategies related to conducting simulations. In a true collaborative effort, the unit manager enlisted nurse faculty facilitators to assist with newly licensed nurses' skill development using simulation. This resource-sharing activity provided opportunities for realistic, simulated learning experiences that benefited faculty, practicing nurses, and students.

Clinical quality scholars: The Clinician Leadership in Quality and Safety Program is a 1-year program that equips doctoral students with skills that they can directly apply in clinical settings. Learning is longitudinal, mentored, and experiential. Throughout the program, students conduct a quality improvement initiative over the course of the year. During the individualization phase, students participate as a member of a clinical improvement team and work closely with a faculty mentor. They meet regularly with their mentors, attend seminars, and create monthly deliverables like project charters, AIM statements, driver diagrams, and run charts. As part of the QI project experience, students join an existing improvement team in the academic medical center and devote at least 130 hours to improvement work. Throughout the program, students are expected to spend time in a clinical setting interacting with patients, learning processes that might be impacted by that work, and executing tasks in support of clinic improvement.

Experiential Learning in Nursing (ELN) elective: During the COVID-19 pandemic, leaders in the academic medical center and undergraduate nursing program partnered to create an Experiential Learning in Nursing Course. The intent of the elective was for pre-licensure nursing students to gain more clinical experience while simultaneously meeting the needs of select nursing units. In this course, students were considered members of a patient care team on an assigned unit and tasked with providing patient care and assisting with other unit responsibilities. All patient care related skills were delegated by an experienced nurse in the unit. Partnering units included cardiac, neuro, surgical and neonatal intensive care, labor and delivery, other pediatrics units, adult acute care medicine, emergency department (ED), and adult orthopedic and trauma. In addition to the clinical experience, the course brought together faculty from various health professions and clinical educators from the academic medical center for seminars. Discussion topics included: examining team-based care, workforce culture, innovative strategies for addressing the workforce shortage, and strategies for maximizing the experiential learning experience.

Nurse residency liaison: One faculty member in the nursing school has assigned workload to collaborate with the academic medical center's new graduate nurse residency program director. The faculty member meets with the Nurse Residency Coordinator for planning, consulting, and collaboration sessions and serves as a liaison to community stakeholders and designs and advocates for learning opportunities for nurse residents.

Clinical Instructor Program: Leaders from the nursing school and the academic medical center implemented a shared vision to fill clinical instructor vacancies and increase retention in bedside nurses. Bedside nurses who have a desire to teach were recruited by the medical center and interviewed by leaders in the nursing school. The nurses selected for the role continued to work two of three 12-h shifts on their respective units. The remaining 12-h shift in their assignment was teaching a pre-licensure clinical group related to their expertise. The nurses report greater job satisfaction and gain skills in teaching and learning practices. Students benefit from the nurse's institutional and clinical expertise. This program promotes the hiring of new graduate RNs at the medical center while allowing students to feel an increased readiness to practice in a rapidly changing healthcare environment.

address safety concerns, as this group was the among the most vulnerable if exposed to COVID-19 [50]. Textbox 3 provides an example of an academic-practice partnership and demonstrates the various ways such a partnership can benefit both the academic partner and the practice partner.

Key Points

- Nursing education is the bridge to improving patient safety.
- Transformative nursing education helps create mindsets for improving patient safety competencies. Integrating evidence-based frameworks like the QSEN competencies, AACN essentials, and IPEC competencies into nursing curricula is the standard by which all nursing schools should be guided.
- Transformative nursing education applications such as experiential learning, simulation, reflective practice, and learning from story are linked to improving patient safety in healthcare settings.
- Leveraging academic-practice partnerships can produce a more practice-ready nursing workforce as healthcare is faced with improving outcomes for complex patients in equally complex healthcare settings.

References

1. Institute of Medicine (IOM, now NASEM). To err is human: building a safer health system. Washington, DC: National Academies Press; 2000.
2. Institute of Medicine (IOM, now NASEM). Health professions education: a bridge to quality. Washington, DC: National Academies Press; 2003.
3. Cronenwett L, Sherwood G, Barnsteiner J, Disch J, Johnson J, Mitchell P, Taylor Sullivan D, Warren J. Quality and safety education for nurses. Nurs Outlook. 2007;55(3):122–31.
4. Cronenwett L, Sherwood G, Gelmon S. Improving quality and safety education: the QSEN learning collaborative. Nurs Outlook. 2009a;57(6):304–12.
5. Cronenwett L, Sherwood G, Pohl J, Barnsteiner J, Moore S, Taylor Sullivan D, Ward D, Warren J. Quality and safety education for advanced practice nursing practice. Nurs Outlook. 2009b;57(6):338–48.

6. American Association of Colleges of Nursing. The essentials: core competencies for professional nursing education. Washington, DC: American Association of Colleges of Nursing; 2021.
7. Barnsteiner J. Safety. In: Sherwood ING, Barnsteiner J, editors. Quality and safety in nursing: a competency approach to improving outcomes. (3rd ed.). ed. Hoboken, NH: Wiley-Blackwell; 2022. p. 213–38, 301–320.
8. Cronenwett L, Barnsteiner J. A national initiative: quality and safety education for nurses (QSEN). In: Sherwood G, Barnsteiner J, editors. Quality and safety in nursing: a competency approach to improving outcomes. 3rd ed. Hoboken, NJ: Wiley-Blackwell; 2022.
9. Day L, Sherwood G. Transforming education to transform practice: using unfolding case studies to integrate quality and safety in subject centered classrooms. In: Sherwood ING, Barnsteiner J, editors. Quality and safety in nursing: a competency approach to improving outcomes. 3rd ed. Hoboken, NH: Wiley-Blackwell; 2022.
10. Johns C. Becoming a reflective practitioner. 6th ed. West Sussex, UK: Wiley-Blackwell; 2022.
11. Spector N, Ulrich B, Barnsteiner J. Improving quality and safety with transition to practice. In: Sherwood G, Barnsteiner J, editors. Quality and safety in nursing: a competency approach to improving outcomes. 2nd ed. Wiley-Blackwell: Hoboken, NJ; 2017. p. 281–300.
12. Johns C. Mindful leadership. A guide for the health care professions. London, UK: Palgrave Macmillan; 2016.
13. Sherwood G, Jones CB, Conklin JL, Dodd A. Quality and safety education for nurses: a bibliometric analysis. J Nurs Scholarsh. 2023;55:914. https://doi.org/10.1111/jnu.12876.
14. Cengiz A, Yoder LH. Assessing nursing students' perceptions of the QSEN competencies: a systematic review of the literature with implications for academic programs. Worldviews Evid Based Nurs. 2020;17(4):275–82. https://doi.org/10.1111/wvn.12458.
15. Altmiller G, Armstrong G. National quality and safety education for nurses faculty survey results. Nurse Educ. 2017;42(5S):S3–7. https://doi.org/10.1097/NNE.0000000000000408.
16. Tanner C. Thinking like a nurse: a research-based model of clinical judgment in nursing. J Nurs Educ. 2006;45(6):204–11.
17. Alteren J. Narratives in learner nurses' knowledge development: a hermeneutical research study. Nurse Educ Today. 2019;76:51–5. https://doi.org/10.1016/j.nedt.2019.01.015.
18. Sherwood G, Day L. Quality and safety in clinical learning environments. In: Sherwood G, Barnsteiner J, editors. Quality and safety in nursing: a competency approach to improving outcomes. 3rd ed. Hoboken, NJ: Wiley; 2022. p. 321–48.
19. Van Schalkwyk SC, Hafler J, Brewer TF, Maley MA, Margolis C, McNamee L, Meyer I, Peluso MJ, Schmutz AM, Spak JM, Davies D, Bellagio Global Health Education Initiative. Transformative learning as pedagogy for the health professions: a scoping review. Med Educ. 2019;53(6):547–58. https://doi.org/10.1111/medu.13804.
20. Kaiafas KN. Emotional intelligence and role-modeling Nursing's soft skills. J Christ Nurs. 2021;38(4):240–3. https://doi.org/10.1097/CNJ.0000000000000881.
21. Kolb D. Experiential learning: experience as the source of learning and development. Upper Saddle River, NJ: Pearson FT Press; 2014.
22. Armstrong G, Sherwood G. Reflective practice: using narrative pedagogy to foster quality and safety. In: Sherwood ING, Barnsteiner J, editors. Quality and safety in nursing: a competency approach to improving outcomes. (3rd ed.). ed. Hoboken, NH: Wiley-Blackwell; 2022. p. 301–20.
23. Cheng SF. Transformation in nursing education: development and implementation of diverse innovative teaching. J Nurs. 2021;68(6):P4–5. https://doi.org/10.6224/JN.202112_68(6).01.
24. McMillan K, Akoo C, Catigbe-Cates A. New graduate nurses navigating entry to practice in the Covid-19 pandemic. Can J Nurs Res. 2023;55(1):78–90. https://doi.org/10.1177/08445621221150946.
25. Graham MM. Navigating professional and personal knowing through reflective storytelling amidst Covid-19. J Holist Nurs. 2022;40(4):372–82. https://doi.org/10.1177/08980101211072289.
26. Horton-Deutsch S, Sherwood G. Reflective practice: transforming education and practice. 2nd ed. Indianapolis: Sigma Theta Tau Press; 2017.

27. Scheel LS, Bydam J, Peters MDJ. Reflection as a learning strategy for the training of nurses in clinical practice setting: a scoping review. JBI Evid Synth. 2021;19(12):3268–300. https://doi.org/10.11124/JBIES-21-00005.
28. Patel KM, Metersky K. Reflective practice in nursing: a concept analysis. Int J Nurs Knowl. 2022;33(3):180–7. https://doi.org/10.1111/2047-3095.12350.
29. Davey CH, Dolansky MA, Harris AT, Singh MK. Integrating a reflective learning activity to ensure quality improvement project success. Nurs Educ Perspect. 2020;41(5):E42–4. https://doi.org/10.1097/01.NEP.0000000000000610.
30. Choperena A, Oroviogoicoechea C, Zaragoza Salcedo A, Olza Moreno I, Jones D. Nursing narratives and reflective practice: a theoretical review. J Adv Nurs. 2019;75(8):1637–47. https://doi.org/10.1111/jan.13955.
31. Hill WE. My wife and my mother-in-law. [Prints and Photographs Division]. Library of Congress. 1915. https://www.loc.gov/resource/ds.00175/.
32. Jaastad TA, Ueland V, Koskinen C. The meaning of reflection for understanding caring and becoming a caring nurse. Scand J Caring Sci. 2022;36(4):1180–8. https://doi.org/10.1111/scs.13080.
33. King S. Josie's story: a mother's inspiring crusade to make medical care safe. New York: Grove Press; 2009.
34. Alderman J. Using a leadership toolkit to teach essential competencies. Nurse Educ. 2023. https://doi.org/10.1097/NNE.0000000000001374.
35. Panda S, Dash M, John J, Rath K, Debata A, Swain D, Mohanty K, Eustace-Cook J. Challenges faced by student nurses and midwives in clinical learning environment—a systematic review and meta-synthesis. Nurse Educ Today. 2021;101:104875. https://doi.org/10.1016/j.nedt.2021.104875.
36. Alderman J, Durham C. In: Sherwood G, Barnsteiner J, editors. Quality and safety in nursing: a competency approach to improving outcomes. 3rd ed. Hoboken, NH: Wiley-Blackwell; 2022. pp. 301–20, 349–84.
37. Mitchell A, Assadi G. Using simulation exercises to improve students' skills and patient safety. Br J Nurs. 2021;30(20):1198–202.
38. Lee S, Quinn B. Incorporating medication administration safety in undergraduate nursing education: a literature review. Nurse Educ Today. 2019;72:77–83. https://doi.org/10.1016/j.nedt.2018.11.004.
39. Interprofessional Education Collaboration (IPEC). 2023. IPEC Core Competencies for Interprofessional Collaborative Practice: Version 3.
40. Marcomini I, Terzoni S, Destrebecq A. Teaching strategies and tools for ensuring safe and quality care: a scoping review. Nurs Educ Perspect. 2021;42(6):339–43. https://doi.org/10.1097/01.NEP.0000000000000809.
41. Bleich M. Quality and safety as a core leadership competency. J Contin Educ Nurs. 2018;49(5):200–2. https://doi.org/10.3928/60220124-20180417-03.
42. Disch J. Leadership in promoting quality and safety. In: Sherwood ING, Barnsteiner J, editors. Quality and safety in nursing: a competency approach to improving outcomes. 3rd ed. Hoboken, NH: Wiley-Blackwell; 2022. p. 268–300.
43. Brewer ML, Flavell HL, Trede F, Smith M. A scoping review to understand "leadership" in interprofessional education and practice. J Interprof Care. 2016;30(4):408–15. https://doi.org/10.3109/13561820.2016.1150260.
44. Hsieh L, Chang Y, Yen M. Improving leadership competence among undergraduate nursing students: innovative objectives development, implementation, and evaluation. Nurs Educ Perspect. 2022;43(1):24–9. https://doi.org/10.1097/01.NEP.0000000000000866.
45. Banks S, Stanley M, Brown S, Matthew W. Simulation-based interprofessional education: a nursing and social work collaboration. J Nurs Educ. 2019;58(2):110–3.
46. Costello M, Prelack K, Faller J, Huddleston J, Adly S, Doolan J. Student experiences of interprofessional simulation: findings from a qualitative study. J Interprof Care. 2018;32(1):95–7. https://doi.org/10.1080/13561820.2017.1356810.

47. American Association of Colleges of Nursing. Guiding principles for academic-practice partnerships. 2012. https://www.aacnnursing.org/Aca-demic-Practice-Partnerships/The-Guiding-Principles.

48. Hahn J, Resha C, Beauvais A, Beckman B, Forte P, Rebeschi L, Snyder M. An innovative academic-practice partnership to support nursing workforce needs and student clinical education. J Nurs Adm. 2023;53(2):88–95. https://doi.org/10.1097/NNA.0000000000001249.

49. Bejster M, Geis A, Cygan H, Ferry-Rooney R, Kalensky M, Moss A. Effects of Covid-19 pandemic on academic-practice partnerships: implications for nursing education. J Nurs Educ. 2022;61(9):533–6. https://doi.org/10.3928/01484834-20220705-09.

50. Gresh A, LaFave S, Thamilselvan V, Batchelder A, Mermer J, Jacques K, Greensfelder A, Buckley M, Cohen Z, Coy A, War-ren N. Service learning in public health nursing education: how COVID-19 accelerated community-academic partnership. Public Health Nurs. 2021;38(2):248–57. https://doi.org/10.1111/phn.12796.

51. Alden K, Coulombe E, Alderman J. You scratch my back; I'll scratch yours: reciprocal intraprofessional collaboration for OB simulation. J Obstet Gynecol Neonatal Nurs. 2013;42(S9):S9. https://doi.org/10.1111/1552-6909.12058.

Nursing Leadership and Patient Safety

Andréa Narvaez and Kelley Kovar

1 Leader Thoughts on Patient Safety and High-Reliability Journey

Nursing leaders support nurses, caregivers, and patient safety daily. This is an essential component to the nurse leader's role. The nurse leader must continuously keep patient safety at the center of every action and decision. "The relationship between leadership and safety plays a pivotal role in creating positive safety outcomes for patient care. A safe culture is one nurtured by effective leadership" [1]. Thus effective nursing leadership contributes to keeping patients and associates safe across the healthcare environment. This relationship of nursing leadership's impact with patient safety has become more critical through the pandemic and moving into the fast-paced post-pandemic healthcare environment. Leadership competencies in patient safety are no longer a nice to have, but a must have for today's nursing leaders. The American Organization of Nursing Leadership [2] defined core patient safety leadership competencies that include active and disciplined listening; engagement and inclusiveness; vigilance for error identification; integrator of people and tasks; interdisciplinary co-leadership and collaboration; action orientation; art of championing; collaborative practice agreements; team leading and participation; and importance of top-down leadership culture of safety (p. 9–10). This list of core competencies is demonstrated in this chapter with the interventions that are practiced by nursing leaders that lead to an increase in patient safety.

A. Narvaez (✉)
AdventHealth Parker, Parker, CO, USA
e-mail: Andrea.narvaez@adventhealth.com

K. Kovar
AdventHealth Littleton, Littleton, CO, USA
e-mail: Kelley.Kovar@adventhealth.com

© The Author(s), under exclusive license to Springer Nature Switzerland AG 2024
C. A. Oster, J. S. Braaten (eds.), *The Nexus between Nursing and Patient Safety*,
https://doi.org/10.1007/978-3-031-53158-3_7

Nursing leaders participate and lead through various processes and activities to achieve the highest levels of patient safety. This chapter highlights several processes that nurse leaders use to create and maintain high-quality and safe care. These processes and activities include:

- Tracking and utilizing data to impact nursing quality indicators
- Maintaining visibility at the front line: suits to scrubs
- Standardized nurse leader rounding (NLR)
- Code Lavender to support staff after stressful events

In addition to these processes, the nurse leader must integrate mentoring, coaching, and succession planning throughout the daily interactions and activities. Finally, caregiver well-being should be considered across the continuum of care to maintain the highest levels of patient safety.

2 Nursing Quality Initiatives, Impact, and Importance: Nursing Sensitive Quality Indicators

Nursing quality indicators, also known as nursing sensitive indicators, include any activity in which nursing can directly positively or negatively impact quality patient outcomes. This directly influences patient safety and overall quality outcomes. Many facilities, especially Magnet facilities, report and obtain nursing quality data through the National Database of Nursing Quality Indicators (NDNQI). This database was originally founded by the American Nurses Association in 1998. "Nursing-sensitive indicators identify structures of care and care processes, both of which in turn influence care outcomes. Nursing-sensitive indicators are distinct and specific to nursing, and differ from medical indicators of care quality. Nursing outcome indicators are those outcomes most influenced by nursing care" [3]. NDNQI collects structure, process, and outcome measures. Nursing facilities may or may not utilize the NDNQI database for collection and trending of data; however, nursing leaders must have a means to collect and trend data impacting patient quality and outcomes.

Some examples of nursing quality indicators include patient falls, patient falls with injury, hospital-acquired pressure injuries (HAPIs), central line-associated bloodstream infections (CLABSIs), and catheter-associated urinary tract infections (CAUTIs). The first step includes collecting and tracking accurate and meaningful data. The data have the greatest impact when collected and followed up on in a timely fashion. For example, discussion of a patient's fall a month after it occurs may not result in the most meaningful conversation with frontline caregivers. These discussions require quick completion to gain the greatest learnings and opportunities for improvement. These learnings then must be shared across shifts, departments, facility, and finally across the system or organization when a greater learning benefit exists. Another example of nursing leaders supporting frontline staff to improve nursing quality indicators includes daily unit-based huddles that discuss any nursing quality event from the previous 24 hours. This quick and effective discussion includes event description, actions taken, and improvement opportunities to prevent the event from occurring again. Nursing leaders may also complete deeper dives on safety events that take more time than a daily unit-based huddle allows. These more in-depth discussions allow for greater learnings at both the frontline and leadership level to provide support for safety improvements.

A nursing leader's role is to observe and identify trends in nursing quality initiatives. Examples of trends to watch include nursing unit, scheduled shift times, or specific caregivers involved in the initiatives. However, the possible trends are endless. The nursing leader is challenged to tease this out with thoughtful process to uncover the actionable trends. Only then can the nursing leader truly influence how a particular nursing quality initiative is impacted and improved. The nursing leader includes discussion with frontline caregivers to determine barriers to successful nursing quality metrics. The answer lies with the front line. The nursing leader then removes or adjusts barriers to create the greatest improvement impact to patient safety. An example of this collaboration of front line and leadership includes the daily safety huddle, which addresses all central lines and catheters on each nursing unit, with an indicator for continued use of the line. This allows for efficient and open discussion to remove these lines timely, to obtain the best patient quality outcomes.

3   Increasing Visibility at the Front Line: Practice of Suits to Scrubs

Nursing leaders frequently hear feedback by frontline nurses about the lack of visibility. With calendars overflowing with meetings and expectations to meet job responsibilities and leading projects, finding time for rounding to focus on quality and patient safety can be complex. The COVID-19 global pandemic resulted in nurses feeling tired, burned out, and experiencing low morale. These conditions can directly impact patient safety. "Nurses struggle with risk exposure to the virus, worries about infecting their families, shortages or personal protective equipment (PPE), longer work hours, and moral distress related to resource allocation" ([4], p. 555). These additional struggles add to anxiety and stress that goes along with working in today's busy and high-paced healthcare environment. Nursing leaders must focus on creating positive connections with frontline nurses to impact staff engagement, patient experience, and patient safety while promoting nurse leader visibility.

Suits to scrubs is an intentional practice for nursing leaders to immerse themselves in the shoes of a frontline nurse. The practice offers an incredible opportunity to see the work that goes on within the facility, understand at a deeper level what nurses and the healthcare team experience, and interact with patients receiving care. By direct interaction and observation, nursing leaders help to identify patient safety issues that might otherwise go unmentioned. "No one knows better than a frontline team member the real-world challenges of patient care in today's tumultuous healthcare environment" ([5], p. 76).

So, what does suits to scrubs look like? Dressed in scrubs, nursing leaders change out of their suits and leave their offices to follow nurses at the bedside. On a monthly basis, rotating through clinical units, this is dedicated time for nursing leaders and the nurses to interact, as well as nursing leaders to interact directly with patients. Nurses are invited to share feedback on what is going well and what are the barriers they are facing to providing excellent patient care. Once barriers and/or opportunities are identified, they can be worked on. "Frontline team members know what's going on" ([5], p. 76). As nursing leaders, it is both a duty and responsibility to listen to what is going on in order to help drive nursing practice and to improve patient care. Suits to scrubs is also an invitation for patients to share feedback. It is a valuable opportunity to connect with patients and to hear firsthand experiences, both good and bad, and patients tend to be more candid and appreciate the time of the nursing leader. Understanding improvement opportunities in real time can lead to increased quality, patient safety, and outcomes.

The practice of suits to scrubs should be considered blocked time on the nursing leaders' calendar and just as important as a finance meeting. By blocking time that is sacred, nursing leaders can both remove barriers to patient care and partner with nurses to improve patient care. It is a time to meet nursing at their level. Dressed in scrubs rather than a business suit, nurses feel more comfortable sharing their feedback, appreciate being involved in decision-making, and develop a deeper level of trust and confidence in their nursing leaders. One experienced ICU nurse stated after experiencing suits to scrubs that she appreciated the chance to show the "real-world challenges of patient care on the front lines."

Nursing leaders have important jobs with many responsibilities. Suits to scrubs should be one of those responsibilities where nursing leaders prioritize and spend their time. The investment to practice suits to scrubs shows that not only you care about nursing but also you care and prioritize patient safety. The practice of suits to scrubs is a unique opportunity to see the work that goes on in the healthcare environment, really listen to understand what nurses experience, and further interact with the patients to help keep them safe.

4 Standardized Nurse Leader Rounding: Improving Patient Safety and Patient Satisfaction

Patients need a nurse leader rounding on them daily to obtain the best quality and safety outcomes. Nurse leader rounding (NLR) is an expectation and basic job function for nursing leaders. However, hard wiring NLR presents challenges. A standardized process is necessary to support this lofty expectation. The standardization includes the time of the day rounding occurs, frequency of NLR, leader completing NLR, and specific discussion points addressed with the patient and family during NLR.

An NLR standardized time of day for all nursing leaders is crucial. The time requires blocking and protecting on all calendars. Nurse managers are often overwhelmed by the prospect of rounding on their entire unit every day. For instance, one nurse manager rounding on their 24-bed nursing unit daily is not reasonable. However, when all nursing leaders within the facility participate in this process, NLR on those 24 patients becomes feasible. All nurse leaders, including the chief nursing officer, directors, managers, and assistant nurse managers, should round at the same time for the greatest efficiency. Some creative ways to add nursing rounders includes adding surgical service leaders. This provides a great opportunity to round on patients postoperatively when they are awake and can provide feedback on their experience. Other creative positions to utilize in rounding include quality directors; regulatory, inpatient therapy leaders; and nursing education and case management leaders. Any clinical leader adds positive impact to standardized daily patient rounding. When coordinating in this manner, NLR on 24 patients utilizing four nursing leaders can be accomplished in 30 min. Blocking just 30 min/day as prioritized time for nursing leaders creates a great impact on patient experience and patient safety.

In addition to the standardized time of day for patient rounding, frequency is key. NLR needs completion daily. On weekdays, when all nursing leaders are present, NLR is essential and therefore treated as the highest priority. On weekends, trained charge nurses can round on all new admissions to the nursing units. This creates daily, standardized NLR. Although less patient rounding is accomplished on the weekends due to decreased leaders on-site, the standardized process is still occurring.

All nursing leaders that conduct NLR need to complete training around the specific discussion points and standardized process for NLR. Nursing leaders are then competency validated to ensure that the standardization is evident across patient areas. This training includes the assessment of the environment for safety, reinforcement of fall risk and precautions, validation of care provided, and recognition opportunities. An experienced nursing leader observes areas of opportunity in the care environment and then follows up with feedback for the frontline caregivers at the bedside. Many of these caregivers are new graduate nurses that need this coaching and loop closure. In addition, nursing leaders can provide in the moment recognition and a job well done with positive reinforcement directly from the nursing leader.

NLR improves patient satisfaction as a main outcome. However, many leaders do not realize, in addition, that NLR also improves patient safety. This includes patient falls and patient falls with injury. Kovar [6] found post-standardized NLR training and implementation, a 48% decrease in patient falls, 100% decrease in patient falls with injury, and a 43% increase in overall patient satisfaction. An experienced nursing leader provides another set of eyes on the patient to ensure that fall precautions are in place, bed alarms are set properly, and patients and families understand fall precautions. Fall precautions include the bed in a low position, call light within reach, side rails in the correct position per facility protocol, and the patient understanding the level of assistance necessary for ambulation.

During the COVID-19 pandemic, NLR was crucial to the safety of patients. Sending an experienced nursing leader to round in the room of a COVID-19 patient allowed for that necessary experienced set of eyes on the patient to assist with identification of safety concerns and solve them while in the room. In addition to ensuring patient safety, the nursing leader was a crucial in-person contact welcomed by the patient and family. All personal protective recommendations were utilized by the nursing leader. This practice also allowed for time the nursing leader could oversee a live interactive call with the patient and family. This connection was crucial during a time when the in-person connection was not possible.

4.1 Use and Implementation of Code Lavender to Promote Nurse Well-Being and Further Patient Safety

Picture this, it has been a stressful day in the intensive care unit with multiple high-acuity patients, a patient that has to return to the operating room emergently, a family that has just received devasting news about their loved one, and the emergency room calling for another bed. This is a contemporary scenario in any hospital. The nurses have had no time for breaks or for lunch, in fact hardly time to even catch their breath, and yet are expected to continue and move on through their shift and perform at the highest level. Nurse leaders have an opportunity to support and invest in nurses in a way that helps support a culture of quality and safety at the same time. Code Lavender is an evidence-based tool that nursing leaders can help put into practice, by implementing and encouraging its use to help support nurse well-being and build positive culture [7]. In review of the literature, there is a theme that compassionate care is not just important for patients but is equally important for healthcare professionals. Emerging interest in nursing self-care and resiliency continues to appear in nursing research and literature. "Decades of research has shown that if a person does not 'refill his or her own cup' that person has little energy available to give to those in his or her care" ([8], p. 289).

Nursing leaders, executives, and educators must sit up and take note of how important this information is for sustainability of nurses working in critical areas. The evidence suggests that there is a need to fuel the spirit of the caregiver. There are major themes that were identified in review of the literature: stress that nurses experience, compassion for healthcare providers, nursing self-care and resiliency, and burnout. The stress that nurses experience can be broken down into themes, which include direct patient care, decisions that must be made, responsibility, and change [7]. Menzies who is credited for identifying the "work stress in nursing" further defined these themes into the personal toll that nurses experience from the work they do [9].

In review of compassionate care specific to healthcare providers, Code Lavender is increasingly evident as a potential tool or action to offer. In original research, a pilot project was completed "to shift the unit-based culture toward encouraging recognition of stressful workplace events and acknowledging colleagues through stressful events with intentional acts of kindness" ([10], p. 182). The pilot introduced and used Code Lavender as the intentional act of kindness, and the results were that 100% of the participants found it helpful and 84% of the participants would recommend the use of Code Lavender to a co-worker.

Code Lavender organizes resource support in real time to help nurses achieve emotional stability and feel supported, so they can provide the best possible clinical care and outcomes for patients. "Healthcare leaders who implement effective strategies to improve nurse retention and engagement can reduce the risk of adverse patient outcomes and retain a highly satisfied and engaged clinical staff" ([11], p. 103). Education needs to be the first step in order to implement the practice of Code Lavender. Education through unit staff meetings includes background on the use of evidence-based tool Code Lavender. Key points are covered on how to initiate a Code Lavender, when and how a Code Lavender can be used, and the introduction of the Code Lavender kit. By taking the time to ask nurses collectively in the staff meeting if they had ever experienced a difficult situation at work that elicited an emotional response but ignored their feelings and just kept pushing through their shift, the response was an overwhelming "yes." This immediately helped to get the nurses' attention and buy-in for explaining that Code Lavender is for these moments. When a Code Lavender is initiated, there is an intentional response that provides "purposeful presence; individual or team support; debriefing and follow-up; prayer and other affectively based interventions" ([12], p. 16).

Recognition of a nurse in need is the first step in a Code Lavender; think of it as a gift of compassion from one nurse to another. Presenting a Code Lavender kit to a nurse begins the Code Lavender. The following framework for implementation of Code Lavender is just one example used by this author, but it is important to note that implementation needs to meet the needs of the organization and/or setting where Code Lavender will be used. The nurse initiating the Code Lavender lets both the charge nurse of the shift and the unit clerk know that a Code Lavender was being initiated. This is a trigger for the unit clerk to send a text message to all of the nurses through Cisco phones. The message sent out to the nurse's phones states Code Lavender followed by a room number, by using a room number and not a name allowed for more privacy, which is preferred by nurses. This message is sent out to all of the nurses working that shift indicating that everyone needs to be alerted to watch the patient in or around this room. The charge nurse who was already made aware that a Code Lavender was being initiated has the Code Lavender toolkit and resource notebook available as a reference and is then able to watch the nurse's patient. The nurse offered the Code Lavender is then provided immediate support through a "menu" of real-time ideas: prayer; take a walk; go outside and get fresh air; have something warm to drink; sit in a calm place (chapel, break room, outside on a bench); listen to music or calming app on phone; talk to a friend or family member; talk with a chaplain; journal; meditate; color; breathe; get something to eat; chocolate or something sweet; or simply go to the bathroom [7].

Code Lavender is an intentional pause letting nurses know that it is okay to take a moment and feel what they are feeling and to further know that they are cared about. The message is that it is important for nurses to take a moment so they can come back and provide safe care to their patients. Unsolicited comments made by nurses who were a part of or experienced a Code Lavender include the following comments: one nurse stated that they "appreciate the permission to take time" and "I have never really had anyone notice me like this," and another nurse stated, "I would highly recommend the use of Code Lavender to a peer." Code Lavender offers intentional and personal care for nurses during a time of need.

5   Mentoring, Coaching, and Succession Planning

Mentoring and coaching are key components of the nursing leader's role. The nurse leader spends significant time in the day talking with the next level of caregivers to provide guidance. There are various levels of mentoring and coaching in every part of a healthcare organization. The most obvious level is nurse manager to frontline associates. This level of coaching keeps patients and associates safe at the front line of care. Nurse leaders listen and assess learning needs, barriers, and opportunities. Mentoring and coaching should occur at every level, including all the way to the top of a great organization. Every associate requires feedback for continuous growth and improvement.

Monthly meetings with direct reports are a critical component to the growth and success of caregivers. This may sound like a daunting task if one leader has many direct reports. However, the opportunity to gain knowledge through mentoring and coaching of associates can only truly be realized with dedicated, individual time directly with the nursing leader. This time allows for discussion of what is going well, possible opportunities, focus areas to work on until the next meeting, and assistance needed in achieving individual growth for the future. The nursing leader cannot possibly answer these questions without individualized time away from distractions. These discussions should not occur at the nurse's station or publicly where anyone else can overhear the conversation. This is an investment in the safety of patients and associates. Allowing a safe place for conversation regarding concerns and celebrating successes creates a safer environment to practice and receive care.

Nursing succession planning in healthcare organizations creates the future of growth and leadership within the nursing organizational structure. This involves the direct planning for mentoring, coaching, and preparing nurses for the next level of leadership. "Healthcare organizations must prioritize support in sustaining the nursing leadership workforce to drive patient-care outcomes, promote patient safety, and preserve a healthy work environment" ([13], p. 40).

Through mentoring and coaching conversations, succession planning naturally occurs. Preparing a nurse for their individual next step in the organization or in healthcare makes transitions smoother for everyone involved. Nursing leaders need to understand the goals and future plans of their associates to create the strategy and road map for the future. A great nursing leader effectively generates a succession plan that is well thought out and discussed regularly. The first level of discussion includes the individual leader to determine their individual plans and goals. The nursing leader then pieces this into the bigger picture of succession planning for the specific organization. Succession planning creates consistency in leaders, culture, and ultimately patient safety and outcomes.

6 Conclusion: Caregiver Well-Being Connected to Patient Safety

Nurse leaders are positioned within healthcare to support and invest in nurses in a way that helps foster and create a culture of quality and safety at the same time. The quality and safety are both for those that deliver care and for those that receive care, of which each are equally important. "Leadership is the cornerstone in the promotion of patient safety" [14]. Taking care and thinking about the well-being of nurses have become increasingly important through the COVID-19 pandemic to present. The global pandemic of COVID-19 and its aftermath have forced nurses to face unimagined stressors and placed them at higher risk for emotional and moral distress.

Through different practices, nurse leaders create visibility and support nurse well-being while actively addressing the importance of quality and patient safety. The pace of change in healthcare is not likely to slow down in the coming months and years, so the importance of nurse leaders' focus on nurse well-being is increasingly important. Providing support, encouraging self-care, and fostering a culture of caring underpin nurses' ability to provide safe patient care.

Key Points

- There is a very important connection between nursing leadership and patient safety.
- Nursing leader's influence is key in supporting nurses to keep patients safe.
- Nursing leaders must track, trend, and utilize data to impact nursing quality indicators.
- Maintaining visibility at the front line with tools and processes creates a great impact on patient safety. Some of these include suits to scrubs, standardized nurse leader rounding, and Code Lavender.
- Coaching, mentoring, and succession planning must be integrated into nursing leader's daily work.
- Caregiver well-being should be considered to maintain patient safety.

References

1. Murray M, Sundin D, Cope V. The nexus of nursing leadership and culture of safer patient care. J Clin Nurs. 2018;27:1287–93.
2. AONE. Role of the nurse executive in patient safety guiding principles toolkit. 2019. https://www.aonl.org/resourcelibrary/guiding-principles-role-nurse-executive-patient-safety.
3. Montalvo I. The national database of nursing quality indicators (NDNQI). Online J Issues Nursing. 2007;12(3)
4. Odom-Forren J. Nursing resilience in the world of COVID-19. J Perianesth Nurs. 2020;35(6):555–6. https://doi.org/10.1016/j.jopan.2020.10.005.

5. Hess V. Nursing leaders: 3 reasons to swap your suit for scrubs. Nurse Lead. 2015;13(1):75–7. https://doi.org/10.1016/j.mnl.2014.05.018.

6. Kovar K. Standardized nurse leader rounding. Doctoral thesis, Regis University; 2020. https://epublications.regis.edu/theses/984/.

7. Narvaez A. Education on the use of code lavender for ICU nurses to decrease turnover and increase engagement. Doctoral thesis, Regis University; 2021. https://epublications.regis.edu/theses/1002/.

8. Priddy M. Confrontation. Crit Care Nurs Q. 2019;42(3):285–91. https://doi.org/10.1097/cnq.0000000000000271.

9. Davey A, Bansal R, Sharma P, Davey S, Shukla A, Shrivastava K. Occupational stress among staff nurses: controlling the risk to health. Indian J Occup Environ Med. 2014;18(2):52. https://doi.org/10.4103/0019-5278.146890.

10. Davidson J, Graham P, Montross-Thomas L, Norcross W, Zerbi G. Code lavender: cultivating intentional acts of kindness in response to stressful work situations. EXPLORE. 2017;13(3):181–5. https://doi.org/10.1016/j.explore.2017.02.005.

11. Hinson T, Spatz D. Improving nurse retention in a large tertiary acute-care hospital. J Nurs Admin. 2011;41(3):103–8. https://doi.org/10.1097/nna.0b013e31820c7242.

12. Stone R. Code Lavender. Nursing. 2018;48(4):15–7. https://doi.org/10.1097/01.nurse.0000531022.93707.08.

13. Chan M. Nurse manager succession planning: an integrative review. Nurs Manag. 2022;53(10):35–51.

14. Charalambous A, Kelly D. Promoting a safety culture through effective nursing leadership in cancer care. Eur J Oncol Nurs. 2018;36:vi–vii. https://doi.org/10.1016/j.ejon.2018.10.002.

Using Implementation Science to Promote Patient Safety in Complex Care Environments

Sharon Tucker and Molly McNett

1   Introduction

Implementation of interventions, care strategies, and surveillance systems are key nursing actions that ensure safety for patients seeking health care. This occurs in all care settings but is particularly important for hospitalized patients who are most vulnerable and at risk for hospital acquired conditions. Nurses are also the only caregivers in hospitals that monitor patients around the clock and thus instrumental to protecting patient safety. The nursing process, fundamental to nursing care, is an important approach to patient safety. This process ensures continuous collection and interpretation of data, planning and implementing actions based on data, and evaluating the effects of the actions and deciding the next course of action. This process is iterative, dynamic, and ongoing and is essential to the mission of providing safe and high-quality nursing care to promote desired patient outcomes. The process also must integrate the best evidence for effective prevention and intervention strategies.

Evidence-based practice (EBP) is a cornerstone to high quality, safe nursing care that advances patient goals and protects them from harm [1]. Yet, implementation of EBP including safety assessments and interventions remains challenging for many reasons especially when new practices must be adopted and old traditional practices replaced. Adopting new practices includes understanding and using change models/ frameworks and processes. Moreover, adopting change in today's healthcare environments is particularly challenging and demanding given the complex workflows, patient multiple comorbidities, aging population, growing infectious disease outbreaks and natural disasters, staffing shortages, changing demographics, state and

S. Tucker (✉) · M. McNett
Helene Fuld Health Trust National Institute for Evidence-based Practice for Nursing and Healthcare, College of Nursing, The Ohio State University, Columbus, OH, USA
e-mail: tucker.701@osu.edu; mcnett.21@osu.edu

federal healthcare regulations, payor and reimbursement limits, and changing healthcare staff values [2, 3]. All these factors contribute to healthcare staff exhaustion, change fatigue, demoralization, burnout, and attrition, which in turn impacts patient and family satisfaction, patient care quality, and patient safety [3]. This chapter reviews the importance of EBP implementation for patient safety, acknowledges the challenges in implementing EBP, and presents change models, implementation models, and implementation strategies to help nurses and inter-professional teams to adopt and implement EBP in complex environments to promote safe patient care.

2 Background

EBP can be viewed as a three-legged stool, whereby the legs include (a) the best evidence identified through research, quality, and other sources; (b) the expertise and experiences of clinicians; and (c) patient preferences, values, and circumstances [1]. Most disciplines teach EBP in their educational programs, albeit the depth and breadth vary among programs [4]. Most clinical agencies today also recognize the value and importance of EBP; however, this does not always translate to dedication of resources to ensure the translation of evidence into practice [5–8]. Clinicians are likewise not often knowledgeable about the EBP process [8] or argue they do not have the time to engage in EBP [9, 10]. Such realities are reflected in many studies and reports that expose gaps with transferring new knowledge to practices. For example, data suggest that only 8% of Americans receive all high-priority, appropriate clinical preventive services [11]. Furthermore, data indicate that it still takes about 15 years to adopt evidence-based cancer clinical guidelines into routine practice by a majority of clinicians and a majority of time [12].

Multiple studies have examined barriers to EBP implementation across settings [13] with similar barrier themes of lack of leadership support, time, lack of agreement among colleagues, knowledge, beliefs/attitudes, administrative support, experts to do the work, information technology support, and financial commitments [14, 15]. Such challenges led to the field of implementation science, defined as the scientific study of methods and strategies that facilitate the uptake of evidence-based practice and research into regular use by practitioners and policymakers [16, 17]. Related terms include translation science and improvement science. A brief description of each term follows, with additional content specific to implementation science in the second half of this chapter.

2.1 Implementation Science vs. Translation Science, and Improvement Science

The field of implementation science emerged in the late twentieth century and grew substantially in the first two decades of the twenty-first century. This field aims to generate science that can help close the gap of "what-is-known" and "what-is-practiced" [16]. The ultimate goal is to develop a knowledge base to guide evidence-based interventions to become normalized within real-world practice settings and patient populations [18]. This field parallels yet differs from translation science, which aims to leverage facilitators and overcome barriers to turning observations from the laboratory, clinic, and community, into interventions that improve the health of individuals and the public [18]. In other words, translation science aims to get the research translated to real health improvements. Implementation science, on the other hand, focuses on how to truncate the gap in adopting evidence from research studies in real-world settings.

Implementation science also differs from quality improvement science, whose historic focus is on generating knowledge for local improvements, rather than producing generalizable scientific knowledge [19]. That said, both focus on bridging the gap between ideal and actual care to improve quality and safety. Tools used in each field also differ, with improvement science using more quality improvement tools, such as process mapping and systems thinking and use of measurement to use the PDSA cycles (plan, do, study, act). In contrast, more traditional experimental and other research methods have been the foundation for implementation science, with pragmatic and hybrid trials surfacing specific to this field.

Implementation science is highly relevant to clinicians given its alignment with the EBP movement. Through developments in information technology, electronic databases, and the internet, implementation science has begun to spread across healthcare settings with growing interest by clinical staff [18]. Like translation science, a first step in the implementation science field is to conduct organizational readiness assessments that assess and identify barriers and facilitators to accelerate the adoption of best practices. This step or a version of it is included in the many theories/models/frameworks (TMFs) that have emerged to guide implementation of EBPs and reduce the knowledge to practice gap [20]. A major underpinning of these TMFs (discussed in detail later) is change principles and processes, borrowed from other scientific fields to guide the mechanisms, processes, and facilitation of change and adoption (and sustainability) of new practices [20]. Indeed, organizational change and organizational culture are recognized as key drivers of implementation science [21]; these origins are discussed next.

2.2   Organizational Change

Organizational theories and models have been developed in several sectors, including business, academia, industry, and healthcare; all having overlapping processes and steps. Organizational change theories and models are essential to quality improvement and EBP, yet have limitations, given the complexity of humans and challenges in changing cultures. Stouten et al. [22] highlighted the long process for change and identified two major reasons that delay change: (1) the lack of scientific literature consensus on basic change processes, and (2) the difficulty in learning from experience. To this point, data suggest that approximately 50–70% of organizational change efforts fail [23], while efforts to change culture average success rates of 19% [24]. The use of TMFs can promote change through systematic processes that include appropriate facilitation and resources. A key principle of all organizational change models is that change will only occur if communicated and accepted by employees and/or project team members; and when support, knowledge, and resources are made available [25]. Three classic organizational change models are reviewed here as examples to guide nurses in understanding factors that can facilitate and inhibit change, as well as systematic steps, for health care organizations: Lewin's Three-Phase Change Management Model, Kotter's Eight-Step Change Management Theory, and Rogers Diffusion of Innovation Theory.

Lewin's Three-Phase Change Management Model. Kurt Lewin is widely recognized for his three-phase change model that grew out of field theory, group dynamics, and action research [26]. Developed in the 1940s as the first major change model, the three phases include unfreezing, changing, and refreezing (Fig. 1). The first phase sets the stage of unfreezing the current practice/way of operating by creating a vision for the needed change, engaging with senior leaders and senior management support, and identifying key concerns (barriers) that will likely emerge. There must be good communication that follows into phase two of the change, that explains the need for the change, addresses miscommunication and any wrong information, and empowers employees to initiate processes to the existing systems that will allow change to occur. The final phase of refreezing aims to align the change with the culture and infrastructure. Strategies are implemented that nurture and sustain the change, including support and training, and recognition of achievements.

Kotter's Eight-Step Change Management Theory. Building on Lewin's change model, Kotter, a Harvard Business School professor, developed an eight-step model (see Fig. 1) for change management that is easy to follow and primarily proposes accepting change and preparing for it ([25]). In the first step, leaders aim to create a sense of urgency, as part of the unfreezing process, among the people to

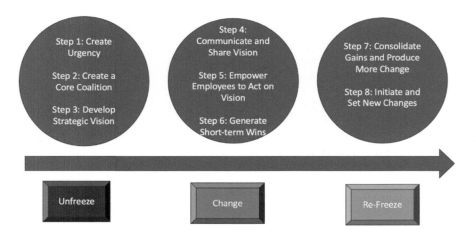

Fig. 1 Lewin change model and Kotter eight-step change model

be affected by the change. The goal is to motivate them to see there are always opportunities in sight and that organizations need to be able to make strategic adjustments in an iterative fashion. Included in the unfreezing is building a team or a coalition of leaders who are committed to the change. This includes ensuring the right people who have a mix of skills, knowledge, and commitment to create a transformative, strategic vision with emotional connection and objectives. The team moves this vision forward in the change phase by communicating accurate information, sharing the need for the change, obtaining support, addressing roadblocks, and seeking feedback. The team empowers employees to try new ideas and approaches, remains focused on short-term wins, and persists with integration into the organizational infrastructure as the refreezing takes place. In this final phase, gains are consolidated to produce more change and ultimately solidify the new change.

A meaningful recent example of application of the Kotter model to quality and safety involves a Canadian group who used the Kotter model during the COVID-19 pandemic to lead quality improvement (QI) in emergency rooms [27]. The well-known issues of insufficient space to meet increased volumes, changing and increased PPE, and lack of EBP knowledge of COVID called for urgent action. The first step of creating an urgency was inherent during the early stages of the pandemic leading to an openness for all front-line staff to get on board quickly. A coalition was created with politicians, administrators, and front-line providers who were able to mobilize change. They created a strategic vision and initiatives that would prioritize essential services without overwhelming the system. Through empowering courageous volunteers, they were able to design, trial, and support new efforts and policies. The empowering also allowed reflection on usual practices that may not work during the crisis as the shift to safety to mitigate against the high levels of morbidity and mortality called for different practices. Short-term wins were celebrated, and changes were consolidated through dynamic protocols and policies that aligned with the strategic vision. This commitment allowed for ongoing change with long-term effects uncertain. Three examples were presented and revolved around repurposing space to manage inequities for care, ensuring use of PPE for maintaining safety for staff, and improving advanced care planning and recommendations for evidence-based goals of care for patients.

Rogers Diffusion of Innovation Theory. The well-known and widely used Diffusion of Innovation Theory was developed by Everett Rogers in the 1960s. Aligned with Lewin's basic concepts, Rogers' theory grew out of his work at Iowa State University where he earned his BA, MS, and PhD degrees in agriculture and rural sociology [28]. While studying with his doctoral advisor, George Beal, Rogers focused on why some farmers adopted high-yielding seed corn and other products and others did not, as well as why adoption took so long to diffuse. These observations led to the theory about innovation diffusion and how innovations are communicated in a social system [29]. Rogers asserted that characteristics of individuals, the internal organizational structure, and the external environment were associated with an organization's level of innovation (Fig. 2). The diffusion of an innovation is considered to go through five main stages: knowledge, persuasion, decision, implementation, and confirmation. Additionally, the innovation itself is influenced by its

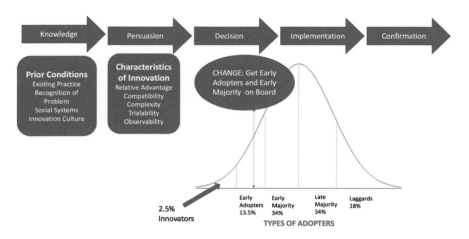

Fig. 2 Rogers' theory of diffusion of innovation

relative advantage, compatibility, complexity, ability to be tested, and observability. Innovations can be adopted and diffused more expeditiously when these characteristics are rated more positively.

Interestingly, Rogers also found that people adopt to change at different rates, which is important as change is rolled out and to its success. Adopters range from innovators, early adopters, early majority, late majority, and laggards. There appears a tipping point once about 35% of individuals are ready to adopt or have adopted the innovation, whereby the speed of adoption accelerates. Thus, leaders of innovations should focus on the first three groups of adopters to promote successful change.

2.3   Complex Adaptive Systems

Another relevant framework that has evolved in healthcare and is important to safety practices is complex adaptive systems (CAS), which emerge from complexity science. Complexity science is the study of complex systems, and complex adaptive systems are "a collection of individual *agents* with freedom to act in ways that are not always predictable, and whose actions are interconnected so that one agent's actions change the context for other agents" ([30], p. 625). Health care systems are not single units as in the past that had limited individuals with whom patients had to interact. They are now large interacting groups often with their unique rules that include instincts, constructs, and mental models [30]. This can create issues when trying to promote consistent and evidence-based standards of care within unique predicaments, context, priorities, and choices of the individual patient. The major features of CAS are nonlinear, emergence or patterns of connections, self-organizing, non-equilibrium (despite efforts to stabilize), co-evolving, and dependent on history [31].

The COVID-19 pandemic provides a clear illustration of how complex adaptive systems have to respond to unexpected change. COVID-19 illustrated a small, surprise event in one part of the world on the daily operations of hospitals and medical practices around the globe [32]. Multiple challenges among large systems emerged, such as lack of capacity to handle the surges of patient volumes, the need for redesign of patient care models, protecting the physical and mental health of front-line workers, and financial losses due to elective and non-urgent procedures and surgeries needing to be canceled. As demonstrated by health systems across the world, they responded and adapted to external environmental changes, largely based on their desire to survive [32]. Complex adaptive systems are adaptable, flexible, and learning systems. Practice changes of any sort will also demand viewing from the lens of complexity and adaptation.

2.4   Nursing Sensitive Indicators

Nurses implement multiple interventions to maintain patient safety. Such practices must evolve and adapt to new information and within complex systems. Although nurses work within teams, they also aim to achieve select outcomes that are uniquely sensitive to nursing interventions. These are often referred to as nursing sensitive indicators or nursing quality indicators [33]. A number of these indicators are related to safe quality care and examples include patient falls with and without injuries, pressure injuries, nosocomial infections, and nursing hours per patient days. While there are a host of other indicators not specifically named by the National Database of Nursing Quality Indicators, nurses should approach all care with the same lens of constantly changing and adapting, using structured approaches to bring about sustained evidence-based changes, and using implementation science to guide the successful uptake of an evidence-based safety practice change.

3   Implementation and Evaluation of Safety Initiatives

As discussed to this point, healthcare teams and researchers have identified the need to be proactive and delineate mechanisms to facilitate implementation of evidence-based safety practices into routine care practices using a science-informed approach. A foundational element of a science-informed approach to implementation is use of a theory, model, or framework (TMF) to guide implementation efforts [34]. As mentioned in the beginning of this chapter, use of a TMF provides a structured and systematic approach to evaluate and address factors that may influence the assessment, planning, implementation, and evaluation of safety initiatives.

Many quality and safety initiatives in healthcare settings have incorporated Donabedian's quality of care model [35]. This model includes three components: structure, process, and outcome. Structure refers to the environment in which implementation of the safety initiative will take place, process is how the practice is put into place, and outcome is a measurable result of the implementation effort. There

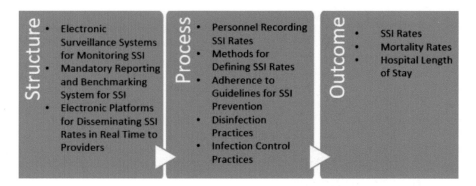

Fig. 3 Examples of structure, process, outcome measures for surgical site infections (SSI)

are many factors that encompass structure and process. Similarly, there are a number of outcomes that can be evaluated as part of any practice change. Figure 3 lists potential structure, process, and outcome measures that may be applicable for safety initiatives related to surgical site infections (SSIs), as one example. Ultimately, Donabedian's model asserts that both structure and process factors directly influence outcomes. As such, for any practice change, and especially when implementing safety initiatives, good structure and good processes are essential in order to achieve the desired outcomes. The change models discussed earlier use different terms, yet follow a structured approach to achieve desired outcomes including patient safety.

In addition to Donabedian's structure, process, and outcome model, a number of TMFs from the field of implementation science (IS) can also be used to plan, implement, and evaluate safety initiatives. An important contribution from the field of IS is development of over 40 theories, models, and frameworks (TMF) to provide structured guidance for implementation efforts [20, 36]. TMFs have been categorized as determinant frameworks, process models, evaluation frameworks, and classic behavior change theories [20].

- Determinant frameworks evaluate factors that can serve as facilitators or barriers (i.e., determinants) influencing the proposed practice change. These frameworks are often used prior to implementation to inform the implementation plan.
- Process models provide a step-by-step approach for implementing the practice change. These models often include phases for implementation, with specific implementation strategies recommended within each phase based on the identified facilitators and barriers to the practice change, as well as other organizational factors.
- Evaluation frameworks provide structure for measuring outcomes of implementation efforts.
- Classic theories include components of organizational and behavior change principles and can be used throughout the implementation process to inform how individuals perceive and respond to the proposed practice change.

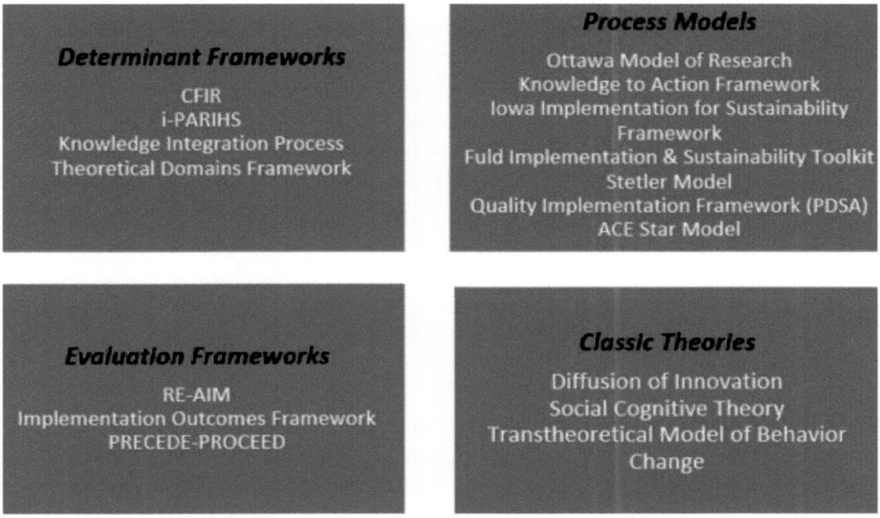

Determinant Frameworks

CFIR
i-PARIHS
Knowledge Integration Process
Theoretical Domains Framework

Process Models

Ottawa Model of Research
Knowledge to Action Framework
Iowa Implementation for Sustainability
Framework
Fuld Implementation & Sustainability Toolkit
Stetler Model
Quality Implementation Framework (PDSA)
ACE Star Model

Evaluation Frameworks

RE-AIM
Implementation Outcomes Framework
PRECEDE-PROCEED

Classic Theories

Diffusion of Innovation
Social Cognitive Theory
Transtheoretical Model of Behavior
Change

Fig. 4 Examples of theories, models, frameworks to guide implementation. Legend: *CFIR* Consolidated Framework for Implementation Research; *i-PARIHS* Integrated-Promoting Action on Research Implementation in Health Services; *PDSA* Plan, Do, Study, Act; *RE-AIM* Reach, Effectiveness, Adoption, Implementation, Maintenance; *PRECEDE-PROCEED* Predisposing, Reinforcing, Enabling Constructs in Educational Diagnosis and Evaluation-Policy, Regulatory, Organizational Constructs in Educational and Environmental Development

When a TMF is used to guide implementation of a practice change, many report greater degree of uptake of the practice change and higher sustainability of the change over time [37]. Examples of the different types of TMFs are displayed in Fig. 4. With any practice change, it is recommended that healthcare teams: (1) perform an assessment of the setting where the practice change will occur, which can often be done with a determinant framework or other organizational assessment tool; (2) use a process model to develop the plan for implementation; (3) consider an evaluation framework to measure outcomes of the practice change, and (4) consider classic behavior theories and change models such as discussed earlier that may inform individual and group behavior in response to the practice change.

3.1   Assessment of the Setting for Implementation

Prior to implementation of a safety initiative, it is important to do an organizational assessment to identify potential facilitators and barriers that may influence implementation and the intended outcomes of the practice change. An organizational assessment can be guided by one of the determinant frameworks identified in Fig. 4, as many of these frameworks have quantitative and qualitative tools to evaluate the presence of facilitators and barriers to implementation. Other tools that can be used to perform organizational assessments include the Implementation Climate Scale

(ICS) (Weiner), the Organizational Readiness to Change Assessment (ORCA) [38], and the Organizational Readiness for Implementing Change (ORIC) [39]. Regardless of the framework or tool used, the assessment must be done prior to implementation of the practice change. Findings should then be reviewed by the team leading the practice change and used to inform the plan for implementation. This information will allow teams to identify factors that will support implementation efforts, and also identify potential barriers prior to implementation that may be mitigated to increase likelihood of implementation success.

3.2 Development of a Plan for Implementation Using a Process Model

Once the initial assessment of the setting for implementation is complete, a process model can then be used to develop an implementation plan. Process models provide a structured and systematic approach to implementation, which often occurs in phases or stages, ranging from pre-implementation and planning to the actual process of implementation, evaluation, and sustainability of a practice change [34]. Within each phase or stage of an implementation process model, there are specific implementation strategies that are performed by the team to promote integration of the practice change among clinicians and leaders.

Implementation strategies are methods and activities to increase the use or "uptake" of a proposed practice change [40]. Implementation strategies can be simple or complex and are often used in combination throughout the phases of implementation to enhance initial and continued use of the practice change among clinicians. Implementation strategies have been labeled and defined to promote a

Implementation Strategies

Assess for Readiness, Access New Funding, Alter Incentive Structures, Assess Workflow, Advisory Board/Workgroups, Auditing & Feedback, Build a Coalition, Capture/Share Local Knowledge, Change Physical Structures/Equipment, Change Record Systems, Change Service Sites, Clear & Consistent Communication, Computerized Reminders, Conduct Ongoing Training, Create Learning Collaborative, Create New Teams, Create Online Learning, Create/Change Credentialing, Cyclical Small Tests of Change, Data Experts, Data Warehouses, Develop Implementation Blueprint, Develop Academic Partnerships, Develop Implementation Glossary, Develop/Implement Quality Monitoring Tools, Develop/Organize Quality Monitoring System, Develop Disincentives, Develop Resource Sharing Agreements, Educational Materials, Educational Meetings, Educational Outreach, Engage Community Resources, Engage Data Experts, Facilitate Relay of Data to Providers, Facilitation of Implementation, Fund the Innovation, Identify Facilitators & Barriers, Identify/Prepare Champions, Identify Early Adopters, Implementation Advisors, Implementation Teams, Increase Demand, Inform Local Opinion Leaders, Intervene with Patients, Involve Executive Board, Involve Patients/Consumers, Local Consensus Discussions, Local Needs Assessment, Make Billing Easier, Make Training Dynamic, Mandate Change, Model/Simulate Change, Obtain Feedback, Obtain Formal Commitment, Ongoing Consultation, Organize Clinical Meetings, Organize Implementation Meeting, Place on Services/Formulary Lists, Prepare Active Participants, Promote Adaptability, Provide Supervision, Provide Technical Assistance, Recruit/Train/Designate Leader, Re-examine Implementation, Remind Clinicians, Revise Professional Roles, Risk Communication, Shadow Experts, Stage Scale Up, Start Dissemination, Tailor Strategies, Use Mass Media, Use Other Payment Schemes, Use Train-the-Trainer, Visit Other Sites, Work With Educational Partners

Fig. 5 ERIC implementation strategies

consistent approach to implementation efforts across teams and settings. Fig. 5 displays the Expert Recommendations for Implementation Change (ERIC) strategies that are used in a number of process models to support the phases or stages of implementation [40]. Strategies can be further categorized as those that address planning, educating, financing, restructuring, managing quality, and policy [40]. When planning for implementation, teams should review findings from the implementation assessment and select strategies aimed at mitigating potential barriers. For example, if the initial assessment indicated the need for education to support the practice change, implementation strategies should include development of educational materials, distribution of educational materials, and conducting educational meetings. Implementation strategies can be a formal part of an implementation plan, as strategies can be assigned to specific team members to oversee that aspect of implementation.

It is important to note that more than one implementation strategy is often used, which is referred to as "bundled" strategies. In addition, selection of strategies should be "tailored" to the site and setting for implementation. For example, the same safety initiative may be implemented in two different settings, but the initial assessment may have indicated different facilitators and barriers at each site. Therefore, the implementation strategies selected for each site may be different, even though the proposed practice change is the same. This "bundled" and "tailored" approach for selection of implementation strategies is commonly used when implementing practice changes in healthcare settings.

Implementation strategies are often embedded within implementation process models and packaged as "toolkits." A toolkit is a compilation of information and resources to guide teams through actionable steps throughout the implementation process [41]. Fig. 6 displays an excerpt from the Fuld Institute Implementation for Sustainability Toolkit [42, 43]. This toolkit includes a process model that has four phases for implementation that align with the Diffusion of Innovation theory: Pre-Initiative, Building Knowledge & Persuasion, Decisions, Implementation & Evaluation, and Confirmability, Sustainment, and Intentional Re-Assessment. Within each phase, there is a listing of implementation strategies that teams can select to develop a customized implementation plan. The toolkit also includes additional resources to provide direction for the implementation team, including a team charter, timeline, and reporting templates. Teams implementing a safety initiative can use a process model to select strategies relevant to their practice change, setting, and resources. The model provides a structure to guide the team through the various phases of implementation. An evaluation model can then be used to select and monitor outcomes during and after implementation.

THE OHIO STATE UNIVERSITY
COLLEGE OF NURSING

Helene Fuld Health Trust National Institute for
Evidence-based Practice in Nursing and Healthcare

FULD ARCC EBP INITIATIVE IMPLEMENTATION AND SUSTAINABILITY GUIDE	
Pre-initiative: Initiative Leader (ARCC Mentor)	
☐ Send summary report for senior leaders - introduction of the initiative° (involve executives)	
☐ Assure EBDM/P Charter° is complete (develop formal implementation plan)	
☐ Link to organizational priorities	
☐ Enlist leadership support (i.e., inform/discuss EBP initiative), educate and obtain formal commitment	
☐ Assemble diverse teams and identify interprofessional collaborators	
☐ Collaborate with Quality (QI/PI) department (quality monitoring tools and monitoring systems)	
☐ Develop implementation plan that includes incremental roll out and subsequent diffusion to other areas as applicable	
☐ Utilize EB Initiative Planner and Timeline*	
☐ Provide introductory information to those who will be impacted by the initiative (staff, stakeholders, opinion leaders)	
☐ Assess and advocate for required resources (funding for the initiative, access new funding if needed)	
Pre-initiative: Organizational Leader	
☐ Assess organizational readiness for EBDM/P initiative (utilize a valid and reliable assessment tool) *	
☐ Ensure leadership engagement (facilitate formal commitments, involve and align executives, advisory boards and workgroups)	
☐ Collaborate on initiative strategy (provide information and obtain local consensus)	
☐ Address and secure resources (budget, protected time, incentives etc.)	
☐ Align EBDM/P work with organizational goals/priorities/data	

* *Organizational Culture & Readiness for System-wide Integration of Evidence-based Practice Survey (OCRSIEP) is an instrument that helps assess the extent to which cultural factors influence the system-wide implementation of EBP in the organization and overall perceived readiness for the integration of EBP. The scale has established face and content validity, with internal consistency reliabilities above 0.85 (Melnyk, Fineout-Overholt, Giggleman, & Cruz, 2010).*

° Use the **Summary report for senior leaders - introduction of the initiative** template

° Use the **Evidence-based Decision Making/Practice (EBDM/P) Charter** template

* Use the **EB Initiative Planner and Timeline** template

Fig. 6 Example of process model with implementation strategies

THE OHIO STATE UNIVERSITY
COLLEGE OF NURSING

Helene Fuld Health Trust National Institute for
Evidence-based Practice in Nursing and Healthcare

FULD ARCC EBP INITIATIVE IMPLEMENTATION AND SUSTAINABILITY GUIDE

Building Knowledge | Persuasion - Initiative Leader (ARCC Mentor) *Raising Awareness, Building Knowledge, and Influencing Beliefs, Persuasion (support engagement/interest)*	
☐Reassess team membership to assure successful implementation	
☐Engage staff, stakeholders, opinion leaders (inter-professional and hierarchy)	
☐Identify and prepare champions (include frontline, inter-professional clinicians and leaders)	
☐Identify potential barriers and plan for them	
☐Organize initiative implementation team meetings	
☐Influence development of favorable attitudes toward the imitative	
☐Identify potential resistance	
☐Highlight advantages and share evidence syntheses	
☐Leverage aspects of the initiative that can promote adoption (compatibility, trial-ability, simplicity/complexity, observability)	
☐Define internal data/outcomes and sources (local needs assessment, baseline data)	
☐Prepare elevator speech	
☐Educate staff on EB initiative (include frontline staff)	
☐Develop informational and educational materials (share evidence syntheses)	
☐Conduct informational and educational sessions and outreach	
☐Distribute initiative information (i.e., unit newsletters/huddles/meetings, visual triggers such as posters/fliers)	
☐Share draft documents for input/review (staff, stakeholders and team) and obtain local feedback/consensus.	
☐Make local adaptations if necessary (promote adaptability)	
☐Activate leadership commitments (executive, senior and mid-level)	
☐Discuss how to make impact observable (Examples: Focus groups, Resource manual, Case studies)	

Fig. 6 (continued)

4 Evaluation of Outcomes of the Practice Change

A critical piece when implementing any safety initiative is ongoing surveillance and evaluation of measures to gauge initial, incremental, and ongoing success. Similar to the assessment and process phases of implementation, the evaluation phase can be guided by an evaluation TMF. Evaluation TMFs include a wide range of outcomes that can be considered beyond solely clinical or patient centric outcomes. Evaluating different types of measures will provide important information throughout early and later stages of implementation and ongoing sustainability of safety initiatives. Measures can be categorized at the process or outcome level, and also as patient, system, provider, and implementation metrics.

4.1   Process Measures

Process measures evaluate the degree to which the practice change is being implemented as intended to achieve target outcomes [44]. These measures are typically evaluated in frequent intervals, as often as daily, weekly, and/or monthly to evaluate implementation progress in real time. By evaluating these measures at frequent intervals throughout the implementation process, teams can make modifications to the implementation plan to promote ongoing engagement in the practice change or safety initiative.

Evaluation of balancing measures is often included with ongoing surveillance of process measures. Balancing measures monitor if implementation of the practice change is causing unintended negative consequences in another part of healthcare system delivery [44]. For example, if a safety initiative focused on reducing restraints for patients on mechanical ventilation, a balancing measure to monitor would be an unanticipated increase in unplanned extubation rates. As teams work to implement any safety initiative, it is important to not only monitor if the safety initiative is achieving the desired outcome, but also to ensure it is not causing other adverse events. Thus, safety initiatives should include both process and balancing measures as incremental evaluations throughout initial and ongoing implementation phases.

4.2   Outcome Measures

Outcome measures are evaluated to determine the impact of the practice change [44]. They are different than process measures in that they are not recorded as frequently, and often align with reportable benchmarks, department or health system goals, and can be linked to return on investment or reimbursement calculations. Outcome measures can occur at the patient, healthcare system, or provider level. Selection of outcomes can be guided by the evaluation framework that is selected and may be dependent on the resources available to evaluate the measure, alignment of the measure with the safety initiative being implemented, and priority areas of the organization or department.

There are a number of outcome measures that are linked to reportable benchmarks for safety initiatives. Measures may be categorized at the patient level, healthcare system level, and/or provider level. Some examples of safety reportable benchmarks at the patient level include [41]:

- Pressure ulcer rate per 1000 admissions
- Death rate among surgical inpatients with serious treatable complications (DVT, pneumonia, sepsis, cardiac arrest) per 1000 admissions
- Retained surgical items
- Central venous catheter related blood stream infection rate, per 1000 admissions
- In hospital fall rate per 1000 admissions
- Perioperative hemorrhage or hematoma rate, per 1000 admissions
- Postoperative sepsis rate, per 1000 admissions

Outcomes at the system level may be specific to safety initiatives but may also encompass more broad measures of overall system performance. Examples of some health system level outcomes include:

- Average hospital length of stay
- Bed occupancy rate
- Treatment costs
- Hospital readmission rates
- Patient satisfaction rates
- Treatment error rates

Lastly, outcome measures at the provider level may be included, depending on the nature of the safety initiative being implemented. Some examples of provider level outcomes include [45]:

- Workplace injury and/or illness rates
- Employee absenteeism
- Employee engagement
- Employee satisfaction
- Employee turnover

These lists of outcome measures are not all inclusive, as there are hundreds of different types of outcomes that may be relevant to safety initiatives at each level. Identification and selection of outcomes relevant to a specific safety initiative can be informed by an evaluation TMF, regulatory and reporting requirements, accreditation standards, and local priorities and resources within the setting for implementation.

4.3   Implementation Outcomes

Outcome measures can also include evaluation of implementation outcomes. Implementation outcomes are the evaluation of the effect of the deliberate actions to implement a new practice [46]. Implementation outcomes ultimately serve as indicators of implementation success, but can also be used as proximal indicators during the implementation process [46]. Implementation outcomes include:

- Acceptability: Perception that the practice change is agreeable among stakeholders.
- Adoption: The initial intention or decision to try the new practice change.
- Appropriateness: The perceived fit or relevance of the practice change for that specific setting or among stakeholders.
- Feasibility: The extent the practice change can be successfully performed within a specific setting.
- Fidelity: The degree to which a practice change was implemented as intended.
- Cost: The financial impact of the practice change.
- Penetration: The integration or spread of a practice change across a setting or group of stakeholders.
- Sustainability: The extent to which a practice change is maintained over time within a specific setting.

Incorporating implementation outcomes into the evaluation plan for a safety initiative can provide valuable information on how well and how often stakeholders (i.e., clinicians) utilize the proposed practice change. Ultimately, if clinicians are not engaging in implementation of the safety initiative (i.e., the implementation outcomes are poor), downstream effects will be poor process metrics and subsequently, poor overall project outcomes.

5 Summary/Case Study: "How to" Application

Lisa (uses she/her pronouns) is a BSN-prepared registered nurse on a 44-bed medical surgical unit in an 800-bed tertiary care center. Staffing shortages have been a major issue for over 12 months. Lisa is frequently the charge nurse and chair of the unit practice committee. She has been assigned to examine and ensure the latest Joint Commission Hospital National Patient Safety Goals. Among the goals is "always use at least two patient identifiers," such as patient's name and date of birth. Data collected on Lisa's unit indicate nurses ask for two separate identifiers inconsistently. This was noted as an issue 1 year ago. At that time, evidence in the literature for best practice was assessed/appraised by one of the evidence-based nurse fellows. An initiative was implemented to ensure the implementation of always using at least two identifiers. Despite this project initiation 1 year ago, random audits with patients and observations indicate that this practice occurs only about 75% of the time; which was a 10% improvement from the year before, but the goal was set at 90% adherence or better as the benchmark. Lisa has 1-h weekly meetings to put forward a plan for addressing this ongoing practice goal. In the beginning, to explore what will sustain the practice, Lisa was encouraged by her manager to learn about implementation science literature and its application and relevance to this project. She attended a conference and read a host of articles to better understand how to sustain this safety practice. Lisa decides to use Rogers' Theory of Diffusion of Innovation along with the i-PARIHS Implementation framework, and Powell's ERIC strategies to work with her practice committee to make this practice stick.

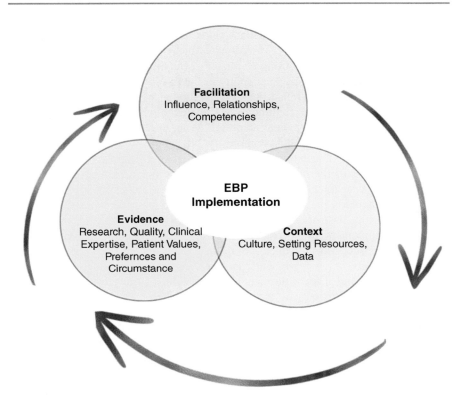

Fig. 7 i-PARIHS model for implementation

The i-PARIHS is considered a broad multidimensional framework that can guide successful EBP implementation [34, 47]. Three main concepts are included in the framework for success: the nature and type of evidence (research as well as clinical experience, patient experience, and local information), the context of the EBP implementation (encompasses culture, leadership, and evaluation), and the way the implementation process is facilitated (using internal facilitator or external person hired) (see Fig. 7). This framework was informed by Roger's diffusion of innovation theory as well as other organizational theories. For Lisa and her team, they will consider the evidence first and re-review the project initially completed by the EBP fellow. They will search the literature for new research findings, consider their clinical experiences and its influences, and the local unit and what might be influencing the implementation. They will then rate the strength of this evidence.

Assuming the strength of the evidence is moderate or greater, they will consider the best practice juxtaposed to their specific practice and workload, patient populations, staffing, leadership, the culture about EBP, and attitudes to the 2-system patient identifier process as a safety practice. This is all about the context that will help identify where there is misinformation, if there are practical issues to discuss, and any concerns with leadership support (also part of the knowledge phase of Rogers' theory—see Fig. 2). They will also look for facilitators they can leverage in the project implementation. This overall assessment will then be used for implementation—which requires a strong facilitator—who they decided will be the assistant nurse manager (with manager support).

Their implementation detailed plan will be guided by Rogers' theory, starting with a plan for building or rebuilding the knowledge regarding the evidence and advantages to the 2-system patient identifier. As an implementation strategy, they will present the practice's limited complexity, how compatible it is with their current practice, and how it can be trialed and observed as beneficial compared to attitudes and barriers to the consistent use. This is the persuasion phase, which is followed by the decision phase. Lisa and her team will strategically engage types of adopters—particularly the innovators, early adopters, and early majority nurses to elevate the practice. Use of technology will be highlighted to make the process easy to recall and implement. In this phase, many implementation strategies will be used including mini education modules, group discussion, incentives, audit and feedback, celebrations for improvements, and announcing and sharing the improvements with staff and leaders throughout organization. During the final phase of confirmation, re-evaluation will occur along with ongoing audit and feedback and opportunities to continuously identify and mitigate barriers. An initial report, interim report, and final report will be generated into an executive summary by Lisa and her committee and shared up the leadership hierarchy. The project and its processes and outcomes will be presented across the health system, along with submission for external conferences and publications.

Key Points

- Nursing practice includes delivering high-quality evidence-based interventions that promote patient safety and optimal outcomes, yet changing practice is not easy, often quite delayed if it occurs at all, and hard to sustain.
- Using systematic approaches and models to change can promote effective adoption, update and sustainment of a new practice in nursing care settings.
- Implementation science is a field that has emerged to help reduce the knowledge to practice gap and accelerate the uptake of research findings and other practice evidence.
- Applying TMF and implementation strategies can help nurses adopt evidence-based practices that can promote patient safety and optimal patient outcomes.

References

1. Melnyk BM, Fineout-Overholt E, Stillwell SB, Williamson KM. Evidence-based practice: step by step: the seven steps of evidence-based practice. Am J Nurs. 2010;110(1):51–3. https://doi.org/10.1097/01.NAJ.0000366056.06605.d2.

2. Ghahramani S, Lankarani KB, Yousefi M, Heydari K, Shahabi S, Azmand S. A systematic review and meta-analysis of burnout among healthcare workers during COVID-19. Front Psych. 2021;12:758849. https://doi.org/10.3389/fpsyt.2021.758849.

3. National Academies of Sciences, Engineering, and Medicine. Taking action against clinician burnout: a systems approach to professional well-being. Washington, DC: The National Academies Press; 2019. https://doi.org/10.17226/25521.

4. Lehane E, Leahy-Warren P, O'Riordan C, Savage E, Drennan J, O'Tuathaigh C, O'Connor M, Corrigan M, Burke F, Hayes M, Lynch H, Sahm L, Heffernan E, O'Keeffe E, Blake C, Horgan F, Hegarty J. Evidence-based practice education for healthcare professions: an expert view. BMJ Evid Based Med. 2019;24(3):103–8. https://doi.org/10.1136/bmjebm-2018-111019.

5. Bianchi M, Bagnasco A, Bressan V, Barisone M, Timmins F, Rossi S, Pellegrini R, Aleo G, Sasso L. A review of the role of nurse leadership in promoting and sustaining evidence-based practice. J Nurs Manag. 2018;26(8):918–32. https://doi.org/10.1111/jonm.12638.

6. Harding KE, Porter J, Horne-Thompson A, Donley E, Taylor NF. Not enough time or a low priority? Barriers to evidence-based practice for allied health clinicians. J Contin Educ Heal Prof. 2014;34(4):224–31. https://doi.org/10.1002/chp.21255.

7. Jiang V, Brooks EM, Tong ST, Heintzman J, Krist AH. Factors influencing uptake of changes to clinical preventive guidelines. J Am Board Fam Med. 2020;33(2):271–8. https://doi.org/10.3122/jabfm.2020.02.190146.

8. Melnyk BM, Gallagher-Ford L, Zellefrow C, Tucker S, Thomas B, Sinnott LT, Tan A. The first U.S. study on nurses' evidence-based practice competencies indicates major deficits that threaten healthcare quality, safety, and patient outcomes. Worldviews Evid-Based Nurs. 2018;15(1):16–25. https://doi.org/10.1111/wvn.12269.

9. Li S, Cao M, Zhu X. Evidence-based practice: knowledge, attitudes, implementation, facilitators, and barriers among community nurses-systematic review. Medicine. 2019;98(39):e17209. https://doi.org/10.1097/MD.0000000000017209.

10. Sadeghi-Bazargani H, Tabrizi JS, Azami-Aghdash S. Barriers to evidence-based medicine: a systematic review. J Eval Clin Pract. 2014;20(6):793–802. https://doi.org/10.1111/jep.12222.

11. Borsky A, Zhan C, Miller T, Ngo-Metzger Q, Bierman AS, Meyers D. Few Americans Receive All High-Priority, Appropriate Clinical Preventive Services. Health Aff (Millwood). 2018;37(6):925–8. https://doi.org/10.1377/hlthaff.2017.1248.

12. Khan S, Chambers D, Neta G. Revisiting time to translation: implementation of evidence-based practices (EBPs) in cancer control. Cancer Causes Control. 2021;32(3):221–30. https://doi.org/10.1007/s10552-020-01376-z.

13. Correa VC, Lugo-Agudelo LH, Aguirre-Acevedo DC et al. Individual, health system, and contextual barriers and facilitators for the implementation of clinical practice guidelines: a systematic metareview. Health Res Policy Sys. 2020;18:74. https://doi.org/10.1186/s12961-020-00588-8.

14. Baatiema L, Otim ME, Mnatzaganian G, de-Graft Aikins A, Coombes J, Somerset S. Health professionals' views on the barriers and enablers to evidence-based practice for acute stroke care: a systematic review. Implement Sci. 2017;12:74. https://doi.org/10.1186/s13012-017-0599-3.

15. Solomons NM, Spross JA. Evidence-based practice barriers and facilitators from a continuous quality improvement perspective: an integrative review. J Nurs Manag. 2011;19:109–20. https://doi.org/10.1111/j.1365-2834.2010.01144.x.

16. Bauer MS, Kirchner J. Implementation science: what is it and why should I care? Psychiatry Res. 2020;283:112376. https://doi.org/10.1016/j.psychres.2019.04.025.

17. Eccles MP, Mittman BS. Welcome to implementation science. Implement Sci. 2006;1:1. https://doi.org/10.1186/1748-5908-1-1.

18. Leppin AL, Mahoney JE, Stevens KR, Bartels SJ, Baldwin LM, Dolor RJ, Proctor EK, Scholl L, Moore JB, Baumann AA, Rohweder CL, Luby J, Meissner P. Situating dissemination and implementation sciences within and across the translational research spectrum. J Clin Transl Sci. 2020;4:152–8. https://doi.org/10.1017/cts.2019.392.

19. Nilsen P, Thor J, Bender M, Leeman J, Andersson-Gare B, Sevdalis N. Bridging the silos: a comparative analysis of implementation science and improvement science. Front Health Services. 2022;1:1–13. https://doi.org/10.3389/frhs.2021.817750.
20. Nilsen P. Making sense of implementation theories, models and frameworks. Implement Sci. 2015;10:53. https://doi.org/10.1186/s13012-015-0242-0.
21. Birken SA, Bunger AC, Powell BJ, Turner K, Clary AS, Klaman SL, Yu Y, Whitaker DJ, Self SR, Rostad WL, Chatham JRS, Kirk MA, Shea CM, Haines E, Weiner BJ. Organizational theory for dissemination and implementation research. Implementation (1988). JAMA. 2017;260:1743–8. https://doi.org/10.1001/jama.260.12.1743.
22. Stouten J, Denise MR, De Cremer D. Successful organizational change: Integrating the management practice and scholarly literatures. Academy of Management Annals 12.2. 2018:752–88.
23. Hughes M. Do 70 Per Cent of All Organizational Change Initiatives Really Fail? Journal of Change Management. 2011;11(4):451–64. https://doi.org/10.1080/14697017.2011.630506.
24. Gibbons P. The science of successful organizational change: How leaders set strategy, change behavior, and create an agile culture. FT Press, 2015.
25. Galli BJ. Change management models: a comparative analysis and concerns. IEEE Eng Manag Rev. 2018;46(3):124–32. https://doi.org/10.1109/EMR.2018.2866860.
26. Hussain ST, Lei S, Akram T, Haider MJ, Hussain SH, Ali M. Kurt Lewin's process model for organizational change: the role of leadership and employee involvement: a critical review. J Innov Knowl. 2018;3:123–7. https://doi.org/10.1016/j.jik.2016.07.002.
27. Hall JN. The COVID-19 crisis: aligning Kotter's steps for leading change with health care quality improvement. Can Med Educ J. 2021;12(1):e109–10. https://doi.org/10.36834/cmej.71165.
28. Singhal A. Forum: the life and work of Everett Rogers—some personal reflections. J Health Commun. 2005;10:285–8. https://doi.org/10.1080/10810730590949978.
29. Rogers E. Diffusion of innovations. 5th ed. Simon and Schuster; 2003.
30. Plsek PE, Greenhalgh T. The challenge of complexity in health care. BMJ. 2001;323(7313):625–8.
31. Reiman T. et al. Principles of adaptive management in complex safety–critical organizations. Safety science. 2015;71:80–92.
32. Begun JW, and Joanna Jiang H. "Health care management during Covid-19: Insights from complexity science." NEJM Catalyst Innovations in Care Delivery 1.5. 2020.
33. Montalvo I. The National Database of nursing quality indicators™ (NDNQI®). Online J Issues Nurs. 2007;12(3):Manuscript 2.
34. Tucker S, McNett M, Melnyk B, Hanrahan K, Hunter S, Kim B, Cullen L, Kitson A. Implementation science: application of evidence-based practice models to improve healthcare quality. Worldviews Evid-Based Nurs. 2021;18(2):76–84. https://doi.org/10.1111/wvn.12495.
35. Donabedian A. The quality of care. How can it be assessed?. JAMA. 1988;260(12):1743–8. https://doi.org/10.1001/jama.260.12.1743.
36. Esmail R, Hanson HM, Holroyd-Leduc J, Brown S, Strifler L, Straus SE, Niven DJ, Clement FM. A scoping review of full-spectrum knowledge translation theories, models, and frameworks. Implement Sci. 2020;15(1):11. https://doi.org/10.1186/s13012-020-0964-5.
37. McNett M, Tucker S, Thomas B, Gorsuch P, Gallagher-Ford L. Use of implementation science to advance nurse-led evidence-based practices in clinical settings. Nurse Leader J. 2021;20(3):297–305. https://doi.org/10.1016/j.mnl.2021.11.002.
38. Helfrich CD, Li YF, Sharp ND, Sales AE. Organizational readiness to change assessment (ORCA): development of an instrument based on the promoting action on research in health services (PARIHS) framework. Implement Sci. 2009;4:38. https://doi.org/10.1186/1748-5908-4-38.
39. Shea CM, Jacobs SR, Esserman DA, Bruce K, Weiner BJ. Organizational readiness for implementing change: a psychometric assessment of a new measure. Implement Sci. 2014;9(1):7. https://doi.org/10.1186/1748-5908-9-7.

40. Powell BJ, McMillen JC, Proctor EK, Carpenter CR, Griffey RT, Bunger AC, Glass JE, York JL. A compilation of strategies for implementing clinical innovations in health and mental health. Med Care Res Rev. 2012;8:123–57. https://doi.org/10.1177/1077558711430690.

41. Agency for Healthcare Research and Quality (AHRQ). Toolkit for Using the AHRQ Quality Indicators. Content last reviewed. Rockville, MD: Agency for Healthcare Research and Quality; 2017. https://www.ahrq.gov/patient-safety/settings/hospital/resource/qitool/index.html.

42. Helene Fuld Health Trust National Institute for Evidence-based Practice in Nursing and Healthcare. Evidence-based implementation and sustainability toolkit. Columbus, OH: Fuld National Institute for EBP; 2020.

43. McNett M, Gorsuch P, Gallagher-Ford L, Thomas B, Melnyk B, Tucker S. Development and evaluation of the Fuld institute evidence-based implementation and sustainability toolkit for healthcare settings. Nurs Adm Q. 2022;47(2):161–72.

44. Institute for Healthcare Improvement (IHI). Science of improvement: establishing measures. 2023. https://www.ihi.org/resources/Pages/HowtoImprove/ScienceofImprovementEstablishingMeasures.asp. Accessed 12 Mar 2023.

45. Sorensen G, Dennerlein JT, Peters SE, Sabbath EL, Kelly EL, Wagner GR. The future of research on work, safety, health and wellbeing: a guiding conceptual framework. Soc Sci Med. 2021;269:113593. https://doi.org/10.1016/j.socscimed.2020.113593.

46. Proctor E, Silmere H, Raghavan R, Hovmand P, Aarons G, Bunger A, Griffey R, Hensley M. Outcomes for implementation research: conceptual distinctions, measurement challenges, and research agenda. Adm Policy Ment Health Ment Health Serv Res. 2011;38(2):65–76. https://doi.org/10.1007/s10488-010-0319-7.

47. Bergström A, Ehrenberg A, Eldh AC, Graham ID, Gustafsson K, Harvey G, Hunter S, Kitson A, Rycroft-Malone J, Wallin L. The use of the PARIHS framework in implementation research and practice-a citation analysis of the literature. Implement Sci. 2020;15(1):68. https://doi.org/10.1186/s13012-020-01003-0.

Part III

Patient Safety at the Frontline

Nursing Workforce Issues and the Impact to Patient Safety

Patricia A. McGaffigan

If your foundation is laid in shifting sand, you may build your house, but it will tumble down (Florence Nightingale) [1].

1 Nurses: Health Care's Indomitable Improvers

Across the continuum of care and in a range of positions that include direct patient care, leadership, quality and safety, academia, public health, industry, and more, nurses play a ubiquitous role in the delivery of safe, reliable, and person-centered care. For centuries, nurses have been at the helm of leading and contributing to the science and improvement work in safety, and the indomitable spirit and contributions of nurses to safety are unparalleled. As the healthcare landscape continues to evolve, the nursing workforce is experiencing both sizeable opportunities and challenges that impact our personal and professional ability to provide and deliver the best care possible. This chapter provides a contemporary review of considerations that foster the safety, well-being, resilience, and contributions of the nursing profession that in turn assure the protection and support of patients and those who care for them.

2 Resilience

Patient safety is directly impacted by the ability to effectively respond to unexpected events and challenges. Resilience, a characteristic of individuals, teams, and organizations, is the ability to adapt and cope with stress, adversity, and change and is a critical factor in promoting patient and workforce safety and well-being in healthcare settings. Ensuring the safety and resiliency of the organization and a workforce that is physically and psychologically safe, joyful, and thriving is a necessary precondition to advancing patient safety. Engineering resilience focuses on

P. A. McGaffigan (✉)
Institute for Healthcare Improvement (IHI), Boston, MS, USA
e-mail: mcgfmin@aol.com

C. A. Oster, J. S. Braaten (eds.), *The Nexus between Nursing and Patient Safety*, https://doi.org/10.1007/978-3-031-53158-3_9

the everyday work of healthcare staff who successfully manage conditions that may necessitate adaptation and ensuring the intentional design and building of capacity of highly complex and dynamic systems.

Individual resilience refers to the ability of healthcare providers to adapt and cope with stress, adversity, and change. More resilient nurses are better able to manage the sociotechnical demands and stressors of their work, prevent errors and mitigate harm, respond to adverse events and natural disasters, and maintain their well-being. A systematic review of nurses and resilience revealed that work-related factors that are negatively associated with nurse resilience include stress, burnout, posttraumatic stress disorder, and workplace bullying. Factors that were positively related to resilience include coping skills, self-efficacy, social support, job satisfaction, job retention, and general well-being [2]. Resilient organizations adapt and respond to unexpected events and challenges and embrace a commitment to safety culture, open communication, and continuous learning and improvement. Organizational resilience enables healthcare organizations to prevent errors and harm to patients, and to respond quickly and effectively when incidents do occur.

Health care safety is often viewed as a state in which as few things as possible go wrong, with a goal to understand causes of errors to prevent future occurrences and eliminate variation caused by human behavior. This Safety 1 "find and fix" approach to minimizing adverse outcomes uses linear cause-effect methods such as root cause analysis, accident reporting, failure assessment, and risk management. Commonly used approaches to "fixing" adverse outcomes emphasize individual compliance and adherence to policies and procedures, training and retraining, and auditing to detect deviations in human performance [3]. While a Safety 1 approach has contributed to progress in safety, such as with circumscribed improvement projects that emphasize human performance, this approach alone is insufficient to achieve and sustain elimination of harm.

Complimentary to Safety 1 is the Safety 2 approach that relates to a system's ability to succeed under varying conditions. With recognition of the highly complex sociotechnical nature of healthcare, the focus is on understanding why most healthcare delivery processes are successful and how they are performed correctly rather than why they fail. Humans are seen as a resource necessary for system flexibility and adaptability and not as liabilities [4].

Resilience engineering emphasizes the ability of a system to adapt to changing conditions and recover from disturbances [5]. Key characteristics of resilient systems include their capacity to anticipate, monitor, respond, and learn [6]. While conversations about resilience and nurses often focus on improving their individual resilience, solutions to address resilience require balanced attention to addressing resilience from both an individual and organizational perspective. This chapter will emphasize contributing factors that may adversely impact resilience, as well as those that foster individual and organizational resilience, from the lens of nursing.

3 The Business Case for Workforce Well-being and Resilience

Years of data from the US Bureau of Labor Statistics provide evidence that health care workers, including nurses, experience higher rates of workplace-related physical injuries and illnesses than professions that are typically considered to be dangerous, including construction and manufacturing. Since the COVID-19 pandemic, reported rates of physical illness and psychological harms including burnout, moral distress, depression, anxiety, and violence have increased across professions and settings of care. Workforce safety and well-being are inextricably linked to patient safety, and workforce harms have a profound toll on patients, families, staff, the ability of organizations to deliver quality of care, and organizational resilience.

Prior to the COVID-19 pandemic, the focus on workforce safety and well-being was relatively inconsistent and fleeting, and largely limited to reportable occupational-related physical illness and injuries, with limited visibility to executives, board members, and safety and quality leaders beyond those working in occupational health. The low awareness and limitations of available and meaningful stratified data on physical and psychological harms have prevented a robust understanding of the costs and consequences to the workforce. Additionally, underreporting of risks, incidents, and harm due to fear of retaliation, job loss, disincentives, and a lack of organizational responsiveness has been common. Other impediments to appreciating the business case for workforce safety and well-being include the lack of integration of occupational health leaders with quality, safety, and other leaders, siloing of patient safety and workforce safety strategies, a lack of transparency and shared learning and improvement practices, and failure to appreciate the direct and indirect costs of workforce harms.

The business case for workforce safety and well-being has been well established [7]. The costs associated with physical illness, injury, and poor well-being include costs of medical and pharmaceutical treatment, short- and long-term workers compensation, indemnity claims, use of premium pay for temporary or overtime staff, and expenses of examining adverse events. The costs associated with absenteeism and presenteeism (where a nurse may be at work, yet is unable perform at their highest capacity), including decreased productivity, often far exceed the direct medical and pharmaceutical costs. Other costs include reassignment and retraining of harmed staff who are unable to continue in their current positions, recruitment, orientation, and onboarding costs of new staff or temporary workers to address turnover and attrition, often at premium rates, loss of experience, impacts on patient safety, experience and coordination of care, and organizational reputation. With heightened focus on workforce well-being, nurses are increasingly taking on roles and responsibilities for workforce well-being using an integrated perspective of physical, mental, emotional, and social well-being of staff.

4 Factors That Impact Nurse Resilience

4.1 Harm to Our Healers

The 2013 Lucian Leape Institute report "Through the Eyes of the Workforce: Creating Joy, Meaning and Safer Health Care" notes the inextricable link between patient and workforce safety and establishes that the basic condition of a safe workplace is the protection of the physical and psychological safety of the workforce. "Unless caregivers are given the protection, respect, and support they need, they are more likely to make errors, fail to follow safe practices, and not work well in teams" [8]. While harms to nurses and other health care workers have been magnified and increasingly recognized since the COVID-19 pandemic, these varied harms long predated the pandemic and have widespread implications for the safety, well-being, and vitality of individuals, organizations, and the healthcare industry.

4.2 Physical Harm

Health care workers experience higher rates of physical harm than industries that are typically considered to be dangerous, including manufacturing and construction, and health workers experience more days lost from work due to an illness or injury compared to these professions [9]. The most common causes of injury experienced by nurses are overexertion injuries due to repetitive motion or strain and excessive physical effort, such as lifting and physical encounters. Nurses are keenly focused on preventing harm to patients from falls, slips, and trips, yet such injuries are common causes of harm to the nursing workforce. Other causes include needlestick and sharps injuries, exposure to hazardous substances such as medications and chemicals, and exposures to bloodborne and respiratory pathogens, including flu, COVID-19, hepatitis, and tuberculosis. The increase in days lost from work by nurses increased nearly 291% from 2019 to 2020, about four times as many cases compared to prior years, driven by a drastic increase in reported cases of COVID-19 during the first year of the pandemic [10].

4.3 Workplace Violence

Workplace violence is experienced by nurses worldwide and has consequences for the safety, well-being and experience of nurses, members of the care team, and patients and families, as well as health care organizations. Workplace violence is defined as an act or threat occurring at the workplace that can include any of the following: verbal, nonverbal, written, or physical aggression; threatening, intimidating, harassing, or humiliating words or actions; bullying; sabotage; sexual harassment; physical assaults; or other behaviors of concern involving staff, licensed practitioners, patients, or visitors [11].

The incidence of violence-related health care worker injuries has steadily increased for at least a decade. Healthcare and social service workers are five times more likely to experience workplace violence than all other workers, accounting for 73% of all nonfatal workplace injuries and illnesses across industries requiring days away from work [12]. While more attention has understandably focused on physical violence, nonphysical violence, which includes bullying, harassment, verbal abuse, incivility, and aggressions, is routinely experienced by nurses.

The National Institute for Occupational Safety and Health (NIOSH) has designated four types of workplace violence (Table 1). Most workplace events in healthcare include Type 2 (client on-worker violence), perpetrated by patients, families, and visitors, as well Type 3 (worker-on worker violence) [13, 14].

Recent surveys have highlighted the prevalence and impact of workplace violence on nurses and the healthcare system. Exposure to workplace violence can impair effective patient care and lead to psychological distress, job dissatisfaction, and turnover among nurses, and the costs associated with increased security measures, injury and compensation claims, replacement staffing, absenteeism, and productivity losses have significant financial implications for health care delivery organizations [15, 16]. Furthermore, workplace violence is underreported. Several reasons predominate, including expectations that it is "part of the job", fear of retaliation and job loss, lack of available reporting systems, concerns that nothing will be done if a report is made, and failure to communicate actions taken to reporting parties. Reported rates are likely much higher.

To address workplace violence, healthcare organizations must prioritize the development and implementation of zero tolerance policies for workers, patients, and visitors for any form of physical and nonphysical violence. Programs must be geared toward identifying and addressing the root causes of workplace violence, such as understaffing, inadequate training, growing mental health realities, and a lack of security measures. Additionally, healthcare organizations can provide education and training on conflict resolution and de-escalation techniques for nurses and other healthcare professionals.

Table 1 National Institute for Occupational Safety and Health types of workplace violence

Types of violence	
Type 1: Criminal intent	Violence is perpetrated by criminals who have no legitimate relationship with the workplace, such as robbery or theft
Type 2: Customer/ client	Violence is directed at employees by customers, clients, and patients
Type 3: Co-worker	Violence is directed at employees by current or former co-workers
Type 4: Personal relationship	Violence is directed at employees by someone with whom they have a personal relationship, such as an intimate partner or family member

4.4　Racism

The National Commission to Address Racism in Nursing defines racism as assaults on the human spirit in the form of actions, biases, prejudices, and an ideology of superiority based on race that persistently cause moral suffering and physical harm of individuals and perpetuate systemic injustices and inequities [17]. In a 2022 survey of 11,863 nurses, 60% reported one or more incidents of bullying or incivility in the past year while 29% reported they had experienced one or more incidents of physical violence with 65% and 40% of nurses reporting bullying and violence, respectively. Sources of violence include patients, families, nursing peers, managers, administration, physicians, and the public [17].

Nearly half of all respondents in a nationwide US survey of 5623 nurses believe that there is "a lot" racism in nursing, 63% reported they had personally experienced racism in the workplace and over half said that racism in the workplace has negatively impacted their professional well-being. Three out of four reported witnessing racism in the workplace and of the 57% who said they had challenged racism in the workplace, 64% said their efforts resulted in no change. Black nurses reported experiencing racist acts from leaders (70%), patients (68%), and peers (66%) [17].

Approaches to addressing racism in nursing include the importance of raising awareness about the prevalence and impact of systemic and individual racism, measuring and monitoring, cultivating safe spaces for dialogue for learning and advancing personal journeys, fostering understanding of the differences between equality and equity, training on implicit bias, microaggressions, and trauma-informed care, and supporting the advancement of diversity, equity, inclusion, and belonging. Ensuring that safety reporting systems are available and allow for anonymous reporting, and stratification of racial, ethnic, sexual identity, gender identification, roles, and other factors is essential to understand the scope and opportunities for improving the experience of the workforce.

4.5　Fatigue

Nurses are especially vulnerable to fatigue and experience physical and emotional exhaustion because of long hours, rotating shifts, and schedules that do not allow for adequate rest, voluntary and mandatory overtime, and high job stress. Fatigue impairs judgment, decreases alertness and attention to details, impairs communication and decision-making quality, increases the risk of burnout, reduces patient satisfaction, and contributes to a higher risk of errors that can harm both patients and nurses.

Studies have found that nurses who work 12 hours or more per shift have a higher risk of making medication errors compared to those who worked shorter shifts and have an increased risk of triggering a near-miss alert compared to those not working extended hours [18]. Nurse fatigue is also associated with increases in patient falls and patient mortality. Nurses who work successive 12-hour shifts experience inadequate sleep between shifts to support physical and cognitive recovery, irrespective of day or night shift and may be especially prone to consequences of fatigue, that include lane deviations and automobile accidents while driving home [19, 20].

Strategies to reduce fatigue include rest and meal breaks during the work shift, ergonomic scheduling to avoid long shifts when possible, prioritization of adequate staffing levels, monitoring of voluntary overtime, and elimination of mandatory overtime. Fatigue Risk Management Systems (FRMS) include policies to reduce risk of fatigue, promoting education for leaders, nurse managers, and nurses, assessing for fatigue as a contributing factor to adverse and near-miss events, ensuring intentional design of systems to minimize the risk of human error, encouraging rest and recovery for nurses, wellness programs, and ensuring sleep hygiene and self-care. Prevention of fatigued drivers and accommodations for emergencies, such as sleep rooms and onsite childcare, are other considerations for fatigue mitigation [21].

5   Burnout, Compassion Fatigue, and Moral Distress and Injury

In addition to nonphysical violence, nurses and other health care workers experience a range of nonphysical harms that take a profound toll on the ability of individuals and teams to provide the highest quality care, and on the joy, meaning, and engagement and retention of the workforce. The stress-injury continuum refers to the range of negative consequences from work-related stress exposure and is inclusive of burnout syndrome, compassion fatigue, moral distress, anxiety, depression, post-traumatic stress disorder (PTSD), and other phenomena [22]. Psychological and emotional harms are often generalized and misclassified into a general heading of "burnout," and nurses are frequently encouraged to improve their individual resiliency. Yet such approaches fail to accurately diagnose, differentiate, and address the unique contributing factors, manifestations, and organization and individual opportunities for prevention and mitigation (Table 2).

5.1   Burnout

The International Classification of Diseases (ICD) defines burnout as a syndrome that results from chronic workplace stress that has not been successfully managed. Burnout syndrome is characterized by three dimensions: energy depletion or exhaustion, increased mental distance or feelings of cynicism related to one's job, and a sense of ineffectiveness and lack of accomplishment. When the term "burnout" was added to the World Health Organization's ICD in 2019, approximately one-third of surveyed nurses reported that they were suffering from burnout. Three years into the pandemic, the rates of reported burnout in surveyed nurses approximately doubled, and burnout is widely reported across other health care professions [23].

Table 2 Burnout, compassion fatigue, and moral distress and injury

	Burnout syndrome	Compassion fatigue [35]	Moral distress (MD) and moral injury (MI) [30]
Definition	Syndrome defined by emotional exhaustion, depersonalization, low personal accomplishment	State of exhaustion that limits one's ability to engage in caring relationships, "cost of caring"	MD: Constrained from acting in accordance with one's ethics and values MI: Experience of distress that leads to harm
Contributing factors	Workplace stressors, including lack of resources, high patient loads, long hours	Caregiving relationship, often associated with but not limited to conditions of suffering and trauma	Clinical decisions or situations that challenges one's deeply held beliefs; inability to provide high quality and healing care
Onset	Spreads gradually and continuously over time	Acute or cumulative following secondary trauma(s)	Situational, acute, or gradual
Manifestations	Physical and mental health challenges, turnover, attrition	Emotional, physical, social, spiritual, and work challenges; turnover	Guilt, shame, anger
Interdependencies	May increase risk of compassion fatigue and moral injury	May be associated with burnout and compounded by moral distress	May contribute to burnout and compassion fatigue
Organizational considerations	Ensure systematic approaches to measuring, monitoring, and addressing burnout. Create positive work and learning environments Engage staff in identifying and creating solutions, including technologies, to reduce turbulence and eliminate non-value-added activity Integrate chief wellness officer roles and programs Provide adequate staffing Foster education, positive and supportive relationships, professional autonomy	Recognize and identify factors to prevent, assess, and minimize consequences Offer onsite counseling, debriefing, recovery programs, and support groups	Recognize and identify the cost and impact of competing demands on what individuals value Foster healthy work environments and cultures that support ethical practice Provide supportive networks that promote collaboration and dialogue

(continued)

Table 2 (continued)

	Burnout syndrome	Compassion fatigue [35]	Moral distress (MD) and moral injury (MI) [30]
Individual nurse considerations	Foster self-care, rest, and mindfulness Limit excessive work hours and set work-life boundaries Identify and participate in initiatives to eliminate low-value work Leverage resources to address stress	Identify risk factors for compassion fatigue Maintain boundaries and work-life balance Augment caring communication practices Leverage available support programs	Build capacity to cultivate ethical competence, ethics in education, self-regulation and mindfulness, and self-care

Burnout is typically associated with chronic workplace stress and is not specific to the caregiving context [24]. Factors that are associated with burnout in nurses include demanding workloads and aspects of the work environment, such as poor staffing ratios, lack of communication between physicians and nurses, and lack of effective organizational leadership within working environments for nurses. In one survey, 84% of nurses say they are stressed or dealing with burnout, with nearly 50% reporting some level of burnout. Leading causes of burnout reported by nurses include not enough staff to adequately do their job (38%), lack of respect from their employer (14%), too many administrative tasks (10%), and insufficient compensation (9%) [16]. The concept of turbulence has been identified as an emerging variable of interest to capture the activities and experience of nurses related to communication and workload, including interruptions, handovers, availability of supplies, and resources [25]. Turbulence may alter communication and lead to breakdowns, distractions, interruptions, loss of information during transitions of care and in tasks, and impaired decision-making [26].

Burnout is associated with a wide range of impacts to individuals, organizations, and care quality. Burnout is a significant predictor of heart disease, chronic pain, gastrointestinal distress, depression, and mortality [24]. In addition to the personal costs, burnout has high social and economic costs for organizations and society, including turnover of nurses from their jobs and the profession.

Magnet hospitals and other hospitals with better work environments, including support for education, positive physician–nurse relationships, nurse autonomy, and nurse manager support, outside of increasing the number of nurses, can lead to improvements in job satisfaction and lower burnout among nurses [27]. Additional strategies to address burnout include managing workload and eliminating non- and low-value added responsibilities, assuring adequate staffing of nurses and nurse support staff, appropriate nurse-to-patient ratios, implementation of healthy work environments, elimination of mandatory overtime, flexible and ergonomic scheduling, and encouragement of self-care. Efforts to address self-care alone place a disproportionate burden on the need for individuals to "become more resilient" and will fail to result in progress in the absence of addressing work stressors.

5.2 Compassion Fatigue

While burnout is a manifestation of a stressful workplace, compassion fatigue is a form of secondary trauma that refers to a state of exhaustion that limits one's ability to engage in caring relationships [28]. Sometimes referred to as the "cost of caring," compassion fatigue occurs when nurses develop declining empathetic ability from repeated exposure to others' suffering and leads to emotional, physical, and spiritual exhaustion. Compassion fatigue may significantly impact professional nursing care and performance and has been in identified as a factor in unsafe and poor quality of care, and results in physical and nonphysical consequences for nurses [29]. Compassion fatigue may be mitigated by systemic and individual strategies that include identification and mitigation of risks, education and awareness, peer and professional support, debriefing, modifying assignments, and self-care.

5.3 Moral Distress and Injury

Moral distress occurs when nurses know the morally ethical course of action to take but have a low degree or no degree of influence and are constrained from doing so by factors that are internal or external, including institutional and social factors. The feeling of unease where the behavior one must take is not aligned with one's moral principles is often triggered by end-of-life care, inadequate staffing and other resources, value conflicts, challenging team dynamics, and when duty conflicts with safety concerns, and may be heightened during natural disasters and crises, such as pandemics. Moral injury, which may occur because of moral distress, refers to the experience of the problem or challenging situation, leading to impaired function or longer term psychological harm, such as profound guilt and shame, a sense of betrayal, profound moral dissonance, and mental health issues. Consequences of unaddressed moral distress and moral injury include increased intention to leave one's job or profession, withdrawal from and loss of connectedness with patients, peers, and others, lack of trust, and a sense of betrayal [30, 31].

Moral resilience is "the capacity of an individual to sustain or restore their integrity in response to moral adversity, including complexity, confusion, distress or setbacks" [32]. While our knowledge and understanding of moral resilience are evolving, strategies have been offered to cultivate individual and organizational capabilities for moral resilience for individuals, nurse leaders, and organizations. Promising areas for building individual capacity include ethical competence, ethics in education, self-regulation and mindfulness, and self-care. Organizations and nurse leaders play a key role in developing strategies for mitigating moral distress and fostering moral resilience that include creating cultures and environments that enable nurses to uphold their commitment to ethical practice [32]. Examples of such strategies include facilitating social connections, promoting positivity, capitalizing on nurses' strengths, nurturing nurses' growth, encouraging nurses' self-care, fostering mindfulness practice, and conveying altruism [33, 34].

6 Healthy Work Environments

The World Health Organization (WHO) defines a healthy environment (HWE) as a place of "physical, mental, and social well-being," supporting optimal health and safety. A HWE is an essential and modifiable organizational characteristic and is crucial for the quality of care and the safety and well-being of patients and the workforce [36, 37]. The Nurses Bill of Rights places emphasis on the nonnegotiable rights for all nurses to meet the increasing complexities of care delivery. Inclusive in the rights are safe work environments that prioritize and protect nurses' safety and well-being and provide support, and resources, and tools to stay psychologically and physically whole. The Bill of Rights also references environments that ensure respect, inclusivity, diversity, and equity; just care settings that facilitate ethical practice, standards, and care; and psychological safety to ensure that nurses may advocate for patients and their own safety without fear of retribution [38].

Two frequently referenced models that address and promote HWEs include the the American Association of Critical-Care Nurses (AACN) Standards for Establishing and Sustaining Healthy Work Environments and the Magnet Recognition Program by the American Nurses Credentialing Center (ANCC). The AACN HWE Standards define six essential standards that are foundational to a HWE and enable nurses to provide the highest standards of compassionate patient care while being fulfilled at work. The standards include skilled communication, true collaboration, effective decision-making, appropriate staffing, meaningful recognition, and authentic leadership [39]. Across five large scale surveys since the development of the HWE Standards in 2005, implementation of the HWE standards has been associated with more engaged nurses, decreased burnout, lower turnover, and better patient care. The most recent survey conducted in 2021 during the COVID-19 pandemic revealed increased concerns about critical staffing levels, declines in care quality and satisfaction with the profession, and an expression of intention to leave the nursing profession within 3 years by 37% of respondents. Nurses who worked in HWE settings reported less moral distress, higher physical and psychological safety, less burnout, job dissatisfaction, and missed care, better staffing and were more likely to report better care quality than survey respondents working in non-HWE environments [39].

The Magnet Recognition Program identifies several elements that contribute to providing a positive working environment for nurses, including transformational leadership, structural empowerment, exemplary professional practice, new knowledge, innovations, and improvements and empirical quality results. Magnet hospitals experience improved patient care, safety, and satisfaction, decreased vacancy rates and turnover, lower burnout, and increased staff satisfaction [40].

Given the amplification of stressors that predated the COVID-19 pandemic and disruptions of the pandemic, including pre-licensure nursing education, and stressors associated with high workloads, stress and burnout that have impacted nurse turnover, retention, and engagement [41], the prioritization, implementation, and monitoring of healthy work environments by nurses, leaders, and health care delivery organizations are essential. The Healthy Work Environment Assessment Tool and Magnet Self-Assessment of Organizational Culture may be used to identify gaps, opportunities, and progress toward improvement [42, 43].

7 Pathways to Resilience: Enhancing Safety, Well-being and Joy

7.1 Safer Together: A National Action Plan to Advance Patient Safety

While most work in safety has centered on reacting to patient and workforce harm, reliance on improvement projects that address downstream harms alone has proven insufficient for advancing and sustaining safety. Like patient safety, optimizing workforce safety and well-being requires an overarching shift from reactive and piecemeal interventions to a total systems approach that balances individual and organizational accountability. Leaders must embrace workforce safety and well-being as a core value, foster the conditions for safety and well-being, partner with the workforce to co-design and support safety and well-being, and promote learning systems for the continuous improvement of workforce safety and well-being. To advance the safety and well-being of patients and the workforce with this reorientation, the National Steering Committee for Patient Safety was convened and chartered with the creation of Safer Together: A National Action Plan to Advance Patient Safety. Created by 27 national organizations, federal agencies, safety experts, nurse leaders, and patient and family advocates, the Plan focuses on four foundational areas that are essential elements of a safety ecosystem. These interdependent foundational areas include culture, leadership, and governance, patient and family engagement, workforce safety and well-being, and the learning system. Steeped in guiding principles inclusive of health equity, the Plan offers practical recommendations, an organizational assessment framework, and implementation resources for constancy of purpose for patient and workforce safety and well-being. The organizational assessment tool offers a pragmatic resource for organizations to assess their commitment, behaviors, and practices associated with workforce safety and well-being [44].

7.2 Clinician Well-being

The National Academy of Medicine's NAM's National Plan for Health Workforce Well-Being calls for immediate and collective action to strengthen health workforce well-being and is based on the vision that people are cared for by a thriving health workforce under conditions that foster their well-being as they improve population health, enhance the care experience, reduce costs, and advance health equity [45]. The seven priority areas of the plan are as follows:

• Create and sustain positive work and learning environments and culture.

- Invest in measurement, assessment, strategies, and research to decrease burnout and improve well-being.
- Support mental health and reduce stigma of seeking services needed to address mental health challenges.
- Address compliance, regulatory, and policy barriers for daily work to prevent unnecessary burdens on health workers.
- Engage effective technology tools to support health workers in providing high quality care that support clinical decision-making and minimize administrative burden.
- Institutionalize well-being as a long-term value and support the resilience of health care.
- Recruit and retain a diverse and inclusive health workforce to promote careers in health professions and vitality of the workforce.

7.3   Joy and Meaning

While mitigating burnout, moral distress, compassion fatigue, and other challenges must be nonnegotiable priorities for health care leaders and nursing, solutions must be reoriented to address the joy and meaning of the health care workforce to foster well-being. Often regarded as sentimental notions, joy and meaning are increasingly recognized as crucial to the safety and well-being of patients, families, the workforce, and the profession and the vitality of organizations. Joy is an attitude, or intellectual, behavioral, and emotional commitment to meaningful and satisfying work, while meaning is a sense of importance of an action or one's purpose [8]. Nurses who find joy and meaning in their work are more likely to provide high-quality care, leading to better patient outcomes, and experience more satisfaction and engagement. The most joyful, productive, engaged staff feel both physically and psychologically safe, appreciate the meaning and purpose of their work, have some choice and control over their time and are part of the solutions for change, experience camaraderie with others at work, and perceive their work life integration to be fair and equitable [46].

The IHI framework for improving joy in work offers four steps to inform organizational initiatives that engage and value employees:

1. Ask staff "What matters to you?": Having conversations that identify what is important to work colleagues are important starting points for improving the work environment and patient care, and promote sharing of needs, preferences, and interest that build connections around shared values. This first step helps define what makes for a good day, minimizes preconceived notions and misconceptions about what matters, and fosters shared goals and purpose.
2. Identify unique impediments to joy in the local context: By building on the "What matters?" conversations, leaders identify impediments that exist in the daily work of nurses to set priorities that can be addressed. This "pebbles in your shoes" conversation enables nurses to provide input on which impediments to address, and builds camaraderie by working together to remove impediments, moving from a "doing to" to a "doing with" experience.

3. Commit to shared responsibility: The third step is to commit to a systems approach to making joy in work a shared responsibility at all levels of the organization, with leaders at all levels looking at processes, issues, or circumstances that are impeding what matters. Central to success is that leaders at all levels dedicate time, attention, skill development, and necessary resources to improving joy in work. This involves meeting the fundamental needs of physical and psychological safety: meaning and purpose: choice and autonomy: camaraderie and teamwork: and fairness and equity.
4. Use improvement science to test approaches to improving joy in work in your organization: The fourth step is to create small tests of change, using principles of improvement science. This enables organizations to evaluate whether the changes they test are leading to improvement, whether they are effective in different departments and settings, and whether they are sustainable. The Model for Improvement [47] is often used to establish an aim for improvement, select measures that can identify whether a change is an improvement, and identify specific changes that can be tested in small, rapid tests of change using PDSA cycles.

7.4 Peer Support

Peer support, a form of psychological first aid, is a critical factor in maintaining and enhancing nurses' mental and emotional health. While especially important for supporting workers in the aftermath of adverse events, peer support is increasingly recognized as an important component of well-being for stressful events and burnout and promoting recovery, well-being, and resilience [48]. Such programs are strategically aligned with a commitment to the safety and well-being of workers and are offered by trained peer supporters to individuals or groups. Distinct from therapeutic relationships, the focus of peer support is on allowing the nurse to recognize how they are doing, realizing they are not alone, identifying that their reactions to traumatic experiences are normal, and providing bridging to other resources, such as behavioral health resources, employee assistance programs, or other organization-sponsored assistance [49].

7.5 Self-Care

The physical, emotional, and professional demands of nursing have a well-documented association with the safety, quality, and experience of patients and necessitate that all nurses prioritize their health and well-being. Yet nearly 70% of nurses report that they prioritize the health, safety, and wellness of patients over their own and across many indicators, nurses of color report worse status [50]. Physical challenges include strenuous tasks such as lifting and repositioning of patients, lengthy shifts, and rotations that impact circadian rhythm and lead to fatigue, fast-paced activities that require endurance, and risks to healthy eating and rest breaks. Heavy workloads, risks of burnout and other secondary traumas, and demands on work-life integration are prevalent. Throughout the pandemic, self-reported declines in mental health revealed increasing odds of feeling sad, depression, and anxiety [51]. While evidence affirms the obligation of leaders, managers, and organizations to prioritize cultures of well-being and safety for nurses to mitigate many of the contributing factors that impact safety and wellness, self-care is a vital component of a nurse's professional obligation. The American Nurses Association Healthy Nurse Healthy Nation is a free nurse health, safety, and wellness program that connects and engages participants with resources and support across six domains for self-care, including physical activity, rest, nutrition, quality of life, safety, and mental health.

Recent research comparing nurses whose workplaces are supportive of wellness and shorter shift lengths with those that provided little, or no wellness support revealed that nurses in supportive organizations were more likely to have better mental and physical health, no burnout, and higher quality of life while nurses who worked in less supportive settings with longer shifts experienced poorer health outcomes [52].

8 Considerations for Recruiting, Interviewing, Hiring, and Supporting the Nursing Workforce

Traditional recruiting, hiring, and interviewing practices in nursing place emphasis on the roles, responsibilities, and competencies associated with the unique needs of specific patient populations and care settings. With the shortages of available nurses that have been exacerbated since the pandemic, more emphasis has focused on the urgency to fill positions with core (employed) or contingent staff. The availability of varied pathways and parties that are involved in the recruitment, vetting and selection of nurses has rapidly expanded beyond classic human resources and unit and department managers to include managed service providers, internal and external agencies, per diem pools, and gig platforms. Given the dearth of data associated with the increased composition of a contingent nurse workforce, the Institute for Healthcare Improvement sought to understand practices associated with patient and workforce safety in exploratory interviews with nurse staffing agencies, nurse leaders, and travel nurses. These qualitative interviews revealed little to no attention to patient and workforce safety in the selection, orientation, onboarding, and support of contingent nurses, and a lack of standardized training standards, practices, and resources associated with patient and workforce reporting systems, feedback mechanisms for understanding and learning about safety events and safety huddles [53].

In an increasingly competitive and complex hiring market, nurse candidates have many more choices for where they will work, and selection of the conditions under which they will work. While compensation continues to be an important factor for nurse candidates, more attention to patient and workforce outcomes and experience, safe, healthy, supportive, and joyful cultures and work environments, and considerations that promote personal and professional well-being, vitality and development will play larger roles for both candidates and employers. Hiring managers and teams and candidates may diversify and expand their respective recruitment, interviewing

Table 3 Considerations for recruitment, interviewing, hiring, and support of the nursing workforce include

Considerations for hiring teams	Considerations for employed or contingent staff
Evaluate and optimize your current state, including retention and attrition rates, data from stay and exit interviews, compensation, current options for flexible staffing, and measures of nursing workforce safety and well-being	Inquire about nurse retention and attrition and seek feedback about what prompts nurses to join and remain within the organization and unit
Analyze and integrate data from culture of safety surveys, patient and workforce safety, engagement and experience, and nurse sensitive quality indicators	Ask about practices and plans to address, monitor, and improve results of recent data from culture surveys and patient and workforce safety dashboards
Stratify data collection and analysis for race, ethnicity, language, sexual orientation, gender identity, employed versus contingent status, length of experience, and shifts/ hours worked	Inquire whether patient and workforce safety and well-being data are stratified, processes for communicating results/gaps, and plans to address gaps
Identify opportunities and create unit and system strategies to attract, retain, recognize, and advance the joy, vitality, and well-being of the nursing workforce	Explore whether strategies and programs are in place and effectively operationalized that foster joy and engagement, eliminate nonvalue added work, recognize, and reward nursing practice, and provide for professional advancement
Create academic-practice partnerships and residency/ transition to practice programs for new nurse candidates	Seek opportunities that offer transition to practice/ residency programs
Establish shared governance, healthy work environment, staffing, and well-being committees	Inquire about shared governance practices, and initiatives related to advancing healthy work environments, staffing, and well-being
Establish and ensure access to programs to support the safety, health, and well-being of the workforce and eliminate harm and stress	Inquire about workforce safety and well-being strategies, systems, and programs, inclusive of assistive devices for repositioning and lifting patients, sharps and needlestick prevention technologies, personal protective device availability, violence prevention and escalation programs, incorporation of fair and just culture frameworks, leadership presence and walk arounds, team communications and debriefing programs, and availability of nursing support team members
Ensure availability of buddy, peer support, mentor, and employee assistance programs	Inquire about peer support and employee assistance programs and request assignment to a support buddy
Provide frequent in-person checkpoints for core and contingent staff. For contingent staff, ensure checkpoints at beginning, middle and end of assignments	Inquire about checkpoints and performance reviews, to include whether and how patient and workforce safety and well-being expectations are evaluated

Table 3 (continued)

Considerations for hiring teams	Considerations for employed or contingent staff
Create interview guides to evaluate competencies and commitment of core and contingent staff for safe, quality, and equitable care and caring	Create your candidate interview guide with questions that address the organization and unit's commitment and practices associated with safe, quality, and equitable care and caring
Establish clear competency requirements to guide selection of core and contingent staff	Ask how clinical, safety, and professional competencies are identified and incorporated into the hiring and selection process, and routinely assessed thereafter
Establish accountability for selection and monitoring of contingent staff for patient and workforce safety events with internal and external staffing partners	Conduct a comprehensive evaluation of your options with staffing agencies and per diem roles to clarify accountability for review, communication, and support for adverse events
Standardize expectations for orientation, onboarding, and related preceptor development programs, inclusive of patient and workforce safety and well-being	Clarify how your orientation and onboarding addresses essential items related to patient and workforce safety
Identify stable preceptor assignments and processes	Inquire about selection and assignment of preceptors, experience and tenure of preceptors, feedback and evaluation processes, and policies for protected time
Transparently communicate the use and proportion, trends and experiences associated with contingent nurses	Identify frequency, use, onboarding, evaluation, and engagement of contingent nurses
Ensure availability of experienced resource, charge, and staff nurses across all shifts and on weekends	Assess for tenure and mix of experienced staff across shifts and on weekends
Engage patient safety leaders to review procedures for onboarding, inclusion, and support for core and contingent staff in safety event reporting and reviews, escalation policies, safety huddles, and rounds	Ask how common safety practices are handled, including patient and safety event reporting and reviews, escalation policies, safety huddles and rounds
Support fully inclusive work environments and experiences for core and contingent staff to include engagement in staff meetings, training, events, participation in shared and clinical governance activities, and improvement initiatives	Invite examples of how core and contingent staff are included in daily operational activities of the unit or department
Ensure that patient assignments are equitably determined and aligned with the competencies of core and contingent staff and needs of patients and families	Evaluate processes and practices for patient-nurse assignments, to include numbers and acuity of patients

(continued)

Table 3 (continued)

Considerations for hiring teams	Considerations for employed or contingent staff
Support innovation to test and scale care delivery solutions and staffing models that promote agility and flexibility	Explore unit and organization's commitments and investments in nurse-led innovation to support safety, well-being, and engagement of nurse workforce
Incorporate practices to reduce fatigue and stress, and support well-being	Confirm practices and expectations related to requests for additional work hours, overtime, sick and vacation time, and shift rotations. Avoid settings that mandate overtime beyond committed hours
Encourage engagement in workforce well-being and support programs and ensure they are readily available and meaningful to all nurses and staff	Seek information on the availability, utilization, and effectiveness of well-being strategies and programs, inclusive of a well-being leader with responsibilities for nursing

and hiring practices to incorporate considerations for attracting, retaining, and supporting the vitality of the nursing workforce (Table 3).

Key Points

- Nurses are key contributors to safe patient care and positive patient outcomes.
- Many challenges exist in the current work environment that inhibit nurses from contributing fully and at their best and also contribute to nurse attrition.
- Challenges, include physical harm, workplace violence, burnout, fatigue, racism, moral distress, and general lack of fulfillment and joy in the workplace.
- Challenges have only intensified since the COVID-19 pandemic.
- Actively promoting a healthy work environment and a focus on caregiver well-being provides the vehicle to assure an adequate nursing workforce that can focus on promoting safety for those receiving care.

References

1. Ulrich BT. Leadership and management according to Florence Nightingale. Norwalk, CT: Appleton & Lange; 1992.
2. Yu F, Raphael D, Mackay L, Smith M, King A. Personal and work-related factors associated with nurse resilience: a systematic review. Int J Nurs Stud. 2019;93:129–40.
3. Braithwaite J, Wears RL, Hollnagel E. Resilient health care: turning patient safety on its head. Int J Qual Health Care. 2015;27(5):418–20.
4. NHS England. Safety I and safety II: The past and future of safety management. 2015. Accessed 27 May 2023.
5. Woods DD, Dekker S, Cook R, Johannesen L, Sarter N. Behind human error: resilience engineering and systems safety. Ashgate Publishing Limited; 2010.
6. Hollnagel E, Woods DD, Leveson N. Resilience engineering: concepts and precepts. CRC Press; 2006.
7. Institute for Healthcare Improvement/National Patient Safety Foundation. Optimizing a business case for safe health care: an integrated approach to safety and finance. Cambridge, MA: Institute for Healthcare Improvement; 2017. Accessed 27 May 2023

8. Lucian Leape Institute. Through the eyes of the workforce: creating joy, meaning, and safer health care. Boston, MA: National Patient Safety Foundation; 2013. Accessed 27 May 2023
9. McGaffigan P, Kingston MB, Schwich RK. Tackling the healthcare acquired condition (HAC) of workforce harm: lessons learned from COVID-19. Manage Healthcare. 2021;6(2):142–54.
10. Bureau of Labor Statistics. Nonfatal injuries and illnesses resulting in days off work among nurses up 291 percent in 2020. May 6, 2022. Accessed 27 May 2023. https://www.bls.gov/opub/ted/2022/nonfatal-injuries-and-illnesses-resulting-in-days-off-work-among-nurses-up-291-percent-in-2020.htm
11. Joint Commission. Workplace violence prevention resources. Accessed 27 May 2023. https://www.jointcommission.org/resources/patient-safety-topics/workplace-violence-prevention/
12. Bureau of Labor Statistics. Fact sheet: workplace violence in healthcare, 2018. Published April 2020. Accessed 27 May 2023. https://www.bls.gov/iif/factsheets/workplace-violence-healthcare-2018.htm
13. Somani R, Muntaner C, Hillan E, Velonis AJ, Smith P. A systematic review: effectiveness of interventions to de-escalate workplace violence against nurses in healthcare settings. Saf Health Work. 2021;12(3):289–95.
14. Phillips JP. Workplace violence against health care workers in the United States. N Engl J Med. 2016;374:1661–9.
15. Byon HD, Sagherian K, Kim Y, Lipscomb J, Crandall M, Steege L. Nurses' experience with type II workplace violence and underreporting during the COVID-19 pandemic. Workplace Health Saf. 2022;70(9):412–20.
16. American Nurses Foundation. Pulse on the Nation's nurses COVID-19 survey series: workplace survey. June-July 2022. Accessed 27 May 2023. https://www.nursingworld.org/~492857/contentassets/872ebb13c63f44f6b11a1bd0c74907c9/covid-19-two-year-impact-assessment-written-report-final.pdf
17. National Commission to Address Racism in Nursing. Racism in nursing report series. November 2021. https://www.nursingworld.org/~49c4d0/globalassets/practiceandpolicy/workforce/commission-to-address-racism/racism-in-nursing-report-series.pdf
18. Bell T, Sprajcer M, Flenady T, Sahay A. Fatigue in nurses and medication administration errors: a scoping review. J Clin Nurs. 2023; https://doi.org/10.1111/jocn.16620
19. Geiger-Brown J, Rogers VE, Trinkoff AM, Kane RL, Bausell RB, Scharf SM. Sleep, sleepiness, fatigue, and performance of 12-hour-shift nurses. Chronobiol Int. 2012;29(2):211–9.
20. James SM, James L. The impact of 12 h night shifts on nurses' driving safety. Nurs Rep. 2023;13(1):436–44.
21. Caruso CC, Baldwin CM, Berger A, Chasens ER, Edmonson JC, Gobel BH, et al. Policy brief: nurse fatigue, sleep, and health, and ensuring patient and public safety. Nurs Outlook. 2019;67(5):615–9.
22. Partners for Nurse Staffing Think Tank. Nurse staffing think tank: priority topics and recommendations. May 2022. Accessed 27 May 2023. https://www.nursingworld.org/~49940b/globalassets/practiceandpolicy/nurse-staffing/nurse-staffing-think-tank-recommendation.pdf
23. American Hospital Association Blog. We need to talk about burnout the same way we talk about benefits. October 2020. Accessed 27 May 2023. https://www.aha.org/news/blog/2020-10-20-we-need-talk-about-burnout-same-way-we-talk-about-benefits
24. Maslach, C, Leiter, MP. 2016. Burnout. In: Fink, G (Ed.), Handbook of stress: Vol. 1. Stress: concepts, cognition, emotion, and behavior. Elsevier Academic Press, 2016, pp. 351–357.
25. Browne J, Braden CJ. Nursing turbulence in critical care: relationships with nursing workload and patient safety. Am J Crit Care. 2020;29(3):182–91.
26. Jennings BM. Turbulence. In: Hughes RG, editor. Patient safety and quality: an evidence-based handbook for nurses. Rockville, MD: Agency for Healthcare Research and Quality (US); 2008. Chapter 29.
27. Shah MK, Gandrakota N, Cimiotti JP, Ghose N, Moore M, Ali MK. Prevalence of and factors associated with nurse burnout in the US. JAMA Netw Open. 2021;4(2):e2036469.
28. Joinson C. Coping with compassion fatigue. Nursing. 1992;22:116–22.
29. Nolte AG, Downing C, Temane A, Hastings-Tolsma M. Compassion fatigue in nurses: a meta-synthesis. J Clin Nurs. 2017;26(23-24):4364–78.

30. American Nurses Association A call to action: exploring moral resilience toward a culture of ethical practice, 2017. https://www.nursingworld.org/~4907b6/globalassets/docs/ana/ana-call-to-action--exploring-moral-resilience-final.pdf
31. Rushton CH, Nelson KE, Antonsdottir I, Hanson GC, Boyce D. Perceived organizational effectiveness, moral injury, and moral resilience among nurses during the COVID-19 pandemic: secondary analysis. Nurs Manag. 2022;53(7):12–22.
32. Rushton CH. Moral resilience: transforming moral suffering in healthcare. New York: Oxford Academic; 2018.
33. American Association of Critical Care Nurses. Position statement: moral distress in times of crisis. March 1, 2020.
34. Wei H, Roberts P, Strickler J, Corbett RW. Nurse leaders' strategies to foster nurse resilience. J Nurs Manag. 2019;27(4):681–7.
35. Boyle DA. Countering compassion fatigue: a requisite nursing agenda. Online J Issues Nurs. 2011;16(1):2.
36. Olds DM, Aiken LH, Cimiotti JP, Lake ET. Association of nurse work environment and safety climate on patient mortality: a cross-sectional study. Int J Nurs Stud. 2017;74:155–61.
37. Institute of Medicine (US). Committee on the work environment for nurses and patient safety. In: Page A, editor. Keeping patients safe: transforming the work environment of nurses. Washington, DC: National Academies Press (US); 2004.
38. American Nurses Association. Nurses bill of rights. 2022. Accessed 27 May 2023. https://www.nursingworld.org/~498d25/globalassets/practiceandpolicy/work-environment/health--safety/nurses-bill-of-rights.pdf
39. Ulrich B, Cassidy L, Barden C, Varn-Davis N, Delgado SA. National nurse work environments—October 2021: a status report. Crit Care Nurse. 2022;42(5):58–70.
40. Kelly LA, McHugh MD, Aiken LH. Nurse outcomes in Magnet® and non-Magnet hospitals. J Nurs Adm. 2012;42(Suppl. 10):S44–9.
41. Martin B, Kaminski-Ozturk N, O'Hara C, Smiley R. Examining the impact of the COVID-19 pandemic on burnout and stress among U.S. nurses. J Nurs Regul. 2023;14(1):4–12.
42. Connor JA, Ziniel SI, Porter C, Doherty D, Moonan M, Dwyer P, et al. Interprofessional use and validation of the AACN healthy work environment assessment tool. Am J Crit Care. 2018;27(5):363–71.
43. American Nurses Credentialing Center. 2019 Magnet® application manual organizational self-assessment. 2019.
44. National Steering Committee for Patient Safety. Safer together: a national action plan to advance patient safety. Boston, MA: Institute for Healthcare Improvement; 2020.
45. National Academy of Medicine. National plan for health workforce well-being. Washington, DC: The National Academies Press; 2022.
46. Perlo J, Balik B, Swensen S, Kabcenell A, Landsman J, Feeley D. IHI framework for improving joy in work. In: IHI White paper. Cambridge, MA: Institute for Healthcare Improvement; 2017.
47. Langley GL, Moen R, Nolan KM, Nolan TW, Norman CL, Provost LP. The improvement guide: a practical approach to enhancing organizational performance. 2nd ed. San Francisco: Jossey-Bass Publishers; 2009.
48. Pelt MV, Morris T, Lilly AC, Pian-Smith MCM, Karasik L, Pelt FV. Supporting caregivers during COVID-19: transforming compassionate care from a way of doing to being. AANA J. 2021;89(1):1–6.
49. Godfrey KM, Scott SD. At the heart of the pandemic. Nurse Lead. 2021;19(2):188–93.
50. American Nurses Association. Healthy nurse, healthy nation: the first 5 years. Am Nurse. 2023;18(4):31–41.
51. Cuccia AF, Peterson C, Melnyk BM, Boston-Leary K. Trends in mental health indicators among nurses participating in healthy nurse, healthy nation from 2017 to 2021. Worldviews Evid-Based Nurs. 2022;19(5):352–8.
52. Melnyk BM, Hsieh AP, Tan A, Teall AM, Weberg D, Jun J, et al. Associations among nurses' mental/physical health, lifestyle behaviors, shift length, and workplace wellness support during COVID-19: important implications for health care systems. Nurs Adm Q. 2022;46(1):5–18.
53. Personal communication, Patricia McGaffigan.

Fostering Psychological Safety on the Frontlines

Mary T. Walsh

Medicine has become a team sport, relying on each individual to interact, communicate, and provide feedback to team members and other departments. In the fast-paced and high-stress environment of healthcare and direct care to patients, psychological safety is foundational to creating a high-performing team. Psychological safety refers to the shared belief that one can raise concerns, ask questions, and challenge the status quo without fear of repercussions [1]. Articulating ideas, concerns, and suggestions are commonly called voice behaviors. This type of communication occurs in meetings and discussions and can contribute to decision-making processes [2]. When individuals feel psychologically safe, they bring their authentic selves to work. When the team feels psychologically safe, members feel a sense of belonging. When the organization feels psychologically safe, departments collaborate and challenge the status quo.

Psychological safety is often present in healthcare, aviation, nuclear power, and military organizations. Its practical significance is apparent as work becomes increasingly team oriented and interdependent [3]. Research conducted on organizations, particularly in healthcare fields that focus on the safety of patients and employees, has documented the importance of psychological safety. Understanding and fostering psychological safety are essential for creating supportive work environments that enhance employee engagement, performance, and overall organizational success. It promotes effective communication and teamwork, as well as individual well-being, and has implications across individual, team, and organizational levels of analysis. Due to a rapidly changing industry and the complexity of nursing, the need for psychological safety in healthcare is rising [4]. In nursing, the

M. T. Walsh (✉)
Mountain Division, CommonSpirit Health, Centennial, CO, USA
e-mail: TracyWalsh.co@gmail.com

C. A. Oster, J. S. Braaten (eds.), *The Nexus between Nursing and Patient Safety*,
https://doi.org/10.1007/978-3-031-53158-3_10

187

need is even more significant due to the increased pressures and challenges due to working long hours, staffing shortages, and, simply put, emotional demands of caring for complex patients.

Research on team dynamics, dating back to the 1960s, described psychological safety as the perception felt by the individual to make suggestions without fear [5]. Many employees found that asking questions and reporting errors threatened their reputation and standing among colleagues [6]. Particularly difficult is speaking up in teams that include different disciplines because differences in status, training, and language can impact communication and shared understanding [7]. Interdisciplinary teams are commonplace in healthcare. Therefore, how the individuals of the team perceive the "interpersonal climate" affects how people work together and the risks they are willing to take [8].

This chapter explores the importance of psychological safety in healthcare settings and studies the link between psychological safety and critical elements such as belonging, learning, collaboration, and communication. Special attention will be paid to the individual healthcare professionals to build their voice behaviors to contribute to the psychological safety of the organization. Creating a psychologically safe work environment impacts all aspects of the nursing experience, from job satisfaction to reducing burnout. Additional considerations will focus on opportunities to enhance employee engagement and improve patient outcomes.

1 The Impact of Psychological Safety

The importance of psychological safety in the healthcare setting has gained attention. Studies have shown that psychological safety improves clinical outcomes and reduces medical errors [9]. Psychological safety is linked to positive outcomes like increased employee engagement, improved psychological health and safety behaviors, and enhanced learning [10, 11]. Trust, privacy, reduced uncertainty, and resistance to change have been associated with psychological safety [12–14].

Research has shown that psychological safety among healthcare professionals, including nurses, is crucial for effective communication, teamwork, and patient-centered care [9]. Studies have shown that it can lead to better patient outcomes, higher job satisfaction, and lower burnout rates in healthcare workers. [9]. Given the demanding and high-stakes nature of healthcare work, creating a psychologically safe environment is essential for the well-being and performance of healthcare professionals and the delivery of quality care.

Psychological safety has become integral to other team attributes like voice behaviors, collaboration, and organizational learning [15]. New research examines psychological safety at different organizational levels (individual, team, and organization), realizing how each level contributes to or is a barrier to this type of culture [16]. Psychological safety in each of these levels is discussed in the next three sections.

2   Psychological Safety in the Individual

Psychological safety at the individual level refers to an individual's perception of feeling safe and comfortable expressing their thoughts, concerns, and ideas without fear of negative consequences or retribution. Creating a supportive work environment is crucial, where individuals feel empowered to use their voices and contribute to the organization [2]. Psychological safety is essential in healthcare, where speaking up can prevent medical errors and improve patient safety [17]. Building skills to effectively communicate concerns and ideas is essential for individuals to exercise their voice and contribute to a psychologically safe workplace.

Speaking up is vital to psychological safety, enabling individuals to share their perspectives, raise concerns, and contribute to decision-making. Research has shown that psychological safety is positively associated with voice behaviors, such as speaking up with suggestions, concerns, and questions [18]. When individuals feel psychologically safe, they are more likely to communicate proactively, share valuable insights, and contribute to problem-solving and innovation [19]. Speaking up fosters a culture of open dialogue, collaboration, and continuous improvement, leading to enhanced individual and organizational outcomes.

2.1   Voice Behaviors

The ways that employees communicate or do not communicate at work are called voice behaviors. Speaking up with ideas and concerns or asking questions demonstrates proactive voice behavior. Remaining silent is often a choice to protect oneself. Using voice behaviors can be predicated by distinct personality traits, i.e., previous experiences using speaking up, and work climates [20]. In the healthcare industry, organizations rely on their employees to contribute to all aspects of the work including active engagement in the change process.

Beginning at the individual level, the person decides whether using voice behaviors is safe and considers the consequences. Past experiences and observed reactions can influence a person's decision to use voice behaviors and speak up. It is the perception of being able to speak up without fear of the consequences to self-image, status, or career [9]. Sometimes, there is an adverse reaction to a person speaking up. Not all environments are conducive to or desire psychological safety—probably not the environments that a person would wish to work, but the threat is real in some organizations.

Employees experiencing burnout use fewer voice behaviors according to recent studies [21]. Burnout symptoms include anger, anxiety, depression, and fatigue and have hindered the willingness of employees to use voice behaviors in the clinical setting [22]. Burnout leads to lack of desire to do anything but the basic tasks, little motivation to report safety concerns, and increased isolation. Burnout affects both the individual and the organization. Burnout impacts the capacity of the person to express or participate in the coordination of patient care, safety behaviors, and innovation [23]. The lack of communication between care team members is often a contributor to errors that can result in harm to patients and employees.

Speaking up and using voice behaviors take energy. When energy is depleted, the individual has little motivation to engage in more than just their assigned duties. In deciding to speak up or to complete an incident report, a person weighs the benefit of exerting what little energy exists or using it for other purposes. It takes energy to speak up. Engaging in the discussion that typically comes with speaking up behavior also takes additional energy. For the depleted employee, it may require too much energy.

As burnout symptoms persist, attitudes toward patients, colleagues, and leaders may change. Positive interactions decrease, leading to a lack of voice behaviors. Healthcare organizations must recognize the intersection between burnout and voice behaviors that impact communication with patients and colleagues [24]. Cultivating a culture of psychological safety where employees feel a sense of belonging leads to greater use of voice behaviors for improved employee well-being and clinical outcomes.

2.2   The Impact of Psychological Safety on Voice Behaviors

Healthcare organizations pay close attention to their employee's perception of psychological safety within the organization. Most training has been directed toward leader development in creating cultures of belonging and inclusion. Recent studies have found that employees identify psychological safety in the organization but also among their teams and leaders. While the employee may feel safe raising concerns with their leader, they may be inhibited from speaking up in front of their colleagues. Individual factors like previous experiences speaking up, personal characteristics, or if they feel valued by the organization may influence their willingness to use voice behaviors [25].

In healthcare settings, psychological safety is critical for nursing teams that work interdependently. Many procedures and processes require two-person checks or team checks to ensure that no errors are made. High-volume, high-risk departments like hospital patient care units depend on team members giving feedback to each other. Nurses who feel psychologically safe give timely feedback, ask questions, and include team members in making care decisions. This leads to better outcomes and reduced harm to patients and colleagues.

However, understanding why healthcare professionals do not speak up is a critical factor in overcoming the lack of use of voice behaviors. Individual factors like fear contribute to a person's willingness to speak up. Fear can encompass many factors: fear of getting into trouble, retribution, and losing status in the peer group. By cultivating emotional well-being and creating a safe space for nurses to express themselves, healthcare organizations can address these fears and improve communication and collaboration among staff, ultimately benefiting the patients they serve.

2.3   Strategies to Build Voice Behaviors in Individuals

At the individual level, each participant joins an organization with unique experiences and perceptions about how voice behaviors are used and will be perceived by leaders. If a team member had a poor experience with asking questions of other team members in a previous role, the team member might not be willing to exercise voice behaviors until it is deemed psychologically safe. The following strategies may help.

1. **Practice giving feedback**
   Building confidence in speaking up takes practice. To build confidence, practice speaking up when nothing is on the line. Providing feedback to colleagues builds relationships and allows one to practice speaking up. John Gottman, a noted psychologist, developed a technique called 5:1 feedback. This technique calls for the individual to provide feedback on an average of five positive comments to every corrective comment. Catching colleagues doing the right thing encourages safe behavior and builds connection. When an error or unsafe behavior is observed, offering feedback to correct the behavior will be taken as constructive because the feedback is trusted.
2. **Ask questions**
   Creating an optimal learning environment constitutes a fundamental cornerstone in cultivating psychological well-being within teams. The practice of asking questions serves not only to enhance individual growth but also to foster knowledge within the team. When individuals are comfortable voicing questions, critical thinking improves. This particular approach allows the individual to explore ideas where doubt exists. It also encourages others to do the same. Set a goal while working to ask at least three questions each shift. The more you do it, the easier it becomes!

The phenomenon of voice behaviors, encompassing proactive communication, such as expressing ideas and concerns and deciding to withhold communication, plays a pivotal role in workplace dynamics. Factors such as personality traits, past experiences, and organizational climate influence the utilization of voice behaviors, which are integral to active employee engagement and change process. Recent investigations underscore the correlation between burnout and diminished voice behaviors in healthcare professionals, with burnout symptoms leading to reduced engagement, communication, and a lack of curiosity.

This interconnectedness between burnout and voice behaviors highlights the necessity for healthcare institutions to recognize their mutual influence, as burnout adversely affects both individual well-being and expression of critical aspects like patient care coordination and safety initiatives. Overcoming the barriers posed by burnout and fostering a culture of psychological safety within healthcare organizations are imperative to encourage voice behaviors, ultimately promoting employee well-being and enhancing clinical outcomes.

3   Psychological Safety Among Team Members

Building psychological safety among team members begins with the belief that asking questions, giving feedback, and admitting mistakes are okay [8]. When teams have high psychological safety, members experience inclusion, belonging, and diverse thinking, leading to high performance [26]. Individual team members contribute to team success and outcomes when they feel connected to other team members. However, research has shown that psychological safety among team members, especially in the healthcare setting, is lacking [4].

A wealth of scholarly research on organizational psychology and group dynamics underscores the assertion that familiarity and face-to-face communication among team members engender psychological safety [27]. The presence of familiarity, often cultivated through frequent interactions and interpersonal exchanges, humanizes team members, mitigating feelings of isolation and enhancing the likelihood of open and honest communication. Face-to-face interactions, characterized by nuanced cues such as facial expressions and body language, establish a context wherein individuals can better discern and interpret their counterparts' intentions, thereby minimizing miscommunication and fostering trust.

Direct communication promotes the exchange of diverse perspectives and ideas and bolsters cohesion and collaboration among team members. Familiarity, connection, and face-to-face communication contribute to psychological safety. Psychological safety strengthens team dynamics and organizational behavior. Psychological safety cultivates productive and engaged teams.

3.1   Status and Hierarchy

Healthcare institutions have traditionally operated within a hierarchical framework, wherein distinct occupational roles, educational backgrounds, and experience levels contribute to pronounced power differentials. This phenomenon is particularly evident in cases involving professions lower in the hierarchy, nonclinical staff, and recent graduates. Research by Omuri et al. [28] highlights that healthcare practitioners tend to be more inclined to assert their opinions when engaging with individuals possessing lesser experiential insights. Pertinently, the perceived level of psychological safety intertwined with the prevailing power distance dynamics significantly influences the efficacy of collaborative teams [29].

3.2   Strategies to Build Psychological Safety in Teams:

1. **Reduce power distance**
   Fostering a reduction in power distance revolves around appreciating how individuals with perceived authority can employ certain behaviors to temper

hierarchical disparities. When operating as a team, it is crucial to recognize the diverse expertise and varied experiences that each member contributes, enriching the collective effort. By genuinely acknowledging and creating space for every team member's voice, we reinforce the notion that each perspective holds value and importance.

2. **Provide opportunities for collaboration**

Collaboration enhances teamwork by leveraging diverse skills and perspectives to yield innovative solutions, fostering accountability and commitment among members. Working with colleagues toward a common goal allows all members to contribute to the team's success. The exchange of ideas promotes open communication, clarifying misconceptions, and building a common understanding, while group learning contributes to individual growth. Collaborative teamwork also facilitates effective conflict resolution through open dialogue and compromise, ultimately cultivating a culture of trust, respect, and shared success that amplifies team effectiveness.

3. **Promote team checks and team coaching**

The primary objective of conducting a team check is to prevent potential errors. The supplementary scrutiny applied to a task functions as a safeguard, intercepting potential mistakes before they manifest into deleterious outcomes. Team checks provide mutual support. The intention is not to punish but to avoid mistakes altogether. Team checks effectively establish a mechanism by which we collectively ensure the precision of our work, underpinned by a sense of mutual vigilance. Team coaching fosters an environment where each member assumes the role of a coach, directing one another toward correct actions and reducing the possibility of error.

4   Psychological Safety in Organizations

In an era where the healthcare landscape has grown increasingly intricate, demanding enhanced teamwork, organizations emphasize involving personnel at every hierarchical level [30]. Within the realm of healthcare, the identification of medical errors and safety incidents heavily relies on self-reporting. Thus, psychological safety has gained importance in motivating all staff members to express their apprehensions confidently. Establishing an atmosphere of security and openness is a pivotal factor influencing the dynamic between leaders and employees, from routine interactions to managing critical safety scenarios.

Central to this notion is cultivating the individual's confidence that posing questions, raising concerns, or offering suggestions will not result in retribution or ridicule. Healthcare institutions employ a range of frameworks, policies, and protocols designed to nurture these communicative behaviors. Leaders recognize their employees who speak up and encourage others to do the same.

4.1   Organizational Silence

Organizational silence is when employees withhold their thoughts, opinions, concerns, or ideas instead of expressing them within the workplace. Withholding one's voice can stem from various factors, such as fear of repercussions, perceived futility in speaking up, or a lack of psychological safety. In such environments, employees remain quiet, leading to missed opportunities, decreased innovation, and hindered problem-solving. This silence can manifest at different levels, from individual employees to entire teams, and can significantly affect an organization's overall performance and growth.

There are several underlying causes for organizational silence. One common factor is the fear of negative consequences, such as reprimand or job loss for voicing dissenting opinions or highlighting problems. When the perception of large power distances or authority gradients is significant, employees might feel that their voices hold less weight than those of higher-ups. Moreover, if past instances have shown that speaking up is met with indifference or hostility, individuals might remain silent to avoid similar experiences. Organizational silence leads to unresolved concerns, decreased morale, and disengaged employees. Withholding voice behaviors and a culture that reinforces silence result in a lack of innovation, adaptability, and an inability to navigate change in an ever-changing industry like healthcare.

Creating a culture of open communication and psychological safety is crucial to addressing organizational silence. Leaders should actively encourage employees to share their thoughts and concerns, ensuring that their voices are valued and heard. Implementing incident reporting systems, leader rounding, and clear channels for raising concerns can help alleviate fears associated with speaking up. By celebrating diverse viewpoints and acknowledging the contributions of all members, organizations can break down the barriers of silence and unlock the full potential of their workforce [31].

4.2   Measuring Psychological Safety
         in Healthcare Organizations

Measuring psychological safety within healthcare organizations is critical as it directly impacts patients' and healthcare professionals' quality of care, teamwork, and overall well-being. Various approaches can be employed to assess the level of psychological safety within these contexts.

1. Culture of Safety surveys:
   One effective method involves using surveys designed to measure the perception of psychological safety. These tools typically include questions that address fear in response to speaking up, comfort in sharing ideas, and perceptions of leadership responsiveness. Responses are analyzed to generate insights into the prevailing level of psychological safety. To encourage participation, safety

surveys are conducted anonymously. Survey results are shared with leaders and associates to create discussions that lead to improvement strategies.

2. Incident Reporting and Feedback Analysis

Monitoring incident reporting and feedback mechanisms can also offer insights into psychological safety. A lack of reports about safety concerns or errors could indicate a culture of silence and low psychological safety. Conversely, increased reporting could suggest that employees feel comfortable raising concerns and expect follow-up. By analyzing the content of these reports, organizations can better understand the risks to safety and mitigate those risks to protect patients and employees from harm.

3. Team Dynamics and Performance

Another approach involves observing team dynamics and performance indicators. Open discussions, constructive feedback, and collaborative problem-solving reflect high psychological safety. Conversely, teams with low psychological safety might exhibit poor communication, unaddressed conflicts, and decreased participation [32].

Case Study: Safety Huddle
Example when psychological safety is present:
During the safety huddle, each team member openly shared their look back and look ahead, including errors or near misses that occurred or could have occurred without any fear of punishment or retribution. Everyone recognized the importance of learning from each other's mistakes to prevent errors in the future. The team felt comfortable discussing potential safety concerns, and they worked together to come up with solutions.

Example when psychological safety is not present:
During the safety huddle, team members hesitated to share their look back or look ahead, and no one mentioned any errors or near misses. Everyone was afraid of being punished or embarrassed if they spoke up. As a result, the team missed out on valuable insights and learnings that could have prevented future errors. The team failed to identify potential safety concerns and did not work together to find solutions, which put patients and staff at risk.

---

5   Conclusion

The importance of psychological safety in healthcare organizations, specifically in nursing, is the focus of this book chapter. As work becomes more team oriented and interdependent, fostering psychological safety is vital for creating supportive work environments that enhance employee engagement, performance, and overall organizational success. Effective communication and teamwork, as well as individual well-being, are promoted through psychological safety, and it has implications across individual, team, and organizational levels of analysis. Due to the complexity of nursing, the need for psychological safety is rising, given the increased pressures and challenges associated with the field.

Key Points

- Psychological safety is essential in healthcare settings and has been linked to positive outcomes like increased employee engagement, improved psychological health and safety behaviors, and enhanced learning.
- Psychological safety among healthcare professionals, including nurses, is crucial for effective communication, teamwork, and patient-centered care.
- Speaking up, or voice behaviors, is vital to psychological safety, enabling individuals to share their perspectives, raise concerns, and contribute to decision-making.
- Organizational silence is a reflection of a safety culture that is not safe to use voice behaviors regardless of the consequences. Silence is rewarded.
- Burnout symptoms hinder the willingness of employees to use voice behaviors, which can negatively impact psychological safety in the workplace.

References

1. Edmondson A. Psychological safety, trust and learning in organizations: a group lens. In: Kramer RM, editor. Trust and distrust in organizations: Dilemmas and approaches. New York, NY: Russell Sage Foundation; 2004. p. 239–72.
2. Liang J, Farh C, Farh J. Psychological antecedents of promotive and prohibitive voice: a two-wave examination. Acad Manage J. 2012;55:71–92. https://doi.org/10.5465/amj.2010.0176.
3. Edmondson AC, Bransby DP. Psychological safety comes of age observed themes in an established literature. Ann Rev Org Psychol Org Behav. 2023;10:55–78. https://doi.org/10.1146/annurev-orgpsych-120920-055217.
4. O'Donovan R, McAuliffe E. Exploring psychological safety in healthcare teams to inform the development of interventions: combining observational, survey and interview data. BMC Health Serv Res. 2020;20:810. https://doi.org/10.1186/s12913-020-05646-z.
5. Schein EH. Personal and organizational change through group methods: the laboratory approach. New York, NY: Wiley; 1965.
6. Brown R. Politeness theory: exemplar and exemplary. In: Rock, the legacy of Simon Ashe: Essays in cognition and social psychology. Hillsdale, NJ: Erlbaum; 1990. p. 23–37.
7. Edmondson A. Speaking up in the operating room: how team leaders promote learning in interdisciplinary action teams. J Manage Studies. 2003;40(6):1419–52. https://doi.org/10.1111/1467-6486.00386.
8. Edmondson AC. Psychological safety, trust, and learning in organizations: a group-level lens. In: Kramer RM, Cook KS, editors. Trust and distrust in organizations: Dilemmas and approaches. Russell Sage Foundation; 2004. p. 239–72.
9. Grailey KE, Murray E, Reader T, Brett SJ. The presence and potential impact of psychological safety in the healthcare setting: an evidence synthesis. BMC Health Serv Res. 2021;21:773. https://doi.org/10.1186/s12913-021-06740-6.
10. Dollard M, Bakker A. Psychosocial safety climate as a precursor to conducive work environments, psychological health problems, and employee engagement. J Occup Org Psychol. 2010;3(83):579–99. https://doi.org/10.1348/096317909x470690.

11. Kwon C, Han S, Nicolaides A. The impact of psychological safety on transformative learning in the workplace: a quantitative study. J Workplace Learn. 2020;7(32):533–47. https://doi.org/10.1108/jwl-04-2020-0057.
12. Hammond W. Psychosocial correlates of medical mistrust among African American men. Am J Community Psychol. 2010;1–2(45):87–106. https://doi.org/10.1007/s10464-009-9280-6.
13. Seibert M, Pfaff H, Scholten N, Kuntz L. Do trained nurses feel more psychologically safe? Results from a multi-level modelling approach. Nurs Open. 2021;6(8):3024–35. https://doi.org/10.1002/nop2.1015.
14. Bülbül S, İşiaçık S, Aytaç S. Measurement of perceived psychological safety: integration, review, and evidence for the scale in the context of Turkey. J Econ Culture Soc. 2022;65:15–28. https://doi.org/10.26650/jecs2021-974757.
15. Edmondson AC, Lei Z. Psychological safety: the history, renaissance, and future of an interpersonal construct; 2014. Retrieved June 25, 2023, from https://annualreviews.org/doi/full/10.1146/annurev-orgpsych-031413-091305
16. Li H, Chen Y, Zheng J, Fang Y, Yang Y, Skitmore M, Rusch R, Jiang T. The influence of the psychological contract on the safety of performance of construction workers in China. Engineering, Construction and Architectural Management; 2022. https://doi.org/10.1108/ECAM-09-2022-0854.
17. Mendelsohn D. Self in medicine: determinants of physician well-being and future directions in improving wellness. Med Educ. 2022;56(1):48–55. https://doi.org/10.1111/medu.14671.
18. Kerrissey MJ, Hayirli TC, Bhanja A, Stark N, Hardy J, Peabody CR. How psychological safety and feeling heard relate to burnout and adaptation amid uncertainty. Health Care Manage Rev. 47(4):308–16. https://doi.org/10.1097/HMR.0000000000000338.
19. Wawersik DM, Boutin ER Jr, Gore T, Palaganas JC. Individual characteristics that promote or prevent psychological safety and error reporting in healthcare: a systematic review. J Healthc Leadersh. 2023;15:59–70. https://doi.org/10.2147/JHL.S369242.
20. Um-e-Rubbab, Naqvi SMMR. Employee voice behavior as a critical factor for organizational sustainability in the telecommunications industry. PLoS One. 2020;15(9):e0238451. https://doi.org/10.1371/journal.pone.0238451.
21. Lam CF, Johnson HH, Song LJ, Wu W, Lee C, Chen Z. More depleted, speak up more? A daily examination of the benefit and cost of depletion for voice behavior and voice endorsement. J Organ Behav. 2022;43(6):983–1000. https://doi.org/10.1002/job.2620.
22. Mudallal RH, Othman WM, Al Hassan NF. Nurses' burnout: the influence of leader empowering behaviors, work conditions, and demographic traits. Inquiry. 2017;54:46958017724944. https://doi.org/10.1177/0046958017724944.
23. Sherf E, Parke MR, Isaakyan S. Distinguishing voice and silence at work: unique relationships with perceived impact, psychological safety, and burnout. Acad Manage J. 2021;64:114–48. https://doi.org/10.5465/amj.2018.1428.
24. Murthy VH. Confronting health worker burnout and well-being. N Engl J Med. 2022;387(7):577–9. https://doi.org/10.1056/NEJMp2207252.
25. O'Donovan R, DeBrun A, McAuliffe E. Healthcare professionals experience of psychological safety, voice, and silence. Front Psychol. 2021;12:626689. https://doi.org/10.3389/fpsych2021.626689.
26. Bresman H, Edmondson A. Exploring the relationship between team diversity, psychological safety, and team performance: evidence from pharmaceutical drug development. Harvard Business School; 2022. Working Paper, No. 22-055, February 2022
27. Reese J, Simmons R, Barnard J. Assertion practices and beliefs among nurses and physicians on an inpatient pediatric medical unit. Hosp Pediatr. 2016;6:275–81.
28. Omura M, Stone TE, Maguire J, et al. Exploring Japanese nurses' perceptions of the relevance and use of assertive communication in healthcare: a qualitative study informed by the theory of planned behaviour. NurseEduc Today. 2018;67:100–7.
29. Appelbaum NP, Lockeman KS, Orr S, Huff TA, Hogan CJ, Queen BA, Dow AW. Perceived influence of power distance, psychological safety, and team cohesion on team effectiveness. J Interprof Care. 2020;34(1):20–6. https://doi.org/10.1080/13561820.2019.1633290.

30. Murray JS, Kelly S, Hanover C. Promoting psychological safety in healthcare organizations. Mil Med. 2022;187:808–10. https://doi.org/10.1093/milmed/usac041.
31. Shojaie S, Matin HZ, Barani G. Analyzing the infrastructures of organizational silence and ways to get rid of it. Procedia Soc Behav Sci. 2011;30:1731–5. https://doi.org/10.1016/j.sbspro.2011.10.334.
32. Frazier M, Fainshmidt S, Klinger R, Pezeshkan A, Vracheva V. Psychological safety: A meta-analytic review and extension. Pers Psychol. 2017;1(70):113–65. https://doi.org/10.1111/peps.12183.

Interprofessional Teams and Communication as a Foundation for Patient Safety

Lori Lynn Fewster-Thuente and William E. Gordon

1 Interprofessional Teams and Communication as a Foundation for Patient Safety

The first documented interprofessional (IP) healthcare teams began on Dutch maternity wards between physicians and midwives in the 1800s. It was noted at this time that poor collaboration, often due to hierarchical structures, resulted in poor patient outcomes [1]. That remains true to the present day. Interprofessional healthcare teams began in earnest in the USA in the 1980s. The World Health Organization defines interprofessional teams as those who learn about, from, and with one another to obtain optimal patient outcomes [2]. When functioning optimally, IP healthcare teams can reduce patient length of stay and cost, improve patient and provider satisfaction, and decrease provider burnout. The purpose of this chapter is to denote the tools and strategies used by high-performing IP teams (HPIPTs) and their impact on patient safety.

L. L. Fewster-Thuente (✉)
Rosalind Franklin University of Medicine and Science, College of Nursing, College of Health Professions, North Chicago, IL, USA
e-mail: lori.thuente@rosalindfranklin.edu

W. E. Gordon
Rosalind Franklin University of Medicine and Science, College of Health Professions, North Chicago, IL, USA
e-mail: william.gordon@rosalindfranklin.edu

© The Author(s), under exclusive license to Springer Nature Switzerland AG 2024
C. A. Oster, J. S. Braaten (eds.), *The Nexus between Nursing and Patient Safety*, https://doi.org/10.1007/978-3-031-53158-3_11

2   Background

2.1   Teams

Like all teams, interprofessional teams are intentional in their composition, the ways in which the team members agree to operate, and the values they hold. The distinguishing composition of interprofessional teams is that their membership is composed of people holding diverse viewpoints, skills, and training. Professionally, such teams are made up of members of more than one profession, which in healthcare means a diversity of licenses, scopes of practice, and expertise.

Interprofessional teams are focused on positive patient outcomes and are organized with that goal or a series of goals in mind. To achieve those outcomes, interprofessional teams must first acknowledge the value of team members and their contributions to the overall team goals. To achieve equity among professions, particularly in a culture that seems to value some healthcare professions over others, the structure of the team is very important.

In systems thinking, behavior is believed to follow structure. This point can be illustrated by the hypothetical that in a room with no doors or windows, egress would be difficult. To leave the confines of this room, one would potentially break through a wall. Systems thinking suggests that if the structure of the room includes a doorway that passes through one of the walls, it will shape the behaviors of those inside as they choose to leave. They are most likely to exit the room utilizing the doorway. In other words, a doorway influences the behaviors of people in ways that are predictable. People will pass through the doorway because, within the room's structure, it is the simplest, most logical course of action.

This would suggest that when teams are formed by hierarchical structures where some individuals are valued more than others (or where power is unequally distributed), the manner in which that team is organized will impact every team member. Depending on the situation, those influences may or may not benefit the team. On a team where a single individual or a group of individuals are designated to be *in charge*, the effects on how the team members function are notable. In an emergent situation, for example in a burning building, having a leader identified who has the skills to lead others to safety validates the hierarchical structure. In that situation, a single leader mitigates assessing who on the team has relevant education or experience. In other, complex situations, however, having a single individual or a small group of individuals who are believed to be uniquely talented or trained or have relevant experience may structurally impede the contributions of others to find solutions. In healthcare in particular, when one provider may not have all of the relevant information or a clear perspective, the patient (as well as the whole team) would benefit from the expression of additional viewpoints. This argument is not to minimize the role of a hierarchical leader who is open to suggestions, but rather is most relevant to those teams in which a leader has conveyed that they may neither listen to nor be interested in other viewpoints. A minimization of top-down hierarchies systemically increases the opportunity and likelihood of divergent ideas and opinions.

If the opportunity to build a nonhierarchical team occurs, such an organizational structure affects the frequency and nature of communication on the team, as well. If open and honest communication is understood to be unwelcome vis-à-vis the structure and positioning of leadership, as with the example of persons attempting to leave an enclosed room, individuals must and will seek their own solutions. This may include non-direct or incomplete communication, undermining the team's effectiveness. If the metaphorical door has been provided (meaning the structure allows or encourages it), communication can flow more freely. If that same door is closed or is nonexistent, team members cannot and will not contribute their knowledge, experience, or wisdom in manners that support the team in reaching its goal(s). This can negatively affect patient outcomes and potential safety.

What Distinguishes a Team?

In order to build more effective interprofessional teams as a foundation for patient safety, it is important to distinguish teams from groups, as they have many similarities, but also some clear distinctions. To envision these differences, let us consider a gathering of people who are at the intersection of two very busy streets. These people all want to get safely to the other side, and they will be watching for traffic signals to indicate when it is safe for them to step off the curb. They have arrived at this point individually or as part of a small contingent, and they share an intention to cross the street at the next available, safe opportunity. How would you classify this gathering? One option would be to say that they all have the same intention and are watching for the same signals and will, by convention, step off the curb at approximately the same time. If we were satisfied that these conditions were met, we might conclude that this gathering is in substantial alignment with the definition of a team: they have similar intentions, they are following the same set of signals and are likely to act in near unison when the light changes. Although their alignment with that definition is close, this gathering of individuals has not adopted a goal that they both value and hold in common. That is, while their individual intentions may be similar, they have not collectively negotiated a mutually valued goal, nor have they reached any form of agreement surrounding commitment to that goal.

If we look back at our gathering on the street corner, it becomes evident that each member is committed to getting themselves (or perhaps even their small subgroup) safely across the street when the light changes. Although that goal exists, it is not inclusive of everyone who has gathered there. The people present are not focused on what they will do together and as a unit. They do not hold a commitment that assures that everyone on that street corner will be able to get across the street safely when the light changes. Potentially, in fact, should one member of the gathering trip and fall on the way to the other side of the street, we cannot assume that others will stop and assist someone who has fallen. While the goal to get across the street is present within individuals, there is no apparent commitment to getting everyone across. In the absence of this outcome being valued or even necessarily agreed upon, our gathering of people on the street is classified as a group rather than a team.

For the group crossing the street to be considered a team, they must have a mutual commitment to everyone safely getting across the street, and individuals must set aside their personal goals in favor of the success of everyone present. If everyone present is not successful in reaching safety on the other side, the gathering of people is functioning as a group and not a team.

These fundamentals of team structure and organization, communication, and shared language are also foundations for the development of collaborative teams. By removing the implied power struggles of hierarchy, which changes the team's organizational structure, clearer communication and an agreed-upon transactional language can be implemented. Such changes enable the team members to more easily work together toward their agreed-upon goals. It is this, in the absence of competition and with an understanding that other team members are watching out for one another with the goal of success, that empowers the team to achieve outcomes that might otherwise have been out of reach.

2.2 Evolution of IP Teams

Although the first IP teams were noted in the 1800s, the concept and practice of interprofessional healthcare teams gained traction in the 1980s and 1990s when patient errors began to be counted and categorized through research. The landmark report *To Err is Human* being published in 1999 found that over 98,000 people were dying each year due to medical errors [3]. The Joint Commission, the agency that accredits healthcare organizations, found that over 80% of these errors were due to miscommunication and therefore preventable. This event prompted additional responses, including The Joint Commission's 2003 National Patient Safety Goals as well as the Institute of Medicine's release of "Patient Safety: New Standard for Care" [4, 5]. The reports spotlighted the need for improved efficiencies and effectiveness of communication on teams of all types.

As healthcare systems and accrediting organizations began to understand the scope of human error, and the mitigation of error by IP teams, teaching interprofessional education (IPE) and implementing interprofessional practice models gained popularity. While providers can learn to be high-functioning team members "on the job," those who have IPE in their training program curricula will be team-ready on their first day. Almost every healthcare education accrediting organization now requires IPE to be in the curriculum and for their graduates to be competent as measured by their individual programs and professions.

Unfortunately, most colleges and universities still offer very little in terms of IPE and continue to train their students in silos, where they have few interactions with students in other healthcare programs. Most schools may offer an IPE "day" or "event" in which students are brought together for a limited time and asked to work together on an assignment. Unless IPE is deemed vital to the mission of the college or university and integrated longitudinally throughout each curriculum, students in individual programs fail to see the value in these types of events.

Additionally, it is imperative that an opportunity be provided for students to gain experience in clinical practice in a team-based format. This interprofessional clinical practice (IPCP) provides learners opportunities to operationalize what they know in real-time/real-situation formats and allows them to improve their skills both as individual team members and collectively as teams as a whole. The transition from being a novice learner in a team-based environment to becoming a member of a high-performing interprofessional team (HPIPT) relies on experience as much as it does knowledge. However, this may be difficult as there may be few providers to be role models.

One of the key evolutionary points in present-day HPIPT is that the team structure must change from the hierarchical, physician-led teams to a situational model, in that the healthcare provider most relevant to the current patient problem is the leader at that moment (see textbox – Leadership and Its Impact on Team Behaviors). This facilitative role is dynamic and can change in a moment depending on the situation. IP teams are vital due to the complexity of patients' illnesses. No one provider can have all of the education, knowledge, and experience needed to treat today's complex patients.

Another vital component of HPIPT is trust between team members. Historically, this trust has been based on hierarchy and was between the physician and the nurse in which the physician trusted the nurse to do what they ordered and the nurse trusted that the order was correct. Now, with multiple members on teams, each one must support one another and be confident that the job each one performs is correct. This can be difficult on teams where the providers may change each shift. Members must also feel safe to voice their opinions without fear. If members cannot trust one another, the pursuit of team-based care and the resulting positive patient outcomes is moot.

A distinct change to current teams is that each provider needs to have respect for their teammates and their professions. Healthcare providers are highly educated and trained, and each deserves respect for what they bring to patient care. If a provider feels disrespected by one or more teammates, then they may withhold needed patient information for fear of negative consequences, which in turn can result in a serious error. If it is a safety issue, team members must speak up, without fear of retribution. If someone chooses not to do their part, they not only fail the team, but they also fail the patient.

2.3   Types of Failures

Sadly, team failures still exist. Given that healthcare providers are human beings and not machines, the likelihood of failure remains significant. Errors in communication, memory, skill, communication, and collaboration all continue. Additionally, no two patients are the same so what may have worked previously with one patient may not work on another.

One of the major sources of failure is communication, both expressive and receptive. Lack of communication is the basis for most errors. Providers withholding information, intentionally or not, fail the patient. Unidirectional verbal patient orders often result in errors because it is difficult to look back to double-check. Hierarchical issues can impact the exchange of information, especially if the receiver is afraid to question or repeat back what they heard. Language and cultural barriers can also result in errors.

The emergent nature of patient illness can be a source of error. When patients have life-threatening illnesses or injuries, providers are calling out information and orders, and there is no time for discussion or consensus. Without a standard procedure for providers to deliver care, vital data may be missed and cause undue harm.

Provider deficits such as extreme fatigue, hunger, personal issues, or influence of drugs or alcohol may result in preventable negative outcomes. Occasionally, providers "work around" a safety process because it may be too cumbersome, etc. and inadvertently make a mistake. System issues such as understaffing, lack of proper training, outdated technology, and inefficient processes frequently lead to patient errors.

Sadly, after years of competition within the educational system to achieve the high standards for licensure in healthcare, many team members continue to function as if they are solo providers, rather than being in a team-based environment. The result is that prior experiences and former ways of doing our work tend to creep back into our cadre of tools, skills, and practices. The return of individual members to their own solo practice will most likely negate the commitment of team members to the identified goal(s) for the team. If members can detect a lack of commitment to their shared goal, or those individuals have supplanted the value of that goal with another, the coherence or cohesion of the team is soon lost. In team-based care, a core reality and assumption must be that everyone on the team, working from the same understanding, participates in the team's achievement of its goals. Lack of commitment to that on any individual's behalf may sabotage the entire team's focus and ultimately the positive outcome.

2.4 High-Risk Context for Communication Failures

Depending on the study, the monetary cost of medical errors can be as high as $20B per year with approximately 100,000–250,000 people losing their lives annually. That can be envisioned as the equivalent of two jumbo jets crashing every day. This figure does not take into account the morbidity and emotional harm from permanent injury, inability to work, or death. Consider if a patient were to have surgery to remove a diseased kidney but the surgical team did not communicate clearly and accidentally removed the healthy kidney. The patient is now left without a functioning kidney and will have to be on dialysis multiple times per week for the rest of their life. Between the cost of ongoing treatment, missed work, and emotional toll of chronic illness, the surgical team has unintentionally done the exact opposite of what it set out to do, which was to heal the patient.

These preventable errors are called *never events* or *sentinel events* [6]. These sentinel errors fall under various categories such as:

- Wrong site surgery
- Infant or patient abduction
- Administration of the incorrect blood product leading to harm
- Physical or sexual assault of a patient or provider
- Patient suicide

- Failure to rescue
- Unanticipated death of an infant or mother
- Patient elopement leading to harm or death
- Medication error leading to harm or death

These *never events* may potentially harm the patient physically, mentally, or spiritually. Even if these events do not result in a negative outcome, they may be thought by some to be inconsequential. It is important to affirm that such events have existential overtones. How long will the patient be out of work? How does the experience change perceptions either of oneself within the family system? What are the consequences for their families who now may have to care for the person for the rest of their lives? How long will recovery take, and how does that impact both the current employment and possible future job opportunities for the patient? If they were the primary breadwinner for the household, the remaining family members may have to work multiple jobs to make up the salary difference. Such errors may have catastrophic impacts that we do not see or understand but are of critical importance to the patient and their family. It is vital that we prevent these errors from happening.

2.5   A Culture That Supports Communication Success

While we have traditionally held the relative successes or failures in team performance as an issue of leadership, when we consider high-performance healthcare teams, we must look at the background in which this team has functioned. Institutional culture may profoundly affect the ability and willingness to create teams where all members' knowledge, skills, and experience can be valued. It is vital that when team members commit to working together, they recognize that the team now functions as a coherent unit. By this we mean that all team members are fully responsible for the successes and failures of the team as a whole. There are no single winners or losers. Team members are bound together by their mutually held agreements and must commit themselves fully to its achievement. When the team succeeds, they succeed. When the team fails, they must also acknowledge their contributions in whatever form to that failure.

Systemic issues may impede either the formation or the functioning of a team. In a hierarchical organization, for example, it may appear impossible to create optimized teams. This may be due to a perception that those charged with overseeing the entire organization may not be supportive of the changes required to move toward nonhierarchical collaboration. In truth, because of the ways in which nonhierarchical teams can function and the results they may produce, they will stand out not for their differences in structure, but because of the results they produce. Wise directors in an organization watch for approaches in teamwork that produce the desired results and ask themselves what, if any, of those can be translated to other teams. It is, without question, easier to build a culture of optimized teams if the corporate leadership is outright and initially supportive. Barring that, however, successful teams can influence the course of the organization by their own results.

Leadership and Its Impact on Team Behaviors

It has been said that team structure is the alchemy by which teams learn to function optimally. To understand that adage, we need to distinguish what is meant by this concept in a team-based context and what behaviors help teams to succeed.

The concept of leadership on healthcare teams has changed dramatically over the past few decades. At one time, it was assumed that medical doctors were the *de facto* heads of healthcare teams, given the extensive educational requirements of their discipline. Indeed, physicians were understood to be the only *doctors* on the team, a semantic mistake that continues to change rapidly as healthcare professions increasingly require the achievement of doctoral study within individual disciplines. For example, where it had at one time been assumed that the head of the team was a *Doctor of Medicine*, it is increasingly common for there to be other doctors on the team as well. For example, team members may bear titles such as *Doctor of Physical Therapy*, *Doctor of Pharmacy*, *Doctor of Nurse Anesthesia Practice*, *Doctor of Nursing Practice*, and perhaps *Doctor of Social Work* or *Doctor of Ministry*. These disciplines may have very similar academic profiles to the medical doctor. While this list is not inclusive, it does point to the reality that increasingly healthcare providers are achieving terminal degree status in their disciplines. This means that the *Doctor of Medicine (MD)* stands out not because of their doctorate, per se, but rather because of their discipline or course of study. The ultimate outcome of this new reality is that there are many people on a healthcare team who are equally qualified to lead when their information, education, and experiences are deemed most appropriate to meet the needs of the patient.

Leadership on a healthcare team is thus deemed situational, shifting from person to person as their unique qualifications are called for. It is not determined so much by title as it is by utility.

The second portion of the concept of structure as alchemy to team functioning has to do with the manner in which team members present themselves, defining expectations and parameters that will either encourage or discourage team interactions. The messaging to team members is fairly simple and considerably more transparent than may be anticipated. How a leader reacts, for example, to input or questions by team members (such as responding with eye rolls, sighs, reactivity to be challenged or questioned) may clearly communicate to team members that their opinions and doubts may not matter. Conversely, when one takes the time to invite, listen to, and consider team member input, they convey to participants that not only is what they are attempting to communicate in this instance going to be valued but so will future efforts. Team members will be more likely to provide insights and assistance when they know that they will be well received than they will if their ideas, comments, or suggestions are dismissed either actively or passively. In other words, how leaders react to team member input will determine how much input team members are likely to offer.

Paying attention to how their team acts and reacts is a perfect opportunity for self-reflection, asking ourselves, "In what way(s) am I contributing to these specific team behaviors?" Perhaps more directly to the point, we must ask ourselves how we may need to change to elevate team functioning. Team interactions have a clear context and do not occur in a vacuum.

3   Process: Tools for Success

3.1   IP Teams

There is no single formulation or algorithm that assures optimal team functioning one hundred percent of the time. There are significant things that teams can do to elevate their functioning. In hopes of alleviating these types of errors, healthcare systems have adopted tools and strategies to put preventative safeguards into place. One such strategy is that healthcare systems have been implementing IP teams across their systems:

- Code Red/Blue/Rapid Response Teams: These interprofessional teams are comprised of specifically trained and designated providers, located in the hospital, who are available 24/7 and are called when a patient, employee, or visitor has been found to have cardiac arrest (Red) or respiratory arrest (Blue) or is in imminent danger of doing so. The teams are comprised of nurses, respiratory therapists, physicians, pharmacists, and other pertinent providers. While these teams can be called by anyone, including visitors (for patients), they are usually called by nurses or nursing assistants. Code Teams provide lifesaving treatment, stabilization, and assistance with transfer to the appropriate unit if necessary. Rapid Response Teams are similar, but the goal is to notify the team prior to the arrest, when the patient is decompensating (dropping blood pressure, respiratory or heart rate) in hopes of preventing a cardiac or respiratory arrest. Both of these types of teams have demonstrated significant decreases in cardiac/respiratory arrest and overall mortality [7].
- Behavioral Health Teams: These are Rapid Response Teams for behavioral health issues that arise on nonbehavioral health units. These IP teams are comprised of psychiatrists, psych-mental health nurses and nurse practitioners, therapists, social workers, and patient care technicians. They are trained to assess, intervene, and educate both patients and other providers. These teams are called when a patient has a distinct change in mood. A patient may become extremely agitated, angry, violent, and threatening or express suicidal ideation, which is often more than the current provider is trained to handle. There are several validated measures to use to assess the patient; most are based on age. A Behavioral Health Team is educated in de-escalation techniques and can intervene in safe ways to prevent harm to either the patient or the providers.

- Massive Transfusion Teams: Trauma centers have found that hemorrhage is the most common cause of death of the patient following arrival at the hospital. A specially trained IP team is required to return a patient to normal hemostasis following a massive hemorrhage from either a trauma, labor, or surgical issue. The team members come from anesthesia, surgery, blood bank, intensive care, and often the hospital quality/risk team. The team has been trained to follow an exact, evidence-based protocol to administer packed red blood cell, platelets, and plasma. Each team member has a specific role in the process, including the quality risk team who is there to document the care provided and, upon conclusion, try to find the root cause analysis of the event so as to prevent the incident from occurring again. These events are always emergent and therefore difficult to plan for with both staffing and supplies. Key factors in survival are being able to accurately assess how much blood the patient has lost, as well as the type and amount of products the patient needs. Blood products expire and are not always readily available. In addition, products such as AB type are very rare, and often hospitals do not have enough of one type or another. Teams must communicate across teams, especially in the event of a mass casualty disaster when multiple patients arrive at the hospital simultaneously so as to distribute their blood product supply equitably [8].
- Workplace Violence Teams: Workplace violence in healthcare occurs four times more often than in other settings, and 20% or more of nurses have been its victims. Congress has initiated legislation to mitigate workplace violence, but no bills have yet been passed [9, 10]. The American Hospital Association (AHA) has lobbied against this legislation as it would be very costly to comply. The AHA, however, does want the federal government to implement laws that prosecute and criminalize the perpetrators as it happens in other industries such as the airlines [11].

The Centers for Disease Control have categorized workplace violence into four types:

- Criminal intent—the perpetrator has no connection to the organization (i.e., a nurse getting mugged in the parking lot).
- Patient on provider—the most common type. Usually occurs in emergency rooms, psychiatric facilities, and long-term care organizations.
- Worker on worker—this is generally bullying and often based on a hierarchical system.
- Personal relationship—when a domestic issue (i.e., partner or spouse) crosses over into the workplace [12].

Organizations such as The Joint Commission and Occupational Health and Safety Association are now requiring that healthcare systems put policies into place to prevent these injuries from occurring [13]. Any incident must be thoroughly investigated and reported. Part of the report must state what is being done to prevent this from happening again. In order to maintain accreditation, teams must be trained as to how to identify risk signs, utilize appropriate communication skills to prevent or manage conflict, respond appropriately to victims of violence, and conduct ongoing training for all healthcare employees.

- Newborn/Infant Abduction Teams: A Code Pink is called when there is the suspected abduction of a newborn or infant. The protocol that each hospital has in place might vary slightly, but the overall goal is to prevent the abduction. The first step is to limit access to neonatal and perinatal units to parents and staff. Proper identification is issued to both the parents and the infant upon birth or admission. These units are to remain locked at all times, and only those with proper identification will be admitted. All hospital staff must be trained to require the identification or refuse admittance. The primary IP team members are the staff of the unit from which the infant was taken and the security staff. All unit staff and security are trained to understand the abduction risk factors, which may include:
- Prior abduction of an infant or child by a family member or friend
  - Newborn or infant removed, or prior child, from parental custody due to abuse or neglect
  - Family history of domestic violence
  - Parental custody cases
  - Parental abuse of alcohol, drugs, or known mental illness

The first step the team takes is to call the Code Pink, which alerts the security team and locks down most, if not all, of the hospital exits. This step is intended to prohibit the abductor from leaving the building. Hospital staff communicates and collaborates to thoroughly inspect the unit and adjoining units. All bags large enough to hold an infant will be searched. Should the infant not be found, police will be contacted immediately. A root cause analysis will be conducted following this event to determine where the system broke down and implement changes to ensure that it does not happen again.

- Transitions of Care: Transitions of Care teams are one of the most vital teams a hospital can have to optimize patient outcomes. These IP teams are initiated when patients are transitioning to another care setting or to home. Failure to transition patients successfully causes unnecessary and costly readmission, medication-related errors, and potentially irreversible harm. The members on these IP teams are case managers, nurses, physicians, pharmacists, physical therapists, and transporters. Their primary focus is to create a plan that is fourfold around medication management, education of patient and family, ensuring that all information is communicated to the next level of care, and follow-up care which is scheduled and communicated.

The one thing each of these teams has in common is the goal to keep both patients and providers alive and safe.

3.2   Communication Tools

The issues of team-based care are not limited to the healthcare professions. Similar concerns and issues about team functioning have been raised in other high-risk and high-stakes environments, where inefficient or ineffective team performance could have catastrophic consequences. These concerns have been raised in the aviation, nuclear power, and business industries, as well as within the fields of military and public safety (including police and fire departments). Many of these industries have done an excellent job of decreasing risk and increasing safety. Healthcare is a bit different though in that, unlike airplanes, no two patients are alike and have to be treated as such.

One of the benchmarks of clear communication is when people speak and understand one another in an effective and efficient way. Shared understandings of the meanings of words, acronyms, expectations, and acceptable scripts empower teams to achieve goals. For example, if on a team, multiple members, whom each come from different backgrounds professionally, ineffectively attempt to share information during a patient handoff or transfer; this may lead to confusion, impeding the targeted, positive patient outcome. Thus, in many professions, there are customary formats for sharing information.

In nursing, one example would be **SBAR** (situation/background/assessment/recommendation), in which the speaker utilizes the acronym to remember to include all of the relevant information. This format is useful for the person who is briefing another provider during a patient transfer but is equally valuable for the person who is assuming responsibility for that patient. For the person responsible for the transfer, it is clear what they should be sharing. For the person receiving that patient, and now assuming responsibility, the tool is valuable as a reminder of what information they will need in order to keep the care as seamless as possible.

The use of the acronym **I-PASS** may also be useful for teams to consider. Here the acronym addresses *Illness severity, Patient summary, Action list*, awareness of the *Situation* and any contingency plans, and acknowledgment or readback of the information, indicating synthesis of what has been said.

These tools begin to establish expected rules of communication, a standardization in a format that becomes familiar to team members and guides their interactions. Some of those are not necessarily built around acronyms as memory tools. These additional tools also bring the team into alignment around behaviors and expectations related to the conveying of information. When an order (**callout**) is given to administer a relevant medication during a situation of emergent care, for instance, it can be easy to misunderstand terms due to their similarity in sound. Hearing the distinction between the numbers 15 and 50 in a crowded and noisy trauma bay can be very problematic. Not administering medication or treatments in proper dosages because the sounds are hard to distinguish can be catastrophic. Thus, one of the methods of communication designed to forestall such a tragedy is the use of the **cross-check**, which is when, having heard a **callout**, the information is verified by repeating back what was said. Doing so provides the person making the **callout** with an affirmation that their statement or information was correctly understood. If the **cross-check** does not match directly and specifically with the **callout**, there is an opportunity for correction. When it is understood on a team that this is the expectation of all team members, it clarifies the communication loop.

A third behavior that reinforces those just discussed is when a **checkback** follows the earlier exchange. In a **checkback**, once the information from the **callout** has been verified with a **cross-check** and the request is executed, the person completing the task returns one more time and announces that the task has been completed. The originator of the **callout** thus knows that the information has been acted upon correctly, rather than simply hoping that to be the case. The **checkback** announces the completion of the task, and the originator affirms that they are aware. Such simple routines, although sounding somewhat innocuous, are essential among members of teams which must optimize their behaviors and functioning. Functional teams not only identify and train team members to utilize these simple tools but also expect their use to be consistent.

3.3   Checklists

Much has been written about the use and value of checklists, and yet there remains substantial resistance to their employment. Checklists help us to remember important tasks and yet are too often seen as a sign that we expect failure. Checklists come in many forms and varieties and serve different purposes. Some checklists preemptively remind us of things we need to do, while others are used as a quality control measure to be certain that we have thoroughly completed a task or process. In the first instance, one might utilize the checklists that preemptively remind us of what needs to be done, like a recipe in cooking. By glancing down the list, we can see whether we have all of the necessary supplies and tools as well as the correct people on the team who know how to utilize them. These sorts of lists not only assist us with issues of readiness but can also provide an established process with which to proceed. The second kind of list is a review of what has occurred and is utilized to verify the completion of a task or process. It is utilized to verify that all needed elements of the team's responsibilities have been met.

Whichever format of the list being used, it must be precise and concise. Do not spell out all of the details of the items on the list, but rather create them to prompt the reader to remember a task or process to be completed. The checklist does not contain all the details of that task or process. Effective checklists remind even the most seasoned experts about major elements of the task being attempted. In a sense, checklists augment the sense of discipline to check or double-check one's work.

3.4   Repeat Backs

Repeat backs are very similar to **cross-checks** or **checkbacks**. They are simple to execute but are vital for clarification in communication. Since the nature of nursing is complex in terms of the information being shared and frequently of the urgency in sharing it, clear communication is vital for optimal patient outcomes. Nurses cannot afford to make mistakes without the danger of catastrophic outcomes based on the mishearing of information or on the misunderstanding of a medical order. The use of repeat backs is simply to clarify that what one has heard was indeed accurate. An example of a repeat back is:

- **Callout** by MD: Give 1 mg of epinephrine IV now.
- **Repeat back** by nurse: Order is 1 mg epinephrine IV now.

If there is any misunderstanding in the order given, the **repeat back** provides assurance to both the nurse and the MD that it was received correctly.

3.5   Numeric and Phonetic Clarifications

Numeric and phonetic clarifications are utilized to clarify the use of letters or digits in the conveyance of information. Frequently, we encounter these in public safety and military communications. They serve a similar purpose in healthcare, where environments in communication may be chaotic and noisy but communication must be concise and accurate. The most common variant of this tool is known as the NATO spelling alphabet or the International Civil Aviation Organization alphabet, in which words are used to clarify letters being cited. Examples for A, B, and C would be (in order) Alpha, Bravo, and Charlie, and ending the alphabet with X, Y, and Z being X-ray, Yankee, and Zulu. These words indicate specific letters and are thus used to indicate those letters when spelling out words or acronyms.

3.6   Clarifying Questions

The use of questions to clarify communication indicates an operational style and alignment among team members that the most important aspect of their work together is to achieve patient safety. The culture of the team around this issue is often dictated by how receptive the internal culture is to the asking of questions in the first place. If a leader perceives that the questions being asked somehow threaten their authority, they will most likely convey that concern to the team either intentionally or unintentionally. Because asking questions can be perceived to be a failing of one's own professionalism or professional knowledge, in the wrong environment, asking questions can also involve an element of professional risk. Similarly, depending on the social agreements among team members, asking questions can also have undesirable consequences. If questions are understood by team members to be a tool for better assuring the achievement of positive outcomes, then they are seen as an asset to the team's overall functioning, rather than a detriment. Clearly, however, creating that culture is dependent largely on the attitudes expressed by the team leadership at any given time. A single question to clarify a process or information may be the defining moment between successful patient outcomes and catastrophic ones.

Some Tools, While Accurate, May Not Be That Useful!
Acronyms can serve as useful tools to help remind us of the information to be utilized or exchanged during communication. Such acronyms must be relatively easy to remember as well as clear in their meaning. They are best when they are both concise and memorable.

One example of an acronym which reminds us about useful information, but is itself too cumbersome to be helpful, is the I-PASS-THE-BATON. Once again, as with SBAR, it reminds the speaker of the material to be covered and serves as a template for the receiver in terms of knowing what to expect. Such tools align the communications between team members. In this rather lengthy acronym, the protocol creates a structured handoff of patient care, beginning with the letter "I," which *Introduces* the name of the provider and their role or job. "PASS" indicates the need to identify the *Patient*, using identifiers, gender, and age. The *Assessment*, much like what was found in SBAR, presents the chief complaint or need of the patient, along with data such as vital signs, any presenting symptoms, and, where available, the diagnosis. The double "S" describes the *Situation* (current status, recent changes, responses to treatment, and any uncertainties) as well as *Safety* concerns. The latter include lab values or reports, allergies, alerts (such as falling), and socio-economic factors of relevance.

The last portion of this acronym (BATON) identifies the *Background* (i.e., comorbidities, current medications, relevant family histories, and identification of any previous episodes). Identifying *Actions* that are needed or have occurred is followed by a brief description and possibly the rationale. *Timing* reminds the providers to discuss the level of urgency, clarifying the priority of the actions needed and the explicit timing of occurrences. As this transfer of care occurs (the "passing of the baton"), it is essential that team members identify who will be responsible and may include not only licensed providers, but also the patient or their family members. Lastly, the team discusses what is *NEXT*. Here, the plan of care is clearly presented, including any anticipated changes or contingency plans.

In short, acronyms are of value when they are concise and memorable, having utility or usefulness for the user. Some acronyms are more useful as checklists in that they are too cumbersome to be effective memory aids.

3.7   Team Meetings

Bringing together members of functioning teams facilitates clear communication and accurate understanding. Those in positions of facilitation or leadership of teams are responsible for providing tools that work, which include the types and purposes of meetings.

Types of Meetings

Brief: This meeting is a short session at the beginning of an event or during transfers to articulate and discuss the plan. Team members identify and clarify roles and responsibilities and discuss the dynamics of member interactions. Goals are agreed upon, and expectations and contingencies are identified and discussed. This type of meeting is used to anticipate outcomes.

Huddle: Similarly short, this style of meeting is generally implemented after a plan of care has been launched and is used to reassess and potentially redistribute the resources available. This meeting may occur a number of times over the course of a plan of care and affirms the team's situational awareness, checking in on initiatives and efforts already in place. The huddle is used to collect information and potentially change or adjust previously agreed to plans.

Debrief: At the completion or end of a process to provide care, providers exchange information designed to optimize the team's performance. Identifying lessons learned (both positive and painful) allows team members to utilize those strategies and behaviors that contributed to the likelihood of positive functioning and outcomes.

One of the ways in which they can help their teams align around purpose and goals as well as reach agreements related to tools to utilize is using a briefing meeting. A **briefing** meeting is an informal and relatively short meeting of team members prior to assuming a task to relay relevant information, check in on needed resources, and affirm the team's readiness to move forward. This is also where team members are likely to gauge what the temperament of the leader is going to be like related to such issues as asking questions. It is imperative that the goal(s) of the team be clearly identified and agreed to if the team is to optimize its functioning around a given outcome. The team must understand what goal they hold in common, and team members must be prepared to value that goal above their own personal agendas or desires.

A second type of meeting that is useful to check in around available and needed resources, team alignment toward goals, or plans to pivot toward new goals is called a **huddle**. Given that this term is utilized in sports, it may be clearer as to its purpose. This is again a short and informal meeting where open communication, including the asking of questions, is encouraged by all team members, including the leadership. Once questions are answered and issues are resolved, the meeting ends and the task continues.

The third form of meeting occurs after the task is complete. Normally, particularly with the pressing schedules in healthcare, it is difficult to get team members to stop before going on to their next assignment. The intention of the **debrief** meeting is to capture what has been learned in the previous team encounter. Typically, the debrief begins with the inquiry about what went well so that the team can harvest immediately relevant information designed to improve future (indeed, possibly even their very next) encounters. Here, the principles of interprofessionalism, including the removal of hierarchy as an organizing structure, becomes paramount. If the team leader or a member of a profession is assumed to be in charge (for example, a medical doctor) and that person controls the conversation, potentially others will restrain their comments or suggestions. This type of meeting works only if the conversation is honest and everyone is allowed to participate.

Sadly, it has been reported that debrief meetings fail to occur following a team process approximately 75% of the time, indicating that there is much valuable information that has been lost. What makes this most disturbing is that information that might have been harvested with the potential of saving another patient's life is gone.

4   Summary

Effective healthcare teams are essential to improving patient outcomes. They represent collaborative efforts by providers who are bound together by mutually held understandings, values, and goals, and are to that extent the product of both intention and effort. Effective interprofessional healthcare teams utilize a framework that is based on communication strategies and tools, abandoning structural barriers such as hierarchy which impede both efficacy and efficiency. To create such teamwork and teams requires the honest reflection of providers, involving experiences of personal and professional humility practiced in an environment of transparency. If the ultimate purpose and goal of the healthcare team are to provide patients with the safest and most effective outcomes, providers must invest in operational agreements that bring that about.

5   Case Study

The ER of a local hospital is having a somewhat typical Friday evening, with a steady influx of patients with assorted complaints. Patient acuity has been varied, but the flow into and out of the emergency room has been reasonably orderly, effective, and efficient.

At about 10:00 PM, emergency services providers (EMS) bring in a patient (Patient A) who was one of several people injured in a multiple car accident. Upon arrival, EMS personnel brief the nurse who receives the patient into the care of the ER personnel. That meeting is a short one, with the emergency services personnel utilizing the **SBAR** acronym to convey information. The nurse who is receiving the patient listens to each component of the acronym, assuring that they have been given all of the information they need to begin appropriate care. Patient A is moved into an ER bay. As others respond to the callout for care for this patient, the nurse again utilizes **SBAR** to *brief* team members, remembering to include the elements of **I-PASS**. Again, team members learn quickly what is needed to initiate care. This information and this patient are transferred quickly to providers with expertise in the areas of concern related to this particular and individual patient. Initially, the leader of this team is the nurse who received the patient from the EMS provider.

They have a full awareness that leadership will quickly rotate to the person present who has the most knowledge, education, and experience that are relevant to this patient's care at the moment. As directives are given for care, team members *check back* with lead providers to assure that they have fully understood what is being asked for and, as the team has previously agreed, will ask *clarifying questions* as needed. Given the unfolding needs of the team and the patient, team members will repeatedly *huddle* with one another to assure that the needed resources are either present or being called for and that the team is functioning with a common, valued goal. It may be important for these sorts of clarifying moments to occur multiple times in the care of this patient.

As care begins to unfold for Patient A, a second victim of the car accident has been brought in. Because the team has agreed together about the appropriate protocols to follow, Patient B's arrival begins in much the same way as Patient A's had. Similar tools are used to convey information and to facilitate the transfer of care of the patient from the EMS team to the ER team. Additionally, the ER team is now dealing with two patients, and team members may find themselves functioning in several teams at once based on the demands of the ER. Again, the tools they use may be implemented multiple times in the care of one patient or may be in use in the care of many. The team members trust one another and share the goal of exceptional care and outcomes for the various patients they serve, and they are familiar with various tools to assure that care is both efficient and effective. Working as a team, accessing the expertise of team members when it is needed, these patients can expect optimized outcomes.

Key Points

- Effective interdisciplinary teams are essential in our current context of complexity and high acuity in healthcare.
- Creating an effective team that impacts patient safety and quality requires intentional and consistent effort by all team members and leaders.
- Teams can be challenged by many factors including hierarchy, communication failures, lack of effective leadership, lack of shared group goals, culture, and structural issues.
- Many tools are available to assist with effective teamwork including checklists, communication tools, and structured team meetings.
- Considering the emergent nature and complexity in healthcare, reflection and attention paid to effective and efficient teams will greatly benefit safety and patient outcomes.

References

1. van der Lee N, Driessen EW, Houwaart ES, Caccia NC, Scheele F. An examination of the historical context of interprofessional collaboration in Dutch obstetrical care. J Interprof Care. 2014;28(2):123–7.

2. World Health Organization (CH). Framework for action on interprofessional education and collaborative practice. Geneva: World Health Organization; 2010.
3. Institute of Medicine (US). To err is human: Building a safer health system. Lexington, KY: Institute of Medicine (US); 1999.
4. Joint Commission (US). 2003 National patient safety goals. Jt Comm Perspect. 2002;22(9):1–3. Available from: https://pubmed.ncbi.nlm.nih.gov/12233144/
5. Institute of Medicine. Patient safety: achieving a new standard for care. Washington, DC: The National Academies Press; 2004. https://doi.org/10.17226/10863.
6. Joint Commission. Sentinel event policy and procedures. Available at: https://www.jointcommission.org/resources/sentinel-event/sentinel-event-policy-and-procedures
7. Ko BS, Lim TH, Oh T, Lee Y, Yun I, Yang MS. The effectiveness of a focused rapid response team on reducing the incidence of cardiac arrest in the general ward. Medicine. 2020;99(10):19032. https://doi.org/10.1097/MD.0000000000019032.
8. American College of Surgeons. Mass transfusion in trauma guidelines; 2014. Available at: https://www.facs.org/media/zcjdtrd1/transfusion_guildelines.pdf
9. Congressman Joe Courtney. Workplace violence prevention for health care and social workers act; 2022 Dec 9. Available at: https://courtney.house.gov/media-center/press-releases/following-deadly-shooting-home-health-care-worker-rep-courtney-urges
10. Illinois Health and Hospital Association. Healthcare worker safety; 2023 March. Available at: https://www.team-iha.org/quality-and-safety/emergency-preparedness/healthcare-worker-safety
11. American Hospital Association. Fact sheet workplace violence and intimidation, and the need for federal legislation; 2022 Jun 7. Available at: https://www.aha.org/fact-sheets/2022-06-07-fact-sheet-workplace-violence-and-intimidation-and-need-federal-legislative
12. Center for Disease Control. Workplace violence prevention for nurses. Available at: https://www.cdc.gov/niosh/topics/violence/training_nurses.html
13. Bloomberg Law. Health-worker violence bill wins house passage amid veto threat; 2019 November 21. Available at: https://news.bloomberglaw.com/daily-labor-report/health-worker-violence-bill-wins-house-passage-amid-veto-threat

Effective Clinical Decision-Making and Action for Patient Safety in Acute Care Settings

Christine W. Nibbelink and Jane M. Carrington

1   Introduction

Effective clinical decision-making is the cornerstone of safe patient care. An awareness-raising study conducted by the Institute of Medicine identified that up to 98,000 deaths occur annually due to errors in decision-making [1]. Significant efforts have been instituted to reduce errors in healthcare decision-making. The Health Information Technology for Economic and Clinical Health (HITECH) Act, part of the American Recovery and Reinvestment Act of 2009, was signed into law in 2009 with the goal of improving patient safety [2]. A major objective of the HITECH Act was to support meaningful use of electronic health records (EHR) including the effective use of clinical decision support systems (CDSS) within the EHR. Despite this enormous effort, research identifies that errors continue to be a serious problem in healthcare today. For instance, an estimated 10% of patient deaths each year occur due to error [3]. In addition, adverse events, defined as unintended consequences resulting in negative patient outcomes, occur in 8.6 out of 100 patient admissions [4]. An alarming 52.6% of adverse events have been identified as preventable [4]. Clearly, improving patient safety outcomes needs to be a significant focus in healthcare today.

Nurse decision-making in patient care has been defined as: development of conclusions based on patient needs and health issues, determination to intervene or not

C. W. Nibbelink (✉)
Hahn School of Nursing and Health Science, University of San Diego, San Diego, CA, USA
e-mail: cnibbelink@sandiego.edu

J. M. Carrington
Department of Family, Community and Health System Science, University of Florida College of Nursing, Gainesville, FL, USA
e-mail: janecarrington@ufl.edu

intervene, and reevaluation of patient needs to determine if further intervention is required [5]. Nurses, working closely at patients' bedside, are essential for early recognition and response to significant changes in patient status. Early nurse recognition of signs and symptoms indicating that patient's decline supports early intervention and improved patient outcomes. Alternatively, failure to rescue occurs when nurses fail to recognize patients' signs and symptoms early preventing early intervention [6]. Low rates of failure to rescue are a nurse-sensitive indicator of quality nursing practice [7]. Effective rescue in nursing practice includes surveillance, timely recognition of complications, taking, action, and activating a team response [8]. Understanding individual and contextual factors that contribute to the accurate identification of patients' significant signs and symptoms indicative of patient deterioration and the decision-making processes associated with effective interventions toward patient rescue is essential to improving patient safety.

Nursing leaders play an essential role in the development of a patient safety culture in the clinical environment. Several characteristics of leadership styles that support a culture of patient safety are described in nursing literature. Open communication, empowerment through interventions such as shared governance, and promotion of educational opportunities for all nursing levels support a positive work environment and improved patient safety outcomes [9].

Decision-making in nursing has been defined as the development of a conclusion based on an assessment of patient's needs (including health problems and concerns) leading to a determination that a particular action is required followed by a reassessment of the patient's response [5]. To support understanding of factors influential to decision-making, several decision-making theories or models have been developed with the goal of enhancing patient safety. The purpose of this chapter is to describe theories and models that support understanding of nurse decision-making and apply theories and models to clinical examples.

2   Background

Decision-making theories and models describe individual and contextual factors that may influence nurses' decision-making processes. A theory includes a set of principles that provide structure toward understanding of a phenomenon [10]. A model approaches understanding of a phenomenon with a narrower focus than a theory [10]. One rationale for the use of a theory or model is to support the understanding of underlying factors that contribute to a problem rather than simply focusing on superficial issues [11].

Nurses care for patients within a highly complex environment. Nurses consider and are influenced by many factors when caring for patients including awareness of their patient's current condition, reflection on their previous patient care experiences, routines in practice, a sense of time limits, team support, goals for patient care, and their role responsibilities as nurses within an overall nursing unit [12]. In addition, the types of leadership at the nursing manager and organizational levels also influence nurse decision-making. For instance, transformational leadership has been found to support the interests of employees and encourage employees' acceptance of the broader organizational mission and values [13]. Research identifies that transformational leadership is positively related to environments with strong patient safety cultures [13]. At the organizational level, use of high reliability organizational approaches leads to a focus on safety, excellence, and elimination of all errors [14].The wide range of individual and contextual factors that influence nurses' patient care decision-making must be considered to effectively support nursing practice and patient safety.

3   Early Decision-Making Models for Nursing and Medicine

Early literature on decision-making in nursing and medicine identifies the influence of logic, experience, and uncertainty in decision-making. Coherence and correspondence approaches also include how evaluation of decision-making occurs during different decision-making approaches.

3.1   Analytic and Intuitive

Initially, nursing research includes a focus on strategies used in nurse decision-making processes [15]. Clinical decision-making requires nurses to collect appropriate patient data, use theoretical and clinical knowledge, and incorporate contextual information to support decisions and address patient care needs [15]. Corcoran-Perry and Bungert describe two approaches, analytic and intuitive, that nurses integrate when making patient care decisions [15]. Analytic decision-making follows a logical process to identify a nursing intervention based on patient signs and symptoms [15]. Intuitive decision-making processes integrate the decision-maker's previous experience and the ability to recognize the current patient care situation as similar to a previous patient care situation to guide identification of the appropriate nursing intervention for the patient care situation [15]. An analytic decision process focuses entirely on measurable signs and symptoms such as shortness of breath that could indicate a pulmonary embolus. An intuitive decision-maker enters a patient's room and just get a sense that something is wrong without awareness of having included specific information in their decision-making. The authors identify that nurses use analytic and intuitive processes when making clinical decisions.

3.2   Coherence and Correspondence

An early decision-making model focused on the two areas of research in decision-making, coherence, and correspondence [16]. Coherence and correspondence were described as two divergent theories that supported understanding of medical decision-making. Coherence focused on the "rational" side of decision-making and included understanding that developed from decision-making that could be supported mathematically. The accuracy of a decision, when examined using coherence, was identified through examination of the decision-making process rather than the outcome of the decision [16]. Thus, a physician accurately evaluating lab values and vital signs in their decision-making process is determined to have made the appropriate decision for the patient. Correspondence theory focused on the outcome of the decision without an evaluation of the rationale behind the decision [16]. Correspondence includes a recognition that decision-making involves uncertainty and contextual factors that may influence the individual decision-maker [16]. Decision-making evaluation using correspondence seeks understanding of decision-making conditions that influence judgment according to the decision-maker. Understanding of factors associated with correspondence requires the input of the decision-maker. Hammond stated that coherence and correspondence theories are complementary and not independent in the decision-making process [16].

The analytic/intuitive and coherence/correspondence theories captured important differences between decision-making approaches. One approach to decision-making is more objective and includes a conscious path leading to a decision. The second approach includes the influences of context and experience that includes an awareness of the final decision without following a conscious path toward that decision.

4 Theories Supporting Nurse Decision-Making, Leadership, and Healthcare Organizations

In healthcare today, several decision-making theories are used to support nursing research, education, and practice. These theories include elements described in early literature and expand on previous work. Several decision-making, leadership, and organizational models or theories are described below.

4.1 Classical Decision-Making Model

Classical Decision-Making Model (CDM) is recognizable in nursing practice as it is consistent with the use of evidence-based practice to guide nursing care. CDM requires the decision-maker to select a specific choice from other options based on a comprehensive examination of available evidence to ensure ideal outcomes and predict which option is ideal [17]. CDM follows a formal process without contextual influence [17]. This approach provides a strong basis in evidence to guide decision-making and is consistent with many descriptions of nurse decision-making for patient care. The use of advanced cardiac life support algorithms are examples of CDM application in clinical settings. Much of medical and nursing education in decision-making follows the CDM model. An important limitation of CDM is that this approach requires an exhaustive search of options for decision-making which may be unrealistic during a patient care crisis.

4.2   Novice to Expert Theory

Benner (2001) developed the novice to expert model. This model identifies five stages of skill acquisition in nurses beginning with the novice nurse [18]. The novice nurses' decision-making occurs through strict adherence to rules and without the benefit of experience or understanding of contextual factors. Advanced beginners are identified by their ability to support their decision-making through recognition of current features of a patient care situation that are similar to previous patient care experiences. The competent stage occurs following two to three years of experience and includes the nurses' ability to understand the long-term outcomes of their plan of care. Proficient nurses have developed the ability to view patient care situations as a whole rather than as individual parts and use previous patient care experiences to guide their decision-making. Expert nurses have several years of experience and use their intuition, rooted in previous patient care experience, to guide their decision-making. The novice to expert model provides an important model to understand and guide professional development in nursing [19].

4.3   Dual Process Model and Bias in Decision-Making

Similar to early decision-making research, the dual process model described two types of decision-making. Fast decision-making occurs independent of memory and cognitive ability and relies on intuition and pattern matching [20–22]. Slow decision-making requires systematic comparison and analysis of new information, including patient assessment and evidence, and relies on memory and cognitive abilities [20–22]. Slow decision-making tends to follow normative processes [21]. Fast decision-making may be influenced by individual perceptions, emotions, and other contextual factors that contribute to bias in decision-making [22].

Fast decision-making, in dual processing theory, is described as more likely to include bias [10]. Understanding and addressing the influence of bias on nurse decision-making are essential for patient safety. For instance, implicit bias and the use of stereotyping during decision-making interfere with the development of trusting relationships with patients [10]. Implicit bias is also associated with racism and other types of discrimination in the healthcare environment and has been linked with errors leading to patient death [23]. Confirmation bias, also known as the bandwagon effect, occurs when the decision-maker looks for information that is consistent with their current perspective [23]. When influenced by confirmation bias, the decision-maker searches for information during an assessment that confirms original hypotheses while ignoring other conflicting information [23]. Confirmation bias has been found to influence nurses' decision-making up to 63% of the time regardless of nurses' level of experience [23]. One example of the influence of bias in decision-making occurs when nurses use interventions based on "how it's always been done" rather than incorporating recent evidence to guide their nursing practice.

Education designed to decrease bias has been successful, but few examples are found in the literature [23]. One approach to decrease bias is called unlearning [24]. Unlearning requires a conscious effort to question previously held beliefs in an effort to identify in effective or inappropriate beliefs that may interfere with effective and safe patient care decision-making [24]. Flawed decision-making rooted in bias may influence nurses' ability to recognize clinical deterioration contributing to failure to rescue patient situations [10, 25].

4.4 Transformational Leadership Theory

Transformational leadership describes leaders who provide inspiration and empowerment to employees with the collaborative goal and vision of achieving ideal outcomes [26]. Transformational leaders foster an environment that stimulates ideas and expands on employees potential [26]. Effective transformational leaders mentor their employees, provide clear communication of goals, approach leadership as a democratic process, and support individuals' decision-making and strengths toward success [27, 28]. Through inspiring trust, respect, motivation to achieve organizational goals and supporting nurses' voices in decision-making, successful transformational leaders create a safe environment for nurses to achieve high levels of excellence in nursing practice toward safe patient care [28, 29]. Research indicates that transformational leadership creates positive work environments, improves job satisfaction, and improves patient safety through reduction of adverse patient outcomes [29, 30]. In contrast, transactional leaders are task oriented, autocratic, punitive, and controlling in their leadership style [27].While transactional leadership may, in some circumstances, be appropriate (such as patient care emergencies), when used as an overall leadership style, use of transactional leadership undermines trust in the leader and inhibits cooperation among employees [27].

4.5 High Reliability Organization Theory

Successful high reliability organizations demonstrate a fundamental commitment to quality and safety [14]. The commitment to high level quality begins with engagement of leaders within the organization [14]. To support engagement, leaders must be informed of organizational strategies rooted in budgeting and other priorities as they consider safety plans and potential issues that may arise in the environment

[31]. When leaders are aware of strengths and weaknesses related to safety and quality, they can share these potential concerns with employees and promote planning for contingencies if necessary [31].

Middle managers also provide an essential role in high reliability organizations. Middle managers communicate the messages of executive messaging to employees [14]. The leadership style and behavior of middle managers should demonstrate consistency with the overall work culture [14]. When implementing safety measures, middle managers should be well informed of the scope of the plan including budgeting limitations and the rationale for what is included and what is not included [31]. Employees working in the environment provide a unique source of information regarding potential safety issues for leaders. Therefore, creating a culture in which employees, with direct experience in the environment, feel open to share safety risks in the work environment is essential to provide opportunities for change [31]. Similarly, expertise in particular topics should be recognized and supported by leaders rather than a hierarchical approach to action [31].

In uncertain circumstances, procedures should be examined for their efficacy in the current situation and not simply implemented because the procedure exists [31]. When the procedure is determined to be inappropriate for the current situation, leaders must be present to support employees in their new approach toward safety [31]. Improvising, during uncertain situations in which previous procedures are determined to be inappropriate, requires leadership that builds employees' confidence and supports a nonhierarchical approach [31]. Confidence in the face of uncertainty must be mitigated by a degree of ambivalence to allow for challenges to the new process if needed [31]. Decision-making should be supported though a flexible and adaptable approach allowing new information to influence the process toward effective communication [31].

5   Action

5.1   Clinical Application of Models Supporting Nurse Decision-Making, Leadership, and Organizations

Table 1 provides clinical application examples of several models and transformational leadership described above. Two models, Primed Practice Decision Model (PPDM) and Shared Decision-Making (SDM), will be used to describe decision-making in more depth in Tables 2 and 3. Discussion of PPDM will include contextual factors that may influence decision-making in nursing practice. SDM will include elements of high reliability organizations as described above and integrate bias within the decision-making process.

Table 1 Decision-making theories for nursing

Theory	Theory application example with elements of transformational leadership	Benefits/limitations/considerations of decision-making theory
Novice to expert theory	A clinical educator looking to enhance novice RNs' experience and competency when inserting a nasogastric tube read an article that compared the knowledge and competency of novice RNs in either the intervention group (using simulation as a teaching tool) or the control group (using case studies as the teaching tool) [32]. The study results identified a significant improvement in the simulation participants' competency compared with the case study participants. The clinical educator decided to use simulation in the evaluation and education of new graduate RNs in nasogastric tube placement. The clinical educator knew that novice RNs had varying degrees of experience inserting nasogastric tubes based on their educational experiences. Using this knowledge, the clinical educator decided to make the simulation sessions a collaborative effort with RNs working together to identify lapses in effective nasogastric tube insertion. In the end, all the participating RNs demonstrated high effectiveness with the nasogastric tube insertion technique in simulation and in patient care. The participating RNs described feeling increased confidence in their nasogastric tube insertion abilities and increased trust in their colleagues.	Benefits • Describes stages of development of practical expertise. Limitations • No description of how a RN moves from one stage to another. Considerations • One RN may be in more than one stage at a time based on the clinical situation [33].
Classical decision-making	During care of a patient with COVID-19, the staff RN identifies that the patient exhibits signs and symptoms of respiratory distress. The staff RN calls the charge RN for support. Together, the charge RN and the staff RN review evidence-based guidelines to decide how best to intervene for this patient. Several recommendations are identified in review of the hospital's evidence-based policy and procedures including managing nutrition, treating the cause, mechanical ventilation, suctioning, administering antibiotics as ordered and other nursing interventions. The RN discusses with the charge RN the opinion that many of these interventions have been provided or are not applicable to the current patient care situation. The charge RN agrees and suggests reviewing research on the care of patients with COVID-19 to identify other interventions to support patients in respiratory distress with COVID-19. They find an article describing prone positioning using the CINAHL database. This article describes research results from various studies on the use of prone positioning for COVID-19 patients and describes how prone positioning should be implemented if the care giver determines it is appropriate for their patient [34]. The staff RN reads the article and makes the decision to use (or to discuss with the provider) prone positioning as an intervention for this patient. The charge RN supports the staff RN in this decision. The staff RN implements prone positioning in their patient care based on evidence and following discussion with the patient's provider.	Benefits • Evidence based. Limitations • Takes time, impractical during time limited situations. • If patient care problem is new or not covered in policy and procedure this approach requires, finding, reading, and assimilation of information from research articles. Considerations • Ideally, decision support that pairs patient assessment findings with evidence-based recommendations for nursing interventions are presented at the appropriate time within the RN's workflow would support timely integration of

Theory	Theory application example with elements of transformational leadership	Benefits/limitations/considerations of decision-making theory
Dual process theory and bias	A staff RN had recently cared for a patient who had experienced respiratory arrest. The arresting patient needed intubation and admission to the intensive care unit. Following this experience, the nursing manager of her unit observes that this staff RN appears to over-identify patients as high risk for respiratory arrest. For instance, she described one of her patients at high risk for respiratory arrest. Later, a more experienced RN assessed the patient and determined the patient was breathing comfortably, with a normal respiratory rate, normal oxygen saturation, and clear breath sounds. When asked about high levels of concern for relatively minor symptoms interfering with the RN's ability to care for their patients in a timely manner, the staff RN described feeling a high level of uncertainty in their ability to identify significant respiratory distress and now is concerned that they may miss significant symptoms in other patients. In reading about the dual process model, the nursing manager realized that low self-efficacy may bias future decision-making [22]. The nursing manager identified that decision-making when patients are at significant risk for decline include fast thinking and intuition rather than a slower systematic analysis of evidence to support decision-making due to time limitations. The nursing manager discovered in the research article that encouraging the RN to reflect on a now growing number of patient care experiences that supports the RNs ability to provide auto-feedback [22] may help this staff RN when making fast decisions with less bias during patient crises. Following this approach, the staff RN stated that they developed more confidence in their ability to effectively identify patient decline.	Benefits • Describes fast and slow decision-making approaches that help support understanding of health care decision-making [22]. Limitations • Fast thinking is more likely to be influenced by bias influencing the decision-making process [22]. Considerations • Debiasing strategies that include training designed to heighten awareness of biases and teach techniques to mitigate biases support reduced bias in decision-making [35]. • Lack of consideration of contextual factors may limit the success of debiasing strategies [23].

Table 2 Contextual factors' influencing RN understanding of patient status (perception, comprehension, projection), pattern matching, mental simulation

Contextual factor	Clinical example	Evidence and other factors that could influence effective decision-making
Experience	RN 1 enters patient A's room and begins assessing patient A. RN 1 begins by asking patient A questions about how she is feeling and whether she is experiencing any pain. During conversation with patient A, RN 1 observes patient A's respiratory rate (24 breaths per minute), oxygen saturation (96%), and respiratory rhythm (regular) but somewhat labored. Patient A denies experiencing pain. Based on RN 1's previous patient care experience, RN 1 uses pattern matching to determine that patient A's symptoms indicate a stable patient status. Mental simulation from previous patient care situations and experiences in education indicate to RN 1 that patient A care should follow patient care interventions for a stable patient. RN 1 understanding of patient status begins with the initial interaction with patient A and continues through the time RN 1 provides care for patient A. Patient A's symptoms are perceived by RN 1, RN 1's comprehension of the patient status is that patient A is stable, and RN 1's projection into the future is that patient A will remain stable.	Understanding of patient status begins with assessing patient history including type 2 diabetes and chronic obstructive pulmonary disease as risk factors for cardiac disease [38]. In addition, a higher risk for atypical chest pain or absence of chest pain exists with comorbidities including diabetes and chronic obstructive heart disease [38, 39].
Education (level of education, policies and procedures, evidence-based practice)	As part of on-boarding to the telemetry unit, RN 1 oriented to the unit with an experienced preceptor for 6 weeks and took an electrocardiogram interpretation course. Based on the knowledge gained from previous education and the preceptor's guidance, RN 1 continues to assess patient A (blood pressure 160/80) and asks the telemetry monitor technician to provide an update on patient A's heart rhythm (sinus rhythm, rate 95, with an occasional premature ventricular contractions).	Early perception of deterioration in patient. status is a nursing sensitive issue [6]. Therefore, this initial step in the decision-making process is essential to effective decision-making and patient safety. Increased nurse education (bachelor's degree or higher), along with staffing levels, has been linked with improved patient rescue [6, 40]. Blood pressure and heart rate increase prior to ST segment depression during ischemia [41].

Table 2 (continued)

Contextual factor	Clinical example	Evidence and other factors that could influence effective decision-making
Autonomy/confidence	RN 1 initially felt confident in their assessment findings but watching patient A's labored respirations creates new concerns. The initial confidence partially stemmed from previous experience in patient care, but patient A exhibits unusual symptoms based on RN 1's previous experience. RN 1's understanding of patient status did not change in the early stages as patient A's symptoms evolved. However, patient A respiratory effort seems to be increasing leading to a reevaluation and new understanding of patient status. RN 1 recalls feeling criticized during the last time they had called a rapid response team for a patient.	Confidence and previous experiences with rapid response teams influence future willingness to call rapid response teams [42].
Bias	RN 1's bias, patients with cardiac symptoms present in a typical manner, may be rooted in education, previous experience, and the communication from the emergency department RN (Patient A is a complainer). This bias (confirmation bias: looking for evidence that is consistent with a previous understanding of patient status and ignoring other information) may have inhibited RN 1 from identifying signs and symptoms of a cardiac source for patient A's pain.	Evidence that would help to look beyond bias: • Atypical cardiac symptoms may present without ST elevation and with absence of chest pain [43]. • Women present with atypical chest pain (including absence of pain) more frequently than men [38].

(continued)

Table 2 (continued)

Contextual factor	Clinical example	Evidence and other factors that could influence effective decision-making
Uncertainty	Initially, RN 1 experiences little uncertainty in this situation (however, RN 1 misidentified the significance of findings). The emergency department RN description of patient A as a complainer continues to weigh on RN1's mind. Maybe patient A was just unhappy? As patient A's status begins to decline RN 1 lacks previous experiences to support pattern matching and mental simulation contributing to RN 1's uncertainty.	Lack of structure and non-essential information inhibits effective handoff reports [44]. Early warning systems have had variable success in early perception of failure to rescue leading to a 40% increase in doctor's workload with only a 3% increase in early perception of patient deterioration [6]. Understanding of how to provide alerts at the right time during the workflow is essential for effective clinical decision support [45].
High stakes situation/time limitations	Initially RN 1 did not identify a high stakes, time limited patient care situation. As the clinical situation progresses, Patient A experiences increasing shortness of breath and describes pain in her upper chest and between her scapula [46]. The telemetry monitor technician informs RN 1 that patient A's heart rhythm exhibits ST elevation with frequent premature ventricular contractions, rate 105. RN 1 takes patient A's blood pressure (175/90). RN 1 reevaluates: perceives Patient A's symptoms, comprehends that patient A's status is deteriorating, and projects into the future that there is a potential for a poor outcome for patient A. This is the development of a new understanding of patient status which prompts RN 1 to call the physician and activate the rapid response team.	New graduate nurses' failure to rescue has been linked with their previous clinical experiences in education, the ability to make decisions independently, previous experiences with deteriorating patients, and confidence with many aspects of patient care including communicating with physicians and the ability to address numerous tasks that become overwhelming [47].

(continued)

Table 2 (continued)

Contextual factor	Clinical example	Evidence and other factors that could influence effective decision-making
Unit culture	The unit culture includes valuing accuracy in identification of patient signs and symptoms. Due to a previous experience in which RN 1 felt criticized for calling the rapid response team, RN 1 now wants to be certain that patient A is experiencing a significant problem prior to calling rapid response team. The rapid response team and physician arrived. Patient A is taken to the intensive care unit.	Cultural factors within a nursing unit that can contribute to reluctance when communicating changes in patient status indicative of patient deterioration. These cultural factors include a hierarchical unit culture that discourages effective communication, collaboration, and poor support for unit staff [6] Nurses may not call rapid response teams when concerned about negative responses from colleagues [48].
Team influence, collegial collaboration, communication	RN 1 did not seek collegial collaboration early in the care of patient A due to a failure to recognize a decline in patient status. Following patient A's transition to the intensive care unit, RN1's nursing manager reviews patient A's EHR and identifies several early indicators of atypical chest pain that the nursing manager believes RN1 should have addressed early in the care of patient A.	An experienced nurse rounding on patients has been found to support early identification of patient deterioration for new graduates [47].

Table 3 Factors influencing interprofessional shared decision-making

Steps	Clinical example	Activities to be integrated within the steps of SDM
Step 1	A newly graduated RN assesses their simulated "patient" and identifies signs and symptoms of sepsis. The newly graduated RN begins discussion with the healthcare team, including the physician, to share their nursing knowledge based on patient assessment. The nurse manager and the physician, aware of potential perceived hierarchies within the environment, encourage contributions from all members of the healthcare team and the patient of their understanding and values to the discussion. Discussion within the healthcare team and with patient/family leads to an understanding that a decision is needed.	Patient with a health condition • Decision point with more than one option: potentially no change to treatment plan, change to treatment plan. • Discussion between healthcare team members and patient (family may be engaged in these discussions when patient is unable) includes sharing of knowledge, options for patient care, and identifying a need for a decision [50].
Step 2	Discussion between healthcare team members and the patient/family continues with newly graduated RN contributing based on their nursing knowledge and patient assessment. All team members and the patient are encouraged to exchange information they feel is relevant including information that may conflict with the group's current understanding of the patient care situation with a goal of supporting understanding.	Exchange of information • Discussion between healthcare team and patient/family to provide details of relevant signs and symptoms. • Discussion includes healthcare team members using decision aids to support integration of evidence-based resources. • Discussion of options among health care team and patient/family [50].
Step 3	Patient/family and healthcare members discuss their perspectives while acknowledging their personal and professional values. RNs advocate for the patient/family's needs and values during this process. The discussion includes thoughtful reflection of potential personal and organizational biases that may influence the decision-making process. Evidence is reviewed to support effective decision-making. The patient/family is encouraged to ask questions.	Values clarification • Patient/family values are central to this discussion. • Healthcare team members recognize their values influence their contributions to the decision process [50].
Step 4	Healthcare team members consider the resources needed for various options. These considerations are shared with the patient/family. The patient/family's values continue to provide essential information in consideration of treatment plan options.	Feasibility of options • Consideration of resources, including expertise, within the organization to support proposed options. • Discussion includes patient/family's identification of feasibility of identified options [50].

Table 3 (continued)

Steps	Clinical example	Activities to be integrated within the steps of SDM
Step 5	The patient/family and healthcare team discussion leads to a decision regarding the treatment plan. The nurse continues to contribute based on the nursing perspective and as an advocate for the patient/family.	Decision • Patient/family identifies their decision preference. • The healthcare team may also provide recommendations during this phase. • Ideal: agreement is reached among all members in the discussion. The physician should agree to facilitate the treatment plan [50].
Step 6	Nursing assessment and discussion with the patient/family continues as the treatment plan is implemented. The nurse communicates the patient's response to the treatment plan with the healthcare team and advocates for the patient's needs and values throughout the nursing care process.	Patient/family support during treatment toward ideal outcomes • The patient/family and healthcare team may change the decision based on patient outcomes [50].

5.2   PPDM

The PPDM describes the influence of experience on the decision-making process during critical and time limited circumstances [36]. PPDM includes contextual factors that may influence the decision-making process (see Fig. 1) [36]. PPDM describes nurse decision-making as beginning with assessment of a patient leading to the development of an *understanding of patient status. Understanding of patient status* includes the following stages: perception of patient's needs (physiological and psychosocial), comprehension of the significance of the patient care situation (including level of risk for the patient), and consideration of potential outcomes for the patient based on the current understanding. Nurses reflect on their previous clinical experience, evidence, and specific patient care needs to recognize a patient care situation as similar to a previous patient care experience or patient care policy and *pattern match* based on this recognition to guide their decision-making in the current situation. A *mental simulation* of the perceived patient response to a previously experienced patient care situation or evidence-based protocol occurs leading the nurse to select a particular intervention for the current patient care situation. The nurse then *intervenes or determines no intervention is needed* and continues patient observation based on their understanding of patient status. The nurse *evaluates the patient's response* for a new understanding of patient status which begins the decision-making process again (*feedback loop*). Accurate *understanding of patient status* is essential for an effective response to meet patients' needs. *Understanding of patient status* occurs throughout this process to determine whether a new course

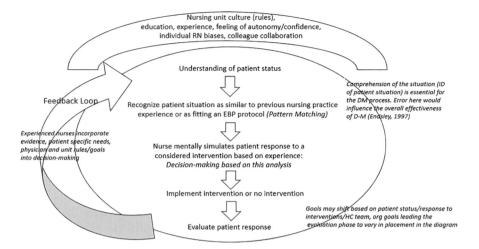

Fig. 1 Practice-primed decision model
Reprinted from: *Applied Nursing Research*, 46, Nibbelink, C. W., & Reed, P. G., Deriving the Practice-Primed Decision Model from a naturalistic decision-making perspective for acute care nursing research, pages 1–10 (2019), with permission from Elsevier. *PPDM with Contextual Factors Influencing Acute Care Nurse Decision-Making*

of action should take place based on a change in patient status. The nurse decision-maker is often aware of formal efforts to understand patient status when considering the evidence but influence of the contextual factors on the nurse's understanding often occurs in an unconscious level [17, 37].

The overall patient care environment also influences the nurse decision-making process. Factors within the overall patient care environment that influence nurse decision-making include *nursing unit culture, education, previous experiences, education, collaboration with colleagues, their personal sense of autonomy and confidence, healthcare team members, and the rules and goals of the overall organization.* Throughout the decision-making process, *bias*, often unconscious, influences the nurse who may use heuristics rather than a systematic approach when making patient care decisions. *Bias* can influence the nurses' understanding of patient status which may interfere with effective patient care decision-making.

The benefits of PPDM include support for the exploration of contextual factors and the influence of experience during high stakes and time limited decision-making situations. Understanding of these factors is important to support nurses as they make decisions during critical patient care circumstances that include time limitations that make integration of evidence-based practice challenging. Leadership considerations include how to best support timely access of evidence-based practice in the EHR during time limited patient care situations.

The PPDM will guide the following discussion of a patient care example. Contextual factors within PPDM will be discussed and applied to the patient care discussion to illustrate how these contextual factors may influence nurse decision-making and practice (see Fig. 1 and Table 2). The case study provides evidence that may support the nurse's decision-making is in the third column of Table 2 but due to contextual factors, the nurse in the case study may not include this evidence in their decision-making.

Clinical Example: Nurse 1 graduated 6 months ago from a nursing program and began working on the telemetry unit following graduation. Today nurse 1 is going to assume care of patient A as a new admission from the emergency department to the telemetry unit. Report from the emergency department nurse indicates that patient A (a 65-year-old female) was admitted for observation/rule out cardiac source for symptoms. Patient A came to the emergency department describing experiencing nausea and vomiting and "difficulty catching my breath" with further test results pending. Patient A's history includes type diabetes and chronic obstructive pulmonary disease. The emergency department nurse reports that patient A's heart rhythm, (rate 85, normal sinus rhythm) is monitored using telemetry, she has 2 L oxygen flowing through his nasal cannula, she has a saline lock in her left forearm. Patient A's respiratory rate was 18, oxygen saturation was 98%, temperature 98.6 degrees Fahrenheit, and her blood pressure was 145/80. The emergency department nurse describes patient A as alert and oriented and a "bit of a complainer."

5.3   SDM

The SDM model supports clinicians' collaboration with patients/family and with other healthcare team members. Furthermore, SDM supports interprofessional and patient/family collaboration in decision-making providing a cohesive approach for patient care [49, 50]. SDM between the clinician and the patient/family emphasizes the importance of effective and ongoing communication of risks and benefits of options to support patient/family participation in the decision-making process. Several factors must be considered in the use of SDM in patient care. Clinicians must consciously acknowledge their biases when describing healthcare options that could otherwise lead to an overly persuasive approach in communication of decision options to patients/family [51]. Excessive persuasion includes selective presentation and timing of information [51]. For instance, if a clinician presents an option positively with minimal presentation of risks to address a current patient need, patients will be more likely to agree with the physician's proposed option [51].

SDM may also be used to support interprofessional communication and collaboration. Several factors may influence interdisciplinary SDM and must be considered when integrating SDM into interprofessional communication and collaboration. These influences include hierarchies within the nursing unit, previous patient care experiences, and cultural and personal values [52]. Ignoring differences in values within the context of the decision-making situation may contribute to imbalanced decision-making and add additional stress between clinicians [52]. SDM is well established, and many examples are available in the literature. SDM has been found to support interdisciplinary, patient, and family communication and collaboration. However, SDM requires users to learn specific behaviors for effective implementation [53].

5.4   SDM Guiding Communication and Collaboration in Acute Care

SDM will guide the discussion in the following clinical example. Through steps that include specific behaviors for SDM integration into clinical practice, communication supporting collaboration of the healthcare team and the patient/family will be demonstrated.

Case Study: Several newly graduated nurses have been hired to work on a medical unit. Following orientation of the new nurses to the unit, identification of symptoms of sepsis in three patients occurred late in their disease process. The newly graduated nurses describe feeling uncomfortable during interprofessional communication with providers due to uncertainty in their patient assessments and feeling intimidated in discussions with physicians.

A clinical nurse educator for the cardiac care unit has been tasked with educating these nurses in their understanding of their patient's status early to prevent failure to rescue situations. The education will include interprofessional communication. The newly graduated nurses state that while they have tried to keep up to date on the latest evidence to support ideal patient outcomes, each patient care situation presents unique challenges, and they struggle to understand the many signs and symptoms each patient presents with. The newly graduated nurses also express uncertainty when communicating with members of the healthcare team.

The clinical nurse educator knows research identifies that effective nursing surveillance supports understanding of patient status [6] and that experience supports identification of patient deterioration [54]. The nurse manager and clinical educator know that patients who are not treated early following the identification of sepsis symptoms experience a mortality rate that is three times higher than patients who receive antibiotics following early identification of sepsis [55]. The clinical nurse educator also knows that the time pressure involved during rapid patient deterioration contributes to less accurate decision-making [56]. Clinical leadership (including the clinical educator) decided to implement standardized training and use of simulation to increase knowledge and also support improved early recognition of patient deterioration [6]. The simulation experience will include opportunities for the newly graduated nurses to communicate interprofessionally. The clinical nurse educator designs simulated patient care scenario sessions to support learning of sepsis assessment signs and symptoms. The simulation scenario includes nurses' communication of assessment findings with actors within the simulation portraying family members, a physician, a nurse manager, and a rapid response team. The simulation mannikin portrays the patient in this simulation.

Expectations during the simulation sessions included calling rapid response team due to early identification of signs and symptoms of sepsis in their simulated "patient." The participant should also effectively communicate the patient's signs and symptoms with the rapid response team members, the nurse manager, and the physician.

6   Summary and Recommendations

Acute care nurses make high stakes decisions for patients under complex circumstances. Effective decision-making includes accurate understanding of patient status to support ideal patient outcomes. Many factors contribute to and influence effective decision-making including nursing unit culture, previous nursing experience, and nurses' support in communication and collaboration. Use of models and theories by nursing leaders in the clinical setting provides consideration of contextual factors that support effective nurse decision-making and collaboration between the healthcare team, patients, and families. Efforts to support nurse decision-making through understanding and incorporation of measures to address contextual factors in the clinical setting could improve patient safety.

Effective nursing surveillance and timely recognition of patient decline are important areas of decision-making research in nursing to support patient safety [6]. While much evidence exists to support nurse decision-making and patient safety, many factors contribute to a challenging decision-making process and may interfere with the integration of evidence into practice and with patient safety. Clearly, much work needs to be done. Future areas of improvement could include design of clinical decision support systems within the EHR that provide decision support at the right time in nurses' workflow, use of artificial intelligence, and machine learning to support early identification of factors indicative of patient decline including early diagnosis of infection and sepsis [57]. Machine learning and artificial intelligence design need to include sociodemographic diversity to provide effective decision support for clinicians in the care of diverse populations [57].

Key Points
- Acute care nurses make decision under high stakes, time limited circumstances.
- Errors in decision-making continue to pose a serious threat to patient safety.
- Understanding contextual factors that influence decision-making processes may support patient safety.
- Several theories and models have been developed and tested that support effective decision-making, leadership, and contextual factors that influence nurse decision-making in acute care settings.
- This chapter links decision-making theories and models with clinical examples to support understanding and integration into practice.

References

1. Kohn LT, Corrigan JM, Donaldson MS. Errors in health care: a leading cause of death and injury; 1999. Available from: http://www.nap.edu/download.php?record_id=9728#.
2. U.S. Department of Health and Human Services. HITECH Act Enforcement Interim Final Rule 2023 [updated 8/31/23]. Available from: https://www.hhs.gov/hipaa/for-professionals/special-topics/hitech-act-enforcement-interim-final-rule/index.html.
3. Committee on Diagnostic Error in Health C, Board on Health Care S, Institute of M, The National Academies of Sciences E. Medicine. In: Balogh EP, Miller BT, Ball JR, editors. Improving diagnosis in health care. Washington, DC: National Academies Press (US). Copyright 2015 by the National Academy of Sciences. All rights reserved; 2015.
4. Sauro KM, Machan M, Whalen-Browne L, Owen V, Wu G, Stelfox HT. Evolving factors in hospital safety: a systematic review and meta-analysis of hospital adverse events. J Patient Saf. 2021;17(8)
5. Tanner CA. Thinking like a nurse: a research-based model of clinical judgment in nursing. J Nurs Educ. 2006;45(6):204–11.
6. Burke JR, Downey C, Almoudaris AM. Failure to rescue deteriorating patients: a systematic review of root causes and improvement strategies. J Patient Saf. 2022;18(1):e140–e55.
7. Mushta J, Rush LK, Andersen E. Failure to rescue as a nurse-sensitive indicator. Nurs Forum. 2018;53(1):84–92.
8. Gephart SM, McGrath JM, Effken JA. Failure to rescue in neonatal care. J Perinat Neonatal Nurs. 2011;25(3):275–82.
9. Murray M, Sundin D, Cope V. The nexus of nursing leadership and a culture of safer patient care. J Clin Nurs. 2018;27(5–6):1287–93.
10. Nilsen P. Making sense of implementation theories, models and frameworks. Implement Sci. 2015;10:53.
11. Verran JA. The value of theory-driven (rather than problem-driven) research. Semin Nurse Manag. 1997;5(4):169–72.
12. Nibbelink CW, Carrington JM. Nurse decision making in acute care. Comput Inform Nurs. 2019;37(3):151–60.
13. Ree E, Wiig S. Linking transformational leadership, patient safety culture and work engagement in home care services. Nurs Open. 2020;7(1):256–64.
14. Lockhart EM, Hill LL, Evers AS. Building high reliability in the healthcare system. In: De Fer TM, editor. The Washington manual of patient safety and quality improvement. Philadelphia: Wolters Kluwer; 2016. p. 24–44.
15. Corcoran-Perry SA, Bungert B. Enhancing orthopaedic nurses' clinical decision making. Orthop Nurs. 1992;11(3):64–70.
16. Hammond KR. How convergence of research paradigms can improve research on diagnostic judgment. Med Decis Mak. 1996;16(3):281–7.
17. Lipshitz R, Klein G, Orasanu J, Salas E. Taking stock of naturalistic decision making. J Behav Decis Making. 2001;14(5):331–52.
18. Benner P. From novice to expert: excellence and power in clinical nursing practice. Upper Saddle River, NJ: Prentice Hall; 2001.
19. Ozdemir NG. The development of nurses' individualized care perceptions and practices: Benner's novice to expert model perspective. Int J Caring Sci. 2019;12(2):1279–85.
20. Thampy H, Willert E, Ramani S. Assessing clinical reasoning: targeting the higher levels of the pyramid. J Gen Intern Med. 2019;34(8):1631–6.
21. Evans JSBT. Dual-process theories of reasoning: Contemporary issues and developmental applications. Dev Rev. 2011;31(2):86–102.
22. Poss-Doering R, Kamradt M, Stuermlinger A, Glassen K, Kaufmann-Kolle P, Andres E, et al. The complex phenomenon of dysrational antibiotics prescribing decisions in German primary healthcare: a qualitative interview study using dual process theory. Antimicrob Resist Infect Control. 2020;9(1):6.

23. Thirsk LM, Panchuk JT, Stahlke S, Hagtvedt R. Cognitive and implicit biases in nurses' judgment and decision-making: a scoping review. Int J Nurs Stud. 2022;133:104284.
24. Helfrich CD, Rose AJ, Hartmann CW, van Bodegom-Vos L, Graham ID, Wood SJ, et al. How the dual process model of human cognition can inform efforts to de-implement ineffective and harmful clinical practices: a preliminary model of unlearning and substitution. J Eval Clin Pract. 2018;24(1):198–205.
25. Lerner JS, Li Y, Valdesolo P, Kassam KS. Emotion and decision making. Annu Rev Psychol. 2015;66:799–823.
26. Bass BM, Riggio RE. Transformational leadership. Psychology Press; 2006.
27. Giltinane CL. Leadership styles and theories. Nurs Stand. 2013;27(41):35–9.
28. Pearson MM. Transformational leadership principles and tactics for the nurse executive to shift nursing culture. J Nurs Adm. 2020;50(3):142–51.
29. Boamah SA, Laschinger HKS, Wong C, Clarke S. Effect of transformational leadership on job satisfaction and patient safety outcomes. Nurs Outlook. 2018;66(2):180–9.
30. Specchia ML, Cozzolino MR, Carini E, Di Pilla A, Galletti C, Ricciardi W, et al. Leadership styles and nurses' job satisfaction. Results of a systematic review. Int J Environ Res Public Health. 2021;18(4)
31. Martínez-Córcoles M. High reliability leadership: a conceptual framework. J Conting Crisis Manage. 2018;26(2):237–46.
32. Karkada S, Radhakrishnan J, Natarajan J, Matua GA, Kaddoura M. Knowledge and competency of novice nursing students in nasogastric tube feeding: is simulation better than case scenario? Oman Med J. 2019;34(6):528–33.
33. Risjord M. Middle-range theories as models: new criteria for analysis and evaluation. Nurs Philos. 2019;20(1):e12225.
34. Sodhi K, Chanchalani G. Awake proning: current evidence and practical considerations. Indian J Crit Care Med. 2020;24(12):1236–41.
35. Ludolph R, Schulz PJ. Debiasing health-related judgments and decision making: a systematic review. Med Decis Mak. 2018;38(1):3–13.
36. Nibbelink CW, Reed PG. Deriving the practice-primed decision model from a naturalistic decision-making perspective for acute care nursing research. Appl Nurs Res. 2019;46:20–3.
37. Nibbelink CW, Carrington JM. Nurse Decision Making in Acute Care. Comput Inform Nurs. 2019;37(3):151–60.
38. Ricci B, Cenko E, Varotti E, Puddu PE, Manfrini O. Atypical chest pain in ACS: a trap especially for women. Curr Pharm Des. 2016;22(25):3877–84.
39. Manfrini O, Ricci B, Cenko E, Dorobantu M, Kalpak O, Kedev S, et al. Association between comorbidities and absence of chest pain in acute coronary syndrome with in-hospital outcome. Int J Cardiol. 2016;217:S37–43.
40. Audet L-A, Bourgault P, Rochefort CM. Associations between nurse education and experience and the risk of mortality and adverse events in acute care hospitals: a systematic review of observational studies. Int J Nurs Stud. 2018;80:128–46.
41. Rehman A, Zalos G, Andrews NP, Mulcahy D, Quyyumi AA. Blood pressure changes during transient myocardial ischemia: insights into mechanisms. J Am Coll Cardiol. 1997;30(5):1249–55.
42. Wood C, Chaboyer W, Carr P. How do nurses use early warning scoring systems to detect and act on patient deterioration to ensure patient safety? A scoping review. Int J Nurs Stud. 2019;94:166–78.
43. Kim I, Kim MC, Park KH, Sim DS, Hong YJ, Kim JH, et al. Prognostic significance of non-chest pain symptoms in patients with non-ST-segment elevation myocardial infarction. Korean J Intern Med. 2018;33(6):1111–8.
44. Galatzan BJ, Carrington JM. Exploring the state of the science of the nursing hand-off communication. CIN: Comput Inform Nurs. 2018;36(10)
45. Olakotan OO, Yusof MM. Evaluating the alert appropriateness of clinical decision support systems in supporting clinical workflow. J Biomed Inform. 2020;106:103453.

46. Joseph NM, Ramamoorthy L, Satheesh S. Atypical manifestations of women presenting with myocardial infarction at tertiary health care center: an analytical study. J Midlife Health. 2021;12(3):219–24.
47. Herron EK. New graduate nurses' preparation for recognition and prevention of failure to rescue: a qualitative study. J Clin Nurs. 2018;27(1–2):e390–401.
48. Nibbelink CW, Brewer BB. Decision-making in nursing practice: an integrative literature review. J Clin Nurs. 2018;27(5–6):917–28.
49. Resnicow K, Catley D, Goggin K, Hawley S, Williams GC. Shared decision making in health care: theoretical perspectives for why it works and for whom. Med Decis Mak. 2022;42(6):755–64.
50. Légaré F, Stacey D, Pouliot S, Gauvin F-P, Desroches S, Kryworuchko J, et al. Interprofessionalism and shared decision-making in primary care: a stepwise approach towards a new model. J Interprof Care. 2011;25(1):18–25.
51. Ozdemir S, Finkelstein EA. Cognitive bias: the downside of shared decision making. JCO Clin Cancer Inform. 2018;2:1–10.
52. Michalsen A, Long AC, DeKeyser GF, White DB, Jensen HI, Metaxa V, et al. Interprofessional shared decision-making in the ICU: a systematic review and recommendations from an expert panel. Crit Care Med. 2019;47(9):1258–66.
53. Légaré F, Thompson-Leduc P. Twelve myths about shared decision making. Patient Educ Couns. 2014;96(3):281–6.
54. White K, Considine J, Currey J. Nurses' recognition and response to clinical deterioration in the cardiac catheterisation laboratory. Aust Crit Care. 2019;32(5):355–60.
55. Andersson M, Östholm-Balkhed Å, Fredrikson M, Holmbom M, Hällgren A, Berg S, et al. Delay of appropriate antibiotic treatment is associated with high mortality in patients with community-onset sepsis in a Swedish setting. Eur J Clin Microbiol Infect Dis. 2019;38(7):1223–34.
56. van der Vegt A, Zuccon G, Koopman B, Deacon A. How searching under time pressure impacts clinical decision making. J Med Libr Assoc. 2020;108(4):564–73.
57. Peiffer-Smadja N, Rawson TM, Ahmad R, Buchard A, Georgiou P, Lescure FX, et al. Machine learning for clinical decision support in infectious diseases: a narrative review of current applications. Clin Microbiol Infect. 2020;26(5):584–95.

Improving Patient Safety by Design: The Role of Human Factors Engineering

Bradley W. Weaver, Paige R. Gannon, and Joel M. Mumma

1   Introduction

A 42-year-old primigravida female at 34 weeks gestation was brought to the obstetric emergency department at midnight with complaints of severe headache, blurry vision, and right upper quadrant pain for the last 5–6 h.

The patient was diagnosed with severe preeclampsia. The senior obstetric resident ordered a loading dose of magnesium sulfate to prevent imminent seizure. The hospital protocol used the intravenous (IV) and intramuscular (IM) regimen where the patient receives a 4 g (20% concentration) intravenous solution bolus and 10 g intramuscular dose (50% concentration), 5 g in each buttock. The senior resident verbally provided the order for magnesium sulfate administration to the junior resident, who subsequently verbally communicated the order to the nurse.

This magnesium sulfate dosing regimen is complex with multiple doses in different locations and was incorrectly prepared by the nurse who felt rushed in an urgent situation. A chart displaying magnesium sulfate's preparation in the drug preparation room had become faded. Therefore, the nurse prepared the medication relying on her memory. Before administering the medicine to the patient, as a part of the protocol, she repeated the dose strength aloud to another nurse who cross-checked it from a printed chart and picked up the error in time. The senior resident also identified the error as the dose was communicated aloud and stopped administering the drug ([1], p. 3–4).

B. W. Weaver · P. R. Gannon
Division of Infectious Diseases, Emory University School of Medicine, Atlanta, GA, USA

Emory Healthcare, Atlanta, GA, USA
e-mail: bradley.weaver@emoryhealthcare.org; paige.gannon@emoryhealthcare.org

J. M. Mumma (✉)
Division of Infectious Diseases, Emory University School of Medicine, Atlanta, GA, USA
e-mail: joel.mumma@emoryhealthcare.org

This vignette illustrates the anatomy of a patient safety event, in which the patient was fortunately unharmed. Such "close calls" are more common than safety events that result in patient harm [2, 3] and are an opportunity to identify strengths and weaknesses in a system, that is, to identify which "defenses" are working and which defenses are failing to prevent harm to patients. To assess the strength of a systems' defenses, however, it is not necessary for a patient safety event to occur. The purpose of this chapter is to discuss how human factors engineering (HFE) can help healthcare systems identify weak defenses and design good defenses both proactively and reactively using principles of good design. This chapter familiarizes you with some of the most established design principles so that you can learn how to evaluate and improve how your workplace is designed.

2   Background

HFE can reduce the likelihood of errors occurring or causing harm in healthcare settings by designing systems to fit people rather than expecting people to adapt to the system [4]. HFE views errors as a symptom of poor system design [4] and consequently believes that errors should be a starting rather than an end point for understanding why safety events occur [5]. James Reason's "Swiss Cheese Model" (SCM) [6], which has popularized this view, argues that work systems contain defenses that prevent hazards (e.g., an incorrect medication concentration being prepared) from leading to harm (i.e., administering a medication of the wrong concentration to a patient). Metaphorically speaking, defenses are layers of cheese and include "hard" defenses, such as barriers (e.g., bed rails or electronic "guardrails" for medication safety), personal protective equipment, or alarms, as well as "soft" defenses, such as training, supervision, or written protocols (i.e., "people and paper") [6].

According to the SCM, harm occurs when a hazard breaches a defensive layer because of a weakness in or failure of that defense (i.e., a layer of Swiss cheese). These weaknesses or failures in a defense create "holes" in that layer, which allow a hazard to move one step closer to causing harm. Typically, multiple layers of defenses are in place so that if one fails, then the other defenses will prevent the hazard from leading to harm. If a failure in each defensive layer occurs, however, then there is little standing in the way of the hazard except for luck.

In the vignette described earlier, the hazard was that the nurse prepared an incorrect dosage of magnesium sulfate. Fortunately, this hazard did not reach the patient because there were several layers of defenses in place, although some defenses failed. One defense was providing a chart with instructions for magnesium sulfate's preparation in the medication preparation room so that nurses do not need to rely on memory. However, this defense failed because the chart had become faded, and the nurse had to instead rely on their memory in an urgent situation. The defense that ultimately blocked the hazard was having a protocol in place for verbally cross-checking a medication dosage before administering that medication.

The SCM implies that adding defenses (i.e., more layers) is one strategy for preventing hazards from resulting in harm. However, adding defenses not only increases the complexity of a system (e.g., adding new protocols upon existing protocols) [6], but additional defenses that are designed or implemented poorly will offer little benefit. Alternatively, the likelihood of a hazard resulting in harm can be reduced by trying to fix the holes in existing layers of defenses. Holes in defenses can by created by poor design [6], for example, an electronic medical record that is difficult to navigate or protocols that were not written by the people most familiar with the work. When poorly designed components (e.g., technology or protocols) are introduced in a work system, they can create what Reason calls "latent conditions" for error, which increase the likelihood of errors occurring or fail to prevent them from causing harm [6]. For example, medical equipment such as patient-controlled analgesia pumps may have a poorly designed user interface that (inadvertently) promotes inefficiencies and errors, such as incorrectly entering a drug concentration [7]. Consequently, the Food and Drug Administration (FDA) requires medical device manufacturers to comply with requirements that are relevant to human factors design principles so that users are not led to err [8].

3   Design Principles

This chapter discusses five principles of good design applied broadly to components such as processes, equipment, signage, and physical environment in healthcare settings. Specifically, good design makes it easier for the people performing the work and reduces the risk of errors. These design principles are called "heuristics" because they are practical and can be used to improve the design of something quickly [9, 10]. These heuristics are usually applied in a method known as "heuristic evaluation," in which someone inspects the design of something (e.g., simple paper forms, a piece of equipment, or a work area such as a nurses' station) against a set of heuristics to identify violations [11].

3.1   Heuristic 1: Minimize Demands on Memory

Inherently, our memory is limited as we can only hold a few things in "working memory" at once [12, 13]. You use your working memory when remembering the name of someone you just met or a phone number you just heard. Although our working memory often serves us well, it can sometimes fail us. How many times have you walked into a room only to forget why you went there in the first place? Or have forgotten the one item you initially went to the grocery store for? Forgetting is a limitation of working memory and is caused by two things: (1) information within working memory decaying over time or (2) "interference" from other information [12]. Although both play a factor, decay plays a larger role in forgetting in the first few seconds, and interference plays a larger role in forgetting after the first few seconds [14, 15]. For instance, you may forget to buy the one grocery item you went to buy because you see other grocery items that you realize you need (or want) before you grabbed the original item; these other grocery items are interfering with your ability to remember to buy the original item.

To keep information available in working memory, the information needs to be "rehearsed" or repeated every so often [12]. Returning to the example of learning a new phone number, we typically need to repeat the numbers until we can write them down. However, rehearsing information can be challenging when faced with competing demands on our limited working memory. In healthcare settings, interruptions and distractions are common occurrences that can tax our working memory heavily. Interruptions affect working memory by interfering with rehearsal or by generating new goals or tasks that "push out" the goals or tasks that are currently front of mind. Consequently, interruptions can lead to errors or forgetting to return to the interrupted task [16, 17].

Whether you are entering information on a computer interface, performing a procedure, or assessing a patient, good design minimizes demands on your working memory. To this end, the first step is to determine whether such demands can be eliminated or at least be reduced. Once a demand on working memory is recognized, one should ask whether it is possible for something else to remember that information instead. This strategy is called "off-loading" memory, of which everyday examples include the blinking cursor in word processing software or the checkmarks in checklists, each of which indicates where one left off if one were to be interrupted. Nurses are bombarded with information that they must hold in memory until that information is needed (e.g., remembering a patient's vital sign before being able to chart it). Given the limitations of working memory, nurses must often use strategies to off-load demands on their memory, such as quickly writing down critical information on sticky notes and report sheets (Fig. 1) or setting alarms on their phones to remind them of critical medication or lab draw times. Strategies for off-loading excessive demands on nurses include reallocating duties (e.g., routine

Fig. 1 Nurses' workstation covered with sticky notes and report sheets, a sign that too many demands are being placed on memory. *Note.* No real patient data is displayed in this photograph

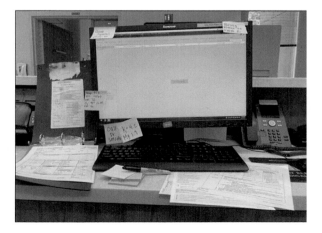

and repetitive tasks) to non-nursing personnel [18] or technological interventions (e.g., by using a single clinical communication and collaboration platform to quickly access and share pertinent information with others on the patient care team) [19].

Another strategy to reduce the demands on working memory is to leverage how our memory stores information; memory stores information in the form of "chunks," which are pieces of information that are related to each other somehow. Hence, if we connect information that we want to remember with something we already know, then it is easier to remember. For example, the mnemonic ABC (airway, breathing, circulation) is easy to remember because "ABC" is a meaningful phrase to many people that refers to the alphabet. Similarly, the mnemonic FAST (face, arm, speech, time) is easier to remember because *fast* is a word, and it relates to the situation (i.e., be fast when responding to an acute stroke).

Working memory allows us to actively use information for short periods of time (e.g., in the order of seconds). In contrast, our "long-term" memory system allows us to store information for indefinite periods of time. Like working memory, information stored in our long-term memory system is also prone to being forgotten. When this occurs, it is more likely that we are unable to retrieve that information (amongst the countless facts stored in long-term memory) rather than it being truly lost [20, 21]. Given this limitation, good design should also limit unnecessary reliance on long-term memory. Much like demands on working memory can sometimes be off-loaded, so too can demands on long-term memory; that is, knowledge can exist in the head or "in the world." [22].

For example, if a task requires supplies to be used in a specific order, having those supplies come prearranged in the correct order transfers knowledge "from the head" to the world. Drews redesigned jumble packs for central line dressing maintenance so that the packs themselves provide "task-intrinsic guidance" for the user (i.e., providing help in context) [23]. Jumble packs are bags of supplies needed to perform a task (e.g., central line dressing maintenance) that have no organization that guides the user as to their sequence of use. Therefore, jumble packs put the burden on the user to remember the correct sequence of use. Drews redesigned the jumble packs to have pockets for individual supplies, which were then arranged in the sequence of use based on best practices and labeled with printed instructions for the contents of each pocket [23]. Tests of the new design in practice found reductions in workload and duration of the procedure as well as increased adherence to best practices. In addition, the new design significantly reduced central line-associated bloodstream infections [24].

Although off-loading demands on long-term memory can be an effective strategy, it is not always possible to do so. In this case, demands on long-term memory may be reduced instead. As a rule of thumb, it is harder for people to recall information (e.g., a fill in the blank test) than it is to recognize information (e.g., a multiple-choice test); one way to leverage this principle is by standardizing common equipment or protocols so that one is not forced to recall how to use a certain piece of equipment or perform a protocol every time it is encountered. For example, a hospital may stock different brands of indwelling urinary catheter kits that contain different supplies or are arranged differently. If a nurse is not as familiar with a particular brand's kit (e.g., because of supply shortages), the risk for error increases as they must now rely on their memory for how to use the kit. By standardizing indwelling urinary catheter kits universally, we can relieve nurses from the burden of having to recall how to use each kit that they encounter. Cartwright standardized the choice of indwelling urinary catheter kit across two acute sites and, concurrently, measured the impact on catheter-associated urinary tract infection (CAUTI) rates at the two sites [25]. An all-in-one kit was chosen, which not only standardized practice but also eliminated the need for staff to recall what products or equipment were needed for the task. Introducing a standardized all-in-one indwelling urinary catheter kit across the two sites was followed by a clinically significant 80% reduction in the CAUTI rate from 2014 to 2016.

3.2 Heuristic 2: Provide Informative Feedback and Clear Closure

To stay aware of what is happening in a situation, we need informative feedback, either from the environment, from a computer interface, or from other people [8, 26]. A good example of this in driving is a backup camera that beeps faster the closer you get to an object. The camera provides visual feedback of what is behind the vehicle, and the beeping provides auditory feedback on how close objects are, which complements the camera view well because depth perception is impaired on a screen. Similarly, some medical devices give auditory feedback to reflect changes in a patient's clinical situation. For example, pulse oximeters change the pulse tone pitch as the heart rate changes, which enables people to detect changes in heart rate. A medication dispensing system has a screen that gives visual feedback about a user's actions, though it would also be beneficial to verbally announce the medication being withdrawn. Such verbal feedback may be helpful as visual warnings on a screen may not be read if they are frequently encountered when withdrawing medications [27]. However, verbal feedback would be heard by the person withdrawing the medication and others in the room.

People working in healthcare can also provide verbal feedback when communicating with each other to catch errors before they reach the patient, particularly closed-loop communication [28]. When someone gives a verbal order or shares an important piece of information (e.g., a medication order), the recipient should immediately repeat back the critical components (e.g., medication, dosage, route). This repeat-back gives the initial sender feedback that they were heard and heard correctly. Then, the initial sender should confirm verbally whether the message was received accurately or correct it if it was misheard. Furthermore, if it takes time to complete the ordered task (e.g., a person must withdraw and prepare a medication before administering it), then the recipient should additionally verbally announce when they are about to execute the order. This provides a second opportunity for other team members to catch errors and provides clear closure to other team members that the order is about to be completed. Altogether, we call this entire process closed-loop communication and closure.

Although the nurse or junior resident in the opening vignette did not verbally repeat back the critical components of the medication order, the nurse announced the medication verbally before administering it, at which point other team members caught the dosage error and stopped it from being given. In this instance, a significant contributing factor to the dosage error was reliance on memory because the poster was faded, but the verbal announcement before administration caught it. In other cases, the initial verbal order may be misheard or misunderstood by the recipient, which can be caused by many factors: the speaker does not speak clearly, the environment is noisy, or the recipient is multitasking. This communication style can (and should!) be used for more than just medication orders. It can also help catch communication errors when the team lead of a code event requests someone to perform a task or when a surgeon requests an item be retrieved—really any time someone gives a verbal order, request, or important piece of information, closed-loop communication and closure should be used to reduce communication errors and keep everyone aware of what is going on in the situation.

3.3   Heuristic 3: Consistency and Standardization

Standardization is important for many components, including the layout of work environments, equipment, controls, displays, and operating procedures. Much of what we interact with in our daily lives is standardized, even if we do not realize it. It may be difficult to notice standardization until you encounter something that does not follow the standard to which one is accustomed. This jarring experience is related to the psychological way in which standardization makes our lives easier— by reducing the need to learn different ways of doing routine things. For example, stop signs are always the same shape and color with the text "STOP" (at least in the United States and most of Europe). Imagine how dangerous it would be if every county or city designed their own stop sign. Standardizing the stop sign makes it quickly recognizable and decreases the demands placed on a driver.

When something is standardized, people develop expectations, which can make behavior faster. In most facilities, for example, the code blue button is located on the wall above the patient's head. This standardized placement enables a person to find and press that button faster than if they had to search for the button—time that is critically needed to stabilize the patient.

Standardization can also help ensure that supplies are compatible with each other. Nasogastric tubes should be able to fit with any syringe, but they do not. Similarly, pulse oximeters (and other vitals cables) should be able to connect to different devices, such as the in-room vitals monitor, portable vitals monitor, and automated external defibrillators (AEDs). If you do not have standardized connectors between devices, it is like needing an iPhone™ lightning connector but only having an Android™ USB-C connector. In an emergency situation between medical devices, this is more than just frustrating—it is also a patient safety issue.

Standardization can also help people distinguish between similar things, facilitating fast and accurate recognition. For example, the oxygen outlet on the wall of an inpatient room is always color-coded green, and the medical air outlet is always color-coded yellow (in the United States) [29]. By differentiating by color, this reduces the likelihood of someone using the medical air outlet erroneously when they needed oxygen. Similarly, fall risk supplies (e.g., fall risk socks, signs, and bands) are often yellow to enable people to quickly recognize that the patient is a fall risk. Another example is when surgical instruments are sterilized, they can be packaged in a tray and "blue wrapped" (i.e., wrapped in a blue fabric that can withstand the sterilization process). The tape used to close the blue wrap around the tray often has chemical-based color-changing ink that serves as a visual indicator that it has been sterilized. The issue is that there are different sterilization methods (e.g., steam sterilization, vaporized hydrogen peroxide sterilization), and the underlying chemical that changes colors is different for these different methods. This can result in chemical tapes that show different colors when sterile, which violates the principle of standardization and consistency.

To illustrate this, consider Fig. 2. The chemical indicator tape on the left changes from green (dirty; not shown) to black (sterile) diagonal lines, whereas the chemical indicator tape on the right changes from red (dirty; not shown) to yellow (sterile) text (i.e., the manufacturer's name). This lack of standardization between different chemical indicator tapes makes it more difficult for the surgical team to recognize when a tray has erroneously not been sterilized. Furthermore, the surgical team

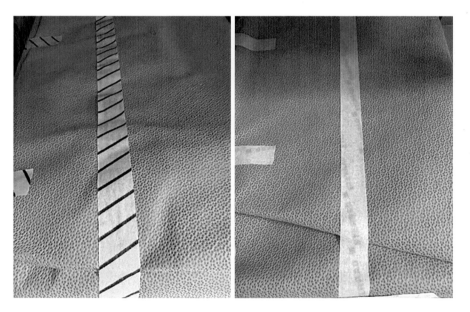

Fig. 2 Chemical indicator tape on blue-wrapped surgical trays in an operating room
Note. Each blue-wrapped tray shown has been sterilized, but due to the different sterilization methods used, different chemical indicator tapes were used that have different colors and patterns to indicate that the trays are sterile

must remember which colors reflect sterility and dirty, which violates the principle of "minimize demands on memory." Ideally, the chemical indicator tape would say "sterile" with high-contrast text only after it has been sterilized (regardless of the sterilization method).

Although standardization clearly has benefits, it also has limitations. Not all tasks lend themselves to standardization. Tasks that are highly dynamic, unpredictable, or complex can be challenging to standardize. Moreover, attempts to standardize such tasks or processes may create, rather than mitigate, problems by taking away one's professional autonomy and diminish the value of their judgment and expertise [30]. Standardization, however, does not need to be applied in all or none fashion. Some steps of tasks, parts of equipment, or parts of the environment can be standardized while still allowing for useful variation or customization. For example, during a cardiac or respiratory arrest, there are standardized algorithms that outline the minimum necessary actions a provider must take for the patient's best chance of survival. These steps provide exact times when medications must be given or when a pulse check should occur. Although these algorithms are standardized, they do allow for more customized care to reverse the cause of the arrest, such as administering medications or performing procedures. Hence, standardization turns a complex scenario into something more organized, yet the standardization still allows for customization to address the various possible causes of the arrest.

3.4   Heuristic 4: Minimalism

Inherently, we as humans can only pay attention to a limited number of things at once [4]. That is, our attention acts as a filter of all the stimuli from our environment, and we usually can only perceive and process things that we attend to. Hence, if we are inundated with information, we will not be able to process all of it. As Wears and colleagues put it, "an abundance of information produces a poverty of attention" ([31], p. 169). Thus, the minimalism principle says that only relevant and important information should be presented or displayed because additional information can be distracting or make it more difficult to find the relevant information [8, 26].

The minimalism principle can be applied in a variety of contexts, such as written and oral communications. Regarding written communications, the more text that a sign, warning, or instructions have, the less likely it is that someone will read them. Precaution signs are a good example of a written communication that should adhere to the minimalism principle because it needs to quickly communicate what precautions to take to minimize the spread of pathogens. Accordingly, these signs should be designed with only the most pertinent information, such as what specific precautions to take (e.g., clean hands, wear gown, keep door shut to maintain negative pressure). Similarly, an organization's policies help inform HCWs how to care for patients. However, if they are written in a way that has excessive details, exceptions, or caveats, it makes it more difficult for people to understand the policy. Importantly, the person looking up the policy may not have a lot of time and just wants to quickly find out the organization's policy to help inform how they will proceed. Thus, if a policy is not to the point, it may not be understood by the nurse in which case people may not follow policy in practice.

We can also apply the minimalism principle to verbal exchanges of information, such as during handoffs between nurses. Handoffs are about preparing the receiving nurse for safe and effective continuity of care for the patient from the offgoing nurse [31]. This should not include *all* the information about the patient, however, because the less relevant information is distracting and makes it harder for the receiving nurse to figure out the most important aspects of the patient's care. Moreover, the electronic medical record should have more comprehensive information about the patient that can be looked through when needed. Hence, handoffs should only include relevant and important information about the care of this patient and their current situation, which is different for each patient. This can be complemented with the offgoing nurse asking whether the receiving nurse understands or has any questions, which helps support understanding and sensemaking [31].

3.5   Heuristic 5: Align with Users' Expectations

Whether you are working with a computer interface (e.g., to document in an electronic medical record), reading a warning sign (e.g., isolation precaution signage), or hearing an overhead page (e.g., code blue), good design means using language and concepts that are familiar to the user. All too often, communication that is aimed at the user makes sense to whomever wrote it, but this offers little assurance that the end users will also understand it. For example, nurses often use their own abbreviations or shorthand when charting. When another user reviews the chart, they may misinterpret the non-standardized abbreviations potentially leading to critical mistakes, such as medication order errors. Even with a highly technical audience, one strategy that is always applicable is to use "plain language," which is the delivery of information in a simple, succinct, and accurate manner [32]. Plain language means using short sentences written in the active (rather than passive) voice and avoiding technical jargon [33]. As an example of using plain language instead of technical jargon, the Joint Commission recommends using the term "daily" instead of the technical abbreviation "q.d." (*quaque die* or "every day") because it has been confused with "q.i.d." (*quater in die* or "four times a day") when the tail of the "q" and period resembles the letter "i" [34, 35].

Communication includes not only verbal information but also visual information. "Icons," or visual symbols, are often used in place of words because of their ability to communicate information quickly, particularly information that is difficult to communicate succinctly with words. Designing effective icons, however, is not trivial. It is easy to design an icon that makes sense to you, but not to other people – just think of the game, Pictionary™! There are several strategies for ensuring that icons will be understandable to users. When creating icons, try to leverage the fact that many icons we encounter every day are already standardized, such as the symbol indicating caution (⚠) or a magnifying glass indicating a search field. Using a standardized icon increases the chances that users will recognize and understand its meaning. When there is not a standard icon to use for your purpose, then it becomes especially important to test your icons on end users to ensure that your icons can be understood quickly and accurately.

Apart from language, it is also important to use concepts or metaphors that are familiar to end users. For example, communicating the severity or urgency of information with the color red (e.g., most urgent or severe), amber (e.g., moderately urgent or severe), or green (e.g., not urgent or severe) is a common practice. A more sophisticated kind of concept that people have is their "mental models" of the world. Mental models are one's concept of how a system works [4], where a "system" refers to anything made up of a set of parts that interact with one another to collectively accomplish a goal(s) or function(s) (e.g., the respiratory system of a patient or an entire healthcare system). Because our mental models help us decide what to do in a situation, designing components to align with people's mental models makes it easier to select appropriate actions quickly and accurately. For example, arranging supplies in a supply room according to their function or physiological system (e.g., vital sign supplies or respiratory-related supplies) aligns with people's mental models of what different supplies are used for (i.e., related to each other), thereby making the search for needed supplies faster and more accurate [36].

Mental models can vary in their accuracy or completeness (e.g., compare your mental model as a clinician to that of a non-clinician when explaining a procedure). Thus, another goal of good design is to support *accurate* mental models. In the context of infection prevention and control (IPC), Clack and colleagues provide an excellent example of how to design isolation precaution signage that improves the accuracy of users' mental models; isolation precaution signage for patients who may be infected or colonized with an infectious organism is important for communicating protocols for providing safe patient care (e.g., what items of personal protective equipment to wear or when and how to clean your hands) [37]. However, one factor that can detract from HCW adherence to such guidelines is their ambiguity surrounding tasks (e.g., not knowing which guidelines apply) and expectations (e.g., not knowing what practice is acceptable or feasible) [37]. Clack and colleagues took a user-centered design approach in which a team of HCWs, infection prevention experts, and human factors engineers iteratively designed and assessed the comprehensibility of signage for contact, droplet, and airborne isolation precautions [37].

Figure 3 shows the final signage for the three types of isolation precautions, each of which supports accurate mental models (i.e., reduces ambiguity) in two ways; firstly, each sign illustrates the mode of transmission, which supports the user's

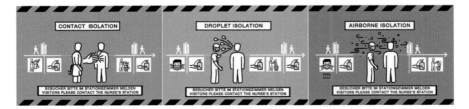

Fig. 3 Final version of signage for contact (left), droplet (middle), and airborne (right) isolation precautions
Note: Credit: Clack and colleagues [37]. Licensed under CC BY 4.0. Figure was converted to grayscale from the original

mental model of how the pathogen is transferred from the patient to the HCW (e.g., touching a patient who is on contact isolation). Additionally, each sign illustrates when specific IPC practices (i.e., donning or doffing personal protective equipment and hand hygiene) should be performed in the user's workflow (i.e., before and after entering the patient's room), which reduces ambiguity about when practices should be performed.

4 Application Discussion

To prevent hazards (e.g., an incorrect dosage of medication or chart documentation errors) from harming patients, healthcare systems use defenses involving technology, processes or protocols, and signage. When defenses fail, a hazard moves one step closer to harming a patient. In this chapter, we illustrate how defenses might be made more robust by adhering to principles of good design (i.e., heuristics). These heuristics can be applied to improve the usability of different components of your workplace, such as the devices you use, processes you follow, or the work areas within which you deliver patient care. To help you apply these heuristics effectively, we provide definitions of each as well as specific components that may benefit from their use below (Table 1).

Table 1 Five heuristics, their definitions, and examples of their application

Heuristic	Definition	Relevant to the design of
Minimize demands on memory	Reduce the amount of information that needs to be remembered by users to complete tasks [8].	Interfaces Equipment and supplies Communication
Provide informative feedback and clear closure	Users should be given useful feedback about their actions as well as a clear indication when something is completed [8].	Interfaces Equipment and supplies Communication
Consistency and standardization	A consistent design should be used throughout a system to make it easier on the user [8].	Interfaces Environment Protocols and policies Equipment and Supplies
Minimalism	Only relevant and important information should be presented or displayed; additional information can be distracting or make it more difficult to find the relevant information [8].	Interfaces Protocols and policies Signage Communication
Align with users' expectations	The language and concepts should be presented in a form understandable by the intended users [8].	Interfaces Signage Communication Environment

Note: Equipment and supplies: Any medical device or item needed to complete a task. Protocol and policies: Information created by an organization to provide direction of a specific procedure. Signage: Visual representation of instructions displayed to users. Communication: Verbal or written language used to exchange information. Environment: The physical design and layout of a space. Interfaces: The way people interact with electronic systems

One opportunity to apply these heuristics is during investigations of a patient safety event, particularly when human error is identified as a contributing factor. Adverse patient safety events are often investigated with a root cause analysis (RCA) to identify contributing factors and corrective actions. However, reviews of RCAs suggest that corrective actions often try to "fix" something about HCWs (e.g., via additional training or reinforcing policies), rather than the larger work system [38, 39]. A poorly designed interface, workplace, process, and signage are all examples of "latent conditions" for human error. How these latent conditions arose can sometimes be understood in terms of the heuristics that they violate. For example, if an error occurred when using a medical device, were there aspects of the equipment that were incongruent with the user's knowledge (e.g., mental model) or were labels and warnings easily understood (i.e., did it align with the user's expectations) [11]? Were there aspects of the device that were inconsistent either internally or with similar or more familiar devices (i.e., was consistency and standardization followed)?

Another opportunity to apply these heuristics is when developing or procuring a new product. Regarding developing a "product," items such as protocols, checklists, and signage (e.g., for isolation precautions) are often created in-house and can thus benefit from the application of heuristics. Heuristics are also relevant to items in healthcare systems that are not designed in-house, such as equipment, devices, or supplies. For example, changing the design of an electronic interface (e.g., on a patient-controlled analgesia pump or intravenous infusion pump) may not be feasible as it may require the manufacturer to make the modification. However, these heuristics can still be applied in the context of procurement decisions for such items. For example, if a hospital were considering purchasing one of the two brands of intravenous infusion pumps, adherence of each device to good design principles could be assessed proactively. Is it easy to tell what the device is doing (i.e., does it provide informative feedback and clear closure)? Does the device require the user to memorize a lot of information to use it or to remember information from screen to screen (i.e., does it minimize demands on memory)? Identifying violations of heuristics can help eliminate candidate products or identify issues that will require additional support or training for end users.

Lastly, these heuristics can be applied proactively to improve an existing product, process, or work area in your workplace. When devices are difficult to learn how to use or signage takes more than one reading, for example, it is tempting to blame ourselves as the reason for our difficulties [22]. Although users are far from being faultless, such difficulties often arise from bad design (particularly when multiple people experience the same difficulty). The next time you find yourself or someone else struggling to use a product, follow a process, or use a work area, then that product, process, or work area might benefit from a heuristic evaluation.

However, it may sometimes be challenging to decide when and how to apply these heuristics. Some heuristics may even come into conflict with each other. One consideration that may help is thinking about how it affects the user and their ability to effectively complete tasks. All heuristics are intended to make it easier on the user and lead to better performance. So, if one design clearly does that, then that is the superior design. Still, it is possible to have different ideas about, for example, what users expect or what constitutes a "minimalist" design. To resolve this, you could elicit feedback from users, which could include asking users to give feedback about designs described or shown to them. It could also involve asking users to perform a task with the proposed design of something and measuring whether one design leads to more errors, was more efficient, or was liked more by users. One could also introduce a new design into one's workflow and obtain data whether it improved things. Existing methods, such as the plan-do-study-act method [40], can do this.

Lastly, we make two recommendations to help ensure that heuristics are applied effectively. The first recommendation is to have more than one person evaluate a component(s) in terms of heuristics. Having more than one person (at least three, ideally) perform a heuristic evaluation increases the number of issues that might be discovered as different evaluators tend to find different violations [41]. Our second recommendation is to involve the input of a human factors engineer in heuristic evaluations of any component. Human factors engineers are skilled at evaluating the heuristics described in this chapter (in addition to other heuristics that were not discussed) [8] as well as in making effective trade-offs when heuristics conflict with one another.

5 Case Study: "How to" Application

The heuristics discussed in this chapter can be used to evaluate the design of things we use to perform tasks, a method known as "heuristic evaluation." In this section, we evaluate the design of a crash cart we have encountered as an illustrative example. Crash carts are mobile containers with supplies and medications needed in emergency situations. There are two ways in which the design of crash carts adheres to the heuristics (i.e., good design). First, the contents of each drawer are often standardized within an organization, making it easier for nurses to learn which drawer to retrieve an item from. Second, only the supplies needed for emergency situations are included in crash carts, which reduces search time by not having extraneous supplies (minimalist design).

There are also several ways in which the design of crash carts violates the heuristics (i.e., bad design). Although the supplies are assigned to specific drawers, the layout of supplies within drawers is not standardized. The supplies should be organized in a standardized way that aligns with users' expectations (e.g., putting supplies for a task together: vacutainer, butterfly needles, tourniquet) to facilitate quick retrieval. Also nurses who are not a part of a rapid response team do not use crash carts often. Therefore, they may not remember which supplies are in which drawers (even with the standardization of supplies in drawers). To minimize demands on memory, each drawer should be labeled. These labels should be minimalistic (i.e., listing the category of supplies instead of every individual supply) and align with users' expectations (e.g., labels that are easily understood by end users, such as visual icons plus text).

Going beyond a heuristic evaluation, steps can be taken to test and validate design changes made based on a heuristic evaluation. For example, an initial set of labels can be created, and then end users can be asked whether they know what the label means if it were on the drawer of a crash cart. Labels that are not quickly identified can then be redesigned and retested. Further, the redesigned crash cart can be tested in a simulation environment to see whether users can more quickly retrieve supplies compared to the original design.

6   Summary

To improve patient safety and quality of care, we should question the design of our workplace and the components therein. This practice helps move us away from the "person perspective" of error (i.e., that error is often the result of people being lazy, incompetent, or unmotivated) towards the "system perspective" of error (i.e., that error is more often the result of bad design) [4]. Ultimately, this practice will help drive us towards systems that work *with* us, rather than *against* us. Work redesign can reduce the workload of nurses, allowing them to focus on delivering quality patient care, directly target the causes of patient safety events (i.e., hazards), or strengthen defenses that prevent hazards from harming the patient. The discussion of heuristics in this chapter should not only prompt you to question the design of things in your workplace but also help you ask the right questions for improving their design.

Key Points
- Errors or inefficiencies are often a symptom of poor design.
- Adhering to principles of good design can reduce the likelihood of errors or inefficiencies occurring.
- A design can be quickly evaluated by comparing the design against a set of design principles, known as heuristics.
- Anyone can learn about principles of good design and start using them to improve their own workplace.

References

1. Singh G, Patel RH, Boster J. Root cause analysis and medical error prevention. In: StatPearls. StatPearls Publishing; 2022. [cited 2023 Apr 8]; Available from: https://www.ncbi.nlm.nih.gov/books/NBK570638/.
2. Williamsen M. Safety stand downs: turning a waste of time into a value added event. In: OnePetro; 2013. Available from: https://onepetro.org/ASSPPDCE/proceedings-abstract/ASSE13/All-ASSE13/77518.
3. Jeffs L, Berta W, Lingard L, Baker GR. Learning from near misses: from quick fixes to closing off the Swiss-cheese holes. BMJ Qual Saf. 2012;21(4):287–94.
4. Lee J, Wickens C, Liu Y, Boyle L. Designing for people: an introduction to human factors engineering. Pearson; 2017.
5. Dekker S. Drift into failure: from hunting broken components to understanding complex systems. CRC Press; 2016. 235 p
6. Reason J. Managing the risks of organizational accidents. Ashgate; 1997. 280 p.

7. Lin L, Isla R, Doniz K, Harkness H, Vicente KJ, Doyle DJ. Applying human factors to the design of medical equipment: patient-controlled analgesia. J Clin Monit Comput. 1998;14(4): 253–63.
8. Zhang J, Johnson TR, Patel VL, Paige DL, Kubose T. Using usability heuristics to evaluate patient safety of medical devices. J Biomed Inform. 2003;36(1):23–30.
9. Kortum P. Usability assessment: how to measure the usability of products, services, and systems. Human Factors Ergonomics Society; 2016. 120 p.
10. Jeffries R, Miller JR, Wharton C, Uyeda K. User interface evaluation in the real world: a comparison of four techniques. In: Proceedings of the SIGCHI conference on human factors in computing systems Reaching through technology—CHI '91. New Orleans, Louisiana: ACM Press; 1991. p. 119–24. [cited 2023 May 15] Available from: http://portal.acm.org/citation.cfm?doid=108844.108862.
11. Gosbee J, Gosbee LL. Usability evaluation in health care. In: Human factors and ergonomics in health care and patient safety. 2nd ed. CRC Press; 2012. p. 543–55.
12. Mathy F, Feldman J. What's magic about magic numbers? Chunking and data compression in short-term memory. Cognition. 2012;122(3):346–62.
13. Chen Z, Cowan N. Core verbal working-memory capacity: the limit in words retained without covert articulation. Q J Exp Psychol. 2009;62(7):1420–9.
14. Berman MG, Jonides J, Lewis RL. In search of decay in verbal short-term memory. J Exp Psychol Learn Mem Cogn. 2009;35(2):317–33.
15. Campoy G. Evidence for decay in verbal short-term memory: a commentary on Berman, Jonides, and Lewis (2009). J Exp Psychol Learn Mem Cogn. 2012;38:1129–36.
16. Westbrook JI, Raban MZ, Walter SR, Douglas H. Task errors by emergency physicians are associated with interruptions, multitasking, fatigue and working memory capacity: a prospective, direct observation study. BMJ Qual Saf. 2018;27(8):655–63.
17. Westbrook JI, Coiera E, Dunsmuir WTM, Brown BM, Kelk N, Paoloni R, et al. The impact of interruptions on clinical task completion. BMJ Qual Saf. 2010;19(4):284–9.
18. Cornell P, Riordan M, Townsend-Gervis M, Mobley R. Barriers to critical thinking: workflow interruptions and task switching among nurses. JONA J Nurs Adm. 2011;41(10):407.
19. Collins R. Clinician cognitive overload and its implications for nurse leaders. Nurse Lead. 2020;18(1):44–7.
20. Conway MA. Episodic memories. Neuropsychologia. 2009;47(11):2305–13.
21. Anderson RC, Pichert JW. Recall of previously unrecallable information following a shift in perspective. J Verbal Learn Verbal Behav. 1978;17(1):1–12.
22. Norman DA. The psychology of everyday things. Basic Books; 1988. 257 p.
23. Drews FA. Adherence engineering: a new approach to increasing adherence to protocols. Ergon Des Mag Hum Factors Appl. 2013;21(4):19–25.
24. Drews FA, Bakdash JZ, Gleed JR. Improving central line maintenance to reduce central line-associated bloodstream infections. Am J Infect Control. 2017;45(11):1224–30.
25. Cartwright A. Reducing catheter-associated urinary tract infections: standardising practice. Br J Nurs. 2018;27(1):7–12.
26. Nielsen J. Enhancing the explanatory power of usability heuristics. In: Proceedings of the SIGCHI conference on Human factors in computing systems celebrating interdependence—CHI '94. Boston, Massachusetts, United States: ACM Press; 1994. p. 152–8. [cited 2023 Mar 23]; Available from: http://portal.acm.org/citation.cfm?doid=191666.191729.
27. Heed This Warning! Don't Miss Important Computer Alerts. Institute For Safe Medication Practices. 2007 [cited 2023 Apr 18]. Available from: https://www.ismp.org/resources/heed-warning-dont-miss-important-computer-alerts
28. Salas E, Wilson KA, Murphy CE, King H, Salisbury M. Communicating, coordinating, and cooperating when lives depend on it: tips for teamwork. Jt Comm J Qual Patient Saf. 2008;34(6):333–41.
29. King D, Houseman B, Decker M. Gas cylinders. In: StatPearls. StatPearls Publishing; 2022. [cited 2023 Apr 25]. Available from: https://www.ncbi.nlm.nih.gov/books/NBK513350/.

30. Sinsky CA, Bavafa H, Roberts RG, Beasley JW. Standardization vs customization: finding the right balance. Ann Fam Med. 2021;19(2):171–7.
31. Wears RL, Perry SJ, Patterson ES. Handoffs and transitions of care. In: Handbook of human factors and ergonomics in health care and patient safety. 2nd ed. CRC Press; 2017. p. 163–71.
32. Warde F, Papadakos J, Papadakos T, Rodin D, Salhia M, Giuliani M. Plain language communication as a priority competency for medical professionals in a globalized world. Can Med Educ J. 2018;9(2):e52–9.
33. Plain Language at AHRQ. [cited 2023 May 15]. Available from: https://www.ahrq.gov/policy/electronic/plain-writing/index.html
34. Do Not Use List Fact Sheet | The Joint Commission. [cited 2023 May 15]. Available from: https://www.jointcommission.org/resources/news-and-multimedia/fact-sheets/facts-about-do-not-use-list/
35. Greenall J. Prescription for safety. Pharm Pract. 2007; [cited 2023 May 15]. Available from: https://www.ismp-canada.org/download/09-Legibility-07-final.pdf
36. Drews FA, Kramer HS. Human-computer interaction design in health care. In: Human factors and ergonomics in health care and patient safety. 2nd ed. CRC Press; 2012. p. 265–77.
37. Clack L, Stühlinger M, Meier MT, Wolfensberger A, Sax H. User-centred participatory design of visual cues for isolation precautions. Antimicrob Resist Infect Control. 2019;8(1):179.
38. Kellogg KM, Hettinger Z, Shah M, Wears RL, Sellers CR, Squires M, et al. Our current approach to root cause analysis: is it contributing to our failure to improve patient safety? BMJ Qual Saf. 2017;26(5):381–7.
39. Peerally MF, Carr S, Waring J, Dixon-Woods M. The problem with root cause analysis. BMJ Qual Saf. 2017;26(5):417–22.
40. Plan-Do-Study-Act (PDSA) Directions and Examples. [cited 2023 May 11]. Available from: https://www.ahrq.gov/health-literacy/improve/precautions/tool2b.html
41. Nielsen J, Molich R. Heuristic evaluation of user interfaces. In: Proceedings of the SIGCHI conference on Human factors in computing systems empowering people—CHI '90. Seattle, Washington: ACM Press; 1990. p. 249–56. Available from: http://portal.acm.org/citation.cfm?doid=97243.97281.

Technology and Patient Safety: A Cause and Solution to Complexity

Jane M. Carrington and Christine W. Nibbelink

1 Introduction

After years of risks to patient safety in healthcare systems, the Institute of Medicine issued reports exposing poor patient outcome data and issued a challenge to address the gaps in patient safety. The Health Information Technology for Economic and Clinical Health (HITECH) Act of 2009 responded to the challenge and began a series of advancements, which were both welcomed to healthcare and challenging for providers. Data has since revealed progress towards patient safety and needed next steps.

With the HITECH Act, the technology system was embedded within the health system forming a system of system. Two systems have added complexity due to individuals within each. Despite advances in data collection from the systems, there remain issues to address. The design of the electronic health record (EHR) has been criticized for not working with nurses and the team to provide care and lacks flexibility for the varied end user. Building on this issue is the volume of data nurses enter or "documentation burden."

Purpose Statement: The purpose of this chapter is to explore the challenge and complexity that technology brings to healthcare as well as the opportunity of harnessing technology to advance patient safety.

J. M. Carrington (✉)
University of Florida, College of Nursing, Gainesville, FL, USA

Health Care Quality, Gainesville, FL, USA
e-mail: janecarrington@ufl.edu

C. W. Nibbelink
Hahn School of Nursing and Health Science, University of San Diego, San Diego, CA, USA
e-mail: cnibbelink@sandiego.edu

C. A. Oster, J. S. Braaten (eds.), *The Nexus between Nursing and Patient Safety*,
https://doi.org/10.1007/978-3-031-53158-3_14

259

2   Background

Healthcare is often conceptualized as a system. As a system, healthcare is further defined as a patient care system. Systems are defined as a collection of "things" that are interconnected working together and produce their own behavior over time [1–3]. This definition works for computer systems, transportation systems, and so forth. These systems are predictable in work and function. When people are included in the system, the system becomes much less predictable. People within a system have different backgrounds and experiences and different priorities in decision-making. This creates a system that lacks predictability and adds complexity. When the system consists of people who can make their own decisions and self-organize their work, the system becomes a complex adaptive system [4, 5]. A patient enters the system through admission into acute care or primary care. For one patient, they can remain in the same local or regional system level with relocation; this same patient can then join another local or regional system. The patient can also be part of a national system. At the lowest level of the system, the patient will receive ongoing primary care with necessary acute care (planned or unplanned). This care trajectory will include members of the care team interacting and communicating to sustain a level of health and to return the patient to their home. This is a very simplistic view of the system.

Ubiquitous in healthcare, technology contains a collection of components that are interconnected that do work together towards a defined output. With conservative beginnings, technology entered healthcare with the thermometer, sphygmomanometer, and stethoscope. These were manual technologies that were used by caregivers and results written into the patient record. Technology became a system when they became interconnected and working together and exhibiting their own behavior. Here, we argue that technology such as patient monitors, glucometers, digital beds, computers (electronic health record), and embedded applications are a system that is within the healthcare system, or this is a "system of systems" [6]. A technology system within the healthcare system shares characteristics of systems of systems as described as heterogeneity, emergent behavior, and large systems [7]. The hypothesis is that systems of systems exhibit the same characteristics as systems; however, these are amplified according to their size and complexity.

Technology in healthcare or systems of systems share a common denominator, people. As stated earlier, individuals collectively providing care to patients in the healthcare system, who can make their own decisions, will add levels of unpredictability to the system. Adding technology to the system with individuals with different levels of technology savviness and experience and lack of unification of design and acceptance for the user adds another element of unpredictability. This chapter focuses on humans using technology within systems of systems to care for patients.

Here, we will take the approach of discussing technology and its role in healthcare as a system within a system or system of system, technology and end user interface, and patient care. The purpose of this chapter is to explore the challenges and complexities that technology brings to healthcare as well as the opportunity of harnessing technology to advance patient safety.

3 Systems

3.1 Healthcare System

According to the Compendium of U.S. Health Systems of 2016, a health system is an organization that includes at least one acute care facility and a group of providers who provide comprehensive care who are connected with each other and the acute care facility [8]. This high-level definition includes some key elements. First, different care settings are included, both acute and primary care. Second, people are included as providers. The term "provider" can be defined to include physicians, advanced practice nurses or nurse practitioners, registered nurses, and physician assistants. Comprehensive care can imply contributions from the interdisciplinary care team and available interventions.

Evaluation of the system is important to understand necessary system adjustments. This is missing from the above general descriptions of systems; however, this is very important for health systems. Foundational research in health system evaluation was done by Donabedian [9] and Mitchell [10]. Both suggested that to evaluate health systems, one studied the quality outcomes or patient outcomes. Donabedian suggested that the physician *Structure* of the health system influenced the *Process* of care delivery, resulting in *Outcomes* or the patient status after care [10]. Mitchell built on this framework and added that the organizational *System* influenced the interventions, *Client*, and *Outcomes*; *Interventions* influenced the *System* and *Client*; *Client* influenced the *Intervention* and *Outcomes*; and the *Outcomes* influenced *Systems* and *Client* [9]. Outcomes are measured using data and quality improvement based on best evidence.

Here, we define health system as a group of providers who provide care for patients in acute and primary care settings that includes evaluations of the system and patient outcomes.

3.2 Technology System

Technology systems are defined as having similar characteristics: input, process, and output [11]. Technology systems without context are without specifics as to purpose, evaluation, or function. The implication is that technology by itself is very flexible to fit into context. Technology system for health systems must take on specific function for patient data. Technology first comes into contact with patients in acute and primary care with the collection of preliminary data consisting of heart rate, temperature, weight, blood pressure, and pulse oxygenation. Within acute care, patients are immediately upon entry connected to patient monitors, and for the critical patients, invasive monitoring devices are connected.

Technology system within the context of health system can be defined then as system with input, process, and output of patient data. Recall that a critical part of the health system definition included individuals. Thus far, the technology system lacks that element. Here, we include individuals with the following definition:

technology systems in health systems have input, process, and output of patient data through the interface with individuals. Technology system now has context and added complexity of individuals.

For example, Fig. 1 illustrates the point. At the top, technology functions with routine input and output. Go below the middle of the figure to add humans, and technology has context for purpose and complexity for user technology interface.

Philosophically, health and technology systems share two important elements, individuals and patients. Patients are the target and purpose of the health and technology systems. Individuals are providers in health system and "end users" in the technology system. End users interact with the technology system or "interface" with the technology system.

Evaluation of the technology system is done using software updates, quality improvement with added text fields, database analysis, and interview and system analysis or survey of end users. Notice that elements of the health system are included in the technology system evaluation. And the same is true for the health system evaluation. This further strengthens the argument that these are systems within or on systems. And the evaluation of one will influence the evaluation of the other.

Here, we define the technology system in the context of health as containing input, process, and output of patient data through the interface with end users, which includes evaluation of the system.

Here, we have explained and defined the health and technology systems. Both are complex with individuals and include evaluation. Together, these are a system of systems together working towards patients and patient outcomes.

Fig. 1 Technology and human context and complex

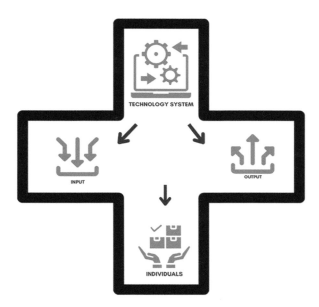

From here, we will take a deeper dive into the technology system and its influence in patient outcomes.

4   Technology System

The Institute of Medicine report "To Err is Human" (2000) revealed that nearly 100,000 patients die in US hospitals due to error in the hospital system [12]. Those doing research in informatics (studying the technology system) used this to emphasize the need for technology system in health system and pushed for requirements to that end. This report was followed up by the report "Crossing the Quality Chasm" (2001) where the challenge was set to increase quality in the US health system by 50% in 5 years [13]. Suggestions to reach the goal were to increase the use of technology, improve billing and payment processes, and develop decision support tools, accountability system, and professional education. Of these, increasing technology and decision support tools were directly part of the technology system. These reports helped to stimulate research in informatics and advance technology system in the health system.

These reports stimulated discussion and helped to inspire the Health Information Technology for Economic and Clinical Health (HITECH) Act of 2009. HITECH Act was signed into law on February 17, 2009, with the goal of adoption and meaningful use of technology in the health system (U.S. Department of Health & Human Services) [14]. Healthcare organizations who fail to comply will have financial penalty and reimbursement issues from the Centers for Medicare & Medicaid Services (CMS). "Meaningful Use" became the shorthand description of the HITECH Act and was divided into phases: (1) electronic health record (EHR) adoption; (2) exchange of patient information; and (3) improve healthcare outcomes. The fourth phase emerged later and involves reducing health disparities and increasing efficiency of billing and physician data entry at the point of care. Another ongoing goal is interoperability of technology systems to exchange patient data.

The HITECH Act and CMS increased the availability of technology in healthcare. While technology had been available, it found an initiative to "land" and hold an important role in healthcare. This is not surprising when through CMS, Meaningful Use of the EHR is now attached to reimbursement, and through HITECH Act, failure to comply would be costly.

A question remains, however: What does Meaningful Use of the EHR mean, and how would it be reported? Table 1 lists the elements of Meaningful Use objectives and measures. Looking at the first round of criteria and evaluation metrics for Meaningful Use Stage 1, take note of the low bar for success and emphasis of structured data, and emphasis on medications. One could argue that a low bar for success encourages success for health organizations with this first stage and raises the question of organizations that exceeded this standard. Second, the emphasis for structured data has other implications. Structured data contrasts with unstructured data in how the data is entered and then entered into the database within the system. The third point to make is the emphasis on medications from legibility of the

Table 1 Meaningful Use objectives and measures, Stage 1

Meaningful use objective	Measure	Implications
Computerized provider order entry (CPOE) for medication orders for any licensed professional per regulations	>30% of different patients with medications have at least one medication entered using COPE	– Seeks to address medication errors due to illegibility
Implement drug-drug interaction check	EHR has this feature enabled	– Turn on, note instances of use or catch of near misses
Generate and transmit e-prescriptions	>40% all permissible prescriptions transmitted electronically	– Address illegibility in prescriptions – Connect primary and acute care and pharmacy
Patient demographic—address, language, gender, race, date of birth, cause of death recorded	>50% patients have recorded demographics as structured data	– Structured data goes directly to the database, straight forward for numbers and addresses – Benefits of data for outcomes from EHR
List of problems and diagnosis is maintained	>80% patients have at least one entry or an indication that problems are known for the patient recorded as structured data	– Problem list in structured format will build the database
Active medication list	>80% patients have at least one entry of prescribed medication as structured data	– Medication list as structured data
Active medication allergy list	>80% have at least one entry of medication allergy or none as structured data	– Medication allergies as structured data
For patients 2–10 years, record VS, height and weight, BMI, and growth charts	>50% 2 years and older have height, weight, and BP recorded as structured data	– Foundational data for children as structured data
Record smoking status for those >13 years old	>50% 13 years and older have smoking status as structured data	– Smoking status as structured data
Implement one clinical decision support rule and method for tracking	Implement one clinical decision support rule	– One decision support rule – Evidence for use and acknowledgement
Report clinical quality measures to CMS or state reporting	2011: provide aggregate numerator and denominator and exclusions through attestation; 2012: quality measures	– Use data for measures
Electronic copy of health record for patients	>50% patients, electronic copy within 3 days of request	– Patients can request their record in the manner of which it is collected

(continued)

Table 1 (continued)

Meaningful use objective	Measure	Implications
Acute care—provide patients electronic copy of discharge instructions at discharge	>50% patients provide copies for those requested	– This is as requested, not required
Provide clinical summaries for office visits	>50% clinical summaries within 3 business days	– Support communication throughout the health system
Exchange clinical information among providers	Complete at least one test of electronic exchange by certified EHR	– Connect providers within health system
Protect EHR information by certified EHR	Perform review security risk analysis, implement updates, and address deficiencies	– Health system responsibility to keep up with technology and address issues

Adapted from http://www.cms.gov/EHRIncentivePrograms

prescription to interactions and allergies. This is consistent with the high medication errors contributing to patient deaths.

Unstructured data is the natural text of the end user using the EHR within the technology system. Natural text cannot go directly into the database. Nurses, for example, may have a finite way of describing a fever, the database does not have that much space, and this would be too cumbersome for extracting data from the database. Two options exist for converting the unstructured to structured text data. First, implement and adopt standardized terminology or language, so everyone uses the same text language that will go directly into the database. Second, use natural language processing to convert free text language to structured language. Numbers or quantitative data is inherently structured data. The emphasis for the data elements to be structured demonstrates the importance of data and the need for data to measure outcomes.

The last point of the Meaningful Use Stage 1 is certified EHR. Vendors develop and sell certified EHRs that are secure and sustain patient data confidentiality. This means that these EHRs include clinical processes, care coordination, quality measures, and privacy and security. At the time of HITECH Act, certified EHRs were a concept. Since then, they are the standard for EHRs.

The focus thus far has been the EHR. For some technology within the system, patient data can move from collection to the EHR as an "auto-feed." For example, from the patient monitor in the intensive care unit, data can be sent to the EHR and to the database. Digital patient data from glucometers, thermometers, and blood pressure devices can all be entered manually into the EHR and then to the database. These are all devices that either directly input or require the end user to input data. Processing takes place getting data to the database and is used to inform algorithms running in the background, such as decision support systems and outcome measures.

Within the Meaningful Use description, there were two concepts: one was meaningful use of the EHR and the second is adoption. Thus far, the discussion has focused on the HITECH Act and Meaningful Use. The important part related to adoption is the end user technology interface.

4.1   The End User Technology Interface

Meaningful Use is about adoption of technology. Adoption follows a long intentional plan of implementation. A traditional implementation plan includes understanding the change to the technology, such as a software upgrade or new application, building it and testing to ensure that it works as intended for the setting, training the end users, rolling out the change or "go live," and evaluating the change. We know that some of the end users will quickly adopt and communicate the change in the technology, while others will lag, and some lag further behind [15]. We also know that end users are more likely to adopt technology or changes in technology when the technology is deemed useful to perform their work and easy to use [16]. Based on the above, successful implementation of technology requires communication informing the end user of how the technology will assist in completing work and not take away from the work. This is a shorthanded way of stating that adoption is aided by the design of the technology.

Remember the earlier discussion about the complex system and the unpredictability due to individuals in the system. Each end user or individual has their background, training, biases, and experiences that will inform their work and decision-making. Look outside; look at the different automobiles in the parking lot or on the street. Different sizes, electric vs. gasoline, fixed roof or convertible or moonroof, dash arrangement of the gauges, and placement of the controls vary for each make and model. Each of us, when preparing to buy a car, seeks the make and model that suits our approach to driving, intuitiveness, comfortability, and perhaps color. The EHR, in comparison, is one application that is inflexible for individual users and in their approach to completing work, in this case, entering data about patient care.

The end user interface has an impact on the approach to work, including data entry. Work, for example, can be admitting a patient. A series of tasks are organized that in total is the work to admit a patient. The series of tasks begin with the patient entering the system or the assigned room, interview for demographics, assessment, vital signs, orders (medications, dietary, activity, tests, procedures, for example), complete admission orders, results, establishing the plan of care, beginning patient teaching, and care coordination. Throughout the process of data entry, workarounds could be used to "shortcut" the process for efficiency. Within the EHR, workarounds could be used to alter the sequence of data entry in a more efficient manner to reduce the "work" reducing the number of mouse clicks to navigate from one template to the next. For the first generation of the clinical systems, designers modeled the templates to be like the trifold flowsheet that were used during the paper system era. The idea was that this design matched what nurses used, so the transition from paper to computer should have been easy. Unfortunately, that plan did not work as intended. This raises a question: What exactly are the issues, and how can they be addressed? Some of the key elements of design for the end user technology interface include the size of the font of the template, sequence of data entry within a template, color of the application, number of mouse clicks from one section to another, speed of processing, minimal typing free text, increased auto fill of data, and organization of information on the "landing page" when signed on the application to name a few.

If using a technology that does not exactly fit your organization of work process, how does one adapt? One choice is to go ahead and use the technology as designed and accept its cumbersome nature. Another is to create work-arounds. End users create informal changes to workflow using technology [17]. Work-arounds are considered to be an unintended consequence of the feature of the technology where end users seek change to workflow. Work-arounds can consist of sequence changes to complete work, shortcuts to a longer process, or alterations in data entry or changes to use of technology. Work-arounds had been discouraged, which then became a learning tool for developers and policy and procedure advocates. One example of a work-around is copy and paste. This is where providers copy notes and patient data from one note or provider and copy as their own. While viewed as a time-saving work-around, the risk of errors is extraordinary due to lack of reviewing the content to verify accuracy for patient status. A common work-around is to ignore alerts or falsely acknowledge them to move on with the task using the EHR. Unfortunately, acknowledging an alert implies that the professional has read it and used decision-making for the patient. Another work-around is not signing the entry to allow for updating and editing. This leads to delays or no "real-time" communication using the EHR.

4.2 Documentation Burden

The pandemic, while tragic, revealed and amplified gaps in the US health and technology systems. Focusing on the technology system, the EHR, and nursing care, the intense work during the COVID pandemic raised questions as to of all the data nurses enter into the system, what is essential and at what frequency. We know that the quantity of data nurses enter into the system has increased [18, 19]. Nurses have perceived that this quantity of data they are directed to enter into the system requires time taken away from patient care [20–23]. Nursing data entry is driven by accreditation and regulatory standards, the philosophy "if it isn't in the EHR it wasn't done," and organizational requirements. We also know that templates share data leading to redundancy.

Building on the documentation burden is cognitive burden. Cognitive burden is the demands of clinical perception, reasoning, recollection, and judgement [24]. These skills are necessary to accurately enter data on the right patient about the right care processes. Cognitive load is related to cognitive burden as work memory actively processes and retrieves information while doing work [25]. Examples of cognitive burden for nurses are the distraction of calls, call lights, families or colleagues asking questions or seeking assistance, alerts within the EHR for repeated clinical decision support flags, or allergy or incompatibility issues of medications that all contribute to increasing cognitive load and 80% of errors, threatening patient safety. Simply put, the very nature of the health and technology systems and their complexities (individuals) contribute to errors.

5   Where We Are Now

Our current healthcare system is a system of system with technology. Together, these systems are fraught with complexity with the inclusion of people or individuals as providers and care team members. These systems together account for 80% of the errors and unforeseen patient deaths. Despite efforts at evaluation and the addition of safety measures, we have made marginal progress to increase patient safety.

Our health and technology systems have applications, EHR, and other applications such as clinical decision support, designed for one user type. The design fails to consider the individual end user and their workflow, decision-making processes, navigation of the stimulation of the environment, and organizational requirements. The application is inflexible to individual end users. Yet, the government mandate has made adoption of the EHR a requirement.

Nurses perceive that they are spending more time entering data and less with patient care. The burden of patient data entry can be linked to the challenges of cognitive load, design of the EHR, and volume of required data entry.

Since the IOM report of 2000, we have experienced a paradigm shift in healthcare and the health and technology systems. This is the result of improved data collection and reporting, and according to Pronovost, errors are not inevitable [26]. Safety indicators are used to quantify safe care, reflecting a 13% decrease in hospital-acquired conditions (conditions developed during the hospitalization); emphasis on safe surgeries and effective handoff communication have all attributed to improved patient outcomes [26]. Notice that these examples are high-level outcomes and are the sum of action taken by members of the healthcare team with patient care, navigating cognitive load and technology with the burden of data entry.

While there is optimism here, there is room for continued improvement. Next, we propose recommendations moving forward to harness technology for patient safety in the complex care environment.

6   Where We Need to Go

Technology system is important for patient safety and measuring outcomes. There are several recommendations to harness technology for patient safety: (1) reconceptualize the EHR as a communication system from a documentation system, (2) examination of quantity of nursing data entry, (3) increased algorithms running in the background through artificial intelligence (AI) to guide decision-making and data entry, and (4) smart rooms.

6.1   Communication System

It could be argued that the technology system is a communication system. The EHR is often referred to as a documentation system, and nurses comment that they document patient data. Documenting care extends well before the EHR to paper systems. According to the American Nurses Association (ANA), nursing documentation includes patient care documents, patient assessments, and outcome measures and meets the criteria of the organization and the profession of nursing [27]. Here, we suggest reconceptualizing the EHR from that of a documentation system to a communication system.

A communication system is a system where information is exchanged between two points, one nurse to the next, and communication is stimulated by an event [28]. Information theory according to Shannon provides insight into shifting the paradigm from documentation to communication [29]. Three elements for information theory are sender, device, and receiver. The sender crafts the message, and the device sends the message to the receiver. Entropy is the uncertainty of information in the message. For example, a message about a change in patient condition instead was a message about something completely different. In this case, entropy is increased, or the message is uncertain or contains less information. Negentropy would be increased when entropy is decreased and occurs when the information in the message is on point as expected. A redundancy is inherent in the English language; however, at a point, redundancy inhibits rather than increases effective communication. Failure of the message to transmit accurately increases uncertainty and is the result of noise. Probability is the likelihood that a message contains specific subject matter. The goal is effective communication with limited noise, controlled redundancy, and reasonable probability resulting in decreased entropy with increased information. Table 2 lists these elements and definitions.

The message is sent from the sender to receiver via communication channel [29]. The channel can be electronic using the EHR or verbal using the handoff. The channel within the system can also be an interface sending patient data to the EHR or

Table 2 Elements of information theory

Concept	Definition	Example
Entropy	Increased entropy-low information in message Decreased entropy-high information in the message (negentropy)	Message is on point as anticipated in the EHR and handoff
Redundancy	Repeated content in message	Same data in multiple places of the EHR
Noise	Failure of the message to reach the receiver as intended	Message disrupted by technical glitch Message not sent Message misunderstood
Probability	Message contains anticipated information specific to event	Message about pain includes essential information for ongoing care

Adapted from Shannon [29]

collecting from the patient to the nurse for data entry such as a digital thermometer or glucometer.

Shifting to communication system from technology system then implies that entering data is crafting a message for the care team and next nurse on shift. And a message about a change in patient condition that is resolved is an example of effective communication. Effective communication also occurs when a problem is anticipated and prevented.

Here, we argue that rather than a technology system of health system, more accurately, communication system is of the health system. The elements of these systems remain true with complexity and individuals. Evaluation remains critical to determine best strategies of communication and patient care.

6.2 Examine Quantity of Nursing Data Entry

We have presented the argument for "document burden" existing in our health system and communication system (formerly technology system). The American Nursing Informatics Association submitted a position paper to the Association Board of Directors, led by Dr. Sengstack where they examined the domains of burden for nurses and data entry [30]. The six burdens examined included those we have already mentioned, regulatory, usability, redundancy, self-imposed (culture of the organization and unit), reimbursement, and quality. This was a good start to the examination, and we need to move forward to quantify nursing data entry and examine for what is essential, nice to have, and unnecessary. This is a brave step requiring nurses to look at what has been added over the years without taking away outdated or unnecessary data points.

6.3 Artificial Intelligence

Artificial intelligence has existed in the EHR with decision support systems, alerting the healthcare team to allergies and medication issues such as incompatibilities. These algorithms have gotten more sophisticated over the years and "smarter" with the use of EHR data, using techniques with EHR data collection (flow sheet templates and free text data in notes and comments). With this data, models can be developed that allow the provision of precision care-specific plans based on precise needs of the patient. Data from the genome has also assisted with targeted medications and dosages. This is only the tip of the iceberg; however, these examples reveal the promise and progress using the data in the EHR to help us understand the health system and patients.

There are other applications using artificial intelligence that could have an impact on the complexity of healthcare and communication. For example, ChatGPT and other applications can be used to automate portions of data entry. Looking at progress notes, there are sections that are routine and could be completed using artificial intelligence applications. Routine assessments may also be done using artificial intelligence. The challenge will be to take the time to check for accuracy to reduce the risk of error in the record and database.

Another application of artificial intelligence is robots. Robots are already in our lives and playing a role in healthcare in surgery, prosthetics, laboratories by automating sample tests, delivering medications and supplies, and social aspects taking the shape of humans and animals. Robots could be used to perform basic tasks that currently take nurses' time. This could increase nurses' time with patients and reduce cognitive load with focus on higher level aspects of care. Robots could enhance nursing care, not reduce nurses.

6.4   Smart Rooms

Smart homes are gaining popularity using applications to control indoor temperature, heating and air conditioning, security, indoor and outdoor lights, and door locks and garage doors. For the application to work, sensors are placed in specific areas of the house, and Bluetooth or Wi-Fi is used to connect the application to the specific device. Simply stated, it includes control functions of the house from a smart phone or tablet.

Imagine sensors in specific areas of a patient room in the hospital. Sensors can detect the activity of the patient, like risk of falling out of bed. Sensors can be placed throughout the room to detect whatever is needed, and data can be transmitted to the EHR. This technology is already being explored in long-term care or nursing homes. Sensors are used for health monitoring, detecting falls, and detection of location [31]. Using an everyday smartwatch can provide much of the same data, and it has been adopted by seniors for the ease of use and function [32].

7   Case Study

Here, we will explore a typical healthcare system which is challenged by many of the same issues described above. Technology was implemented without understanding that the end users understand their work and technology needs. The leadership welcomed the vendor's EHR despite the gaps in how the licensed employees worked and entered data. It was clear that the technology and employees were not working together due to issues with the user technology interface. All the providers (nurses, nurse practitioners, physician assistants, and physicians) were frustrated that the technology did not help them take care of patients, but rather increased their work. Eventually, the frustrations led to increased errors, turnover of licensed personnel, and threats to patient safety.

Leadership sought to understand the problems and identify solutions. They hired a nurse informatics consultant to guide the system towards the needed changes. The leadership was instructed to first establish the goals they wanted to accomplish with this project. Leadership then met with employees of all roles and established goals for the system: (1) each employee will perform work that is within their licensure;

(2) a process will be created to appraise policy and procedures and standards for best evidence; (3) the system will have a change in philosophy that everyone contributes to patient outcomes and data measurement including communication vs. documentation; (4) all technology will be appraised for feature and function to improve the user technology interface; and (5) employees and technology will work together, cooperatively, and the user-tech interface will become "active," rather than passive.

Guided by the nursing process, the leadership started with a system assessment and observed and talked with employees. The system assessment included following a patient from entry to exit, orders from entry to results or completion, creation of assignments for nurses and technicians, handoff at change of shift and patient transfers, and quality improvement process. For each part of the assessment, data was recorded and mapped. Using the information from the system assessment, they talked with employees. They sought to understand the difficulties in doing their work with technology, risks of errors using technology, decision-making using technology, and some work-arounds commonly used by employees while using technology. Changes were then made throughout the system. Changes were guided by change theory and done with the input and feedback from all members of the system.

Goal 1. Each employee will perform work that is within their licensure.

The system assessment and interviews revealed that the greatest violation of this goal was that nurses occasionally left the floor to get laundry or supplies when no one was available. This left patients without direct care of their nurse. The system transport personnel were often stretched beyond capacity transferring patients. This was addressed in two ways. First, additional transportation personnel were added, and second, the system purchased a robot. The robot picked up supplies and nutrition for the units or items that did not require a human to communicate instructions or manage the item. The robot functioned using AI and required 3 months to train. Software is updated regularly.

Goal 2. A process will be created to appraise policy and procedures and standards for best evidence.

An issue emerged that employees often did not trust the technology for decision-making. Data revealed that nurses often acknowledged the alert; however, they either took time to verify the decision support or disagreed and made a different decision. To address this, all policy and procedures and standards were evaluated, and then a process was developed to systematically review and update for best evidence. Secondly, an AI application scans the literature for updated best evidence and incorporates this into the decision support application. It was made clear that the decision support application does not replace the expertise of the nurse or other providers. However, knowing that the application has the most recent research and best evidence, the trust value should increase.

Goal 3. The system will have a change in philosophy that everyone contributes to patient outcomes and data measurement including communication vs. documentation.

The healthcare system adopted a practice theory of communication to guide entering patient information in the EHR and handoffs. Each person is a sender and receiver of a message, and each is responsible to facilitate effective communication. All employees attended training to learn effective communication strategies using the EHR and handoffs. Each learned the pitfalls of miscommunication and how to address or avoid them. All employees shifted their language from documentation to communication.

Goal 4. All technology will be appraised for feature and function to improve the user technology interface.

There were times when nurses perceived that they cared for the computer, not the patient. And a common work-around identified was the use of copy and paste of messages in the EHR. A list was made of all technologies used in the system. Each was then defined as communication channels or means of transferring messages from sender to receiver, consistent with the system philosophy. Each was analyzed for their ability to support communication and common work-arounds. Those that were outdated were updated with improved user design. Work-arounds that were defined as helpful and not putting undue risk to the employee or patient were adopted by the system. The EHR was also appraised, and a list of items that interfered with the user was shared with the vendor. What could be adjusted was adjusted. The goal was to reduce the number of clicks to navigate screens and reduce the number of repeated data or information.

Goal 5. Employees and technology will work together, cooperatively, and the user-tech interface will become "active," rather than passive.

Building on the fourth goal, the user-tech interface is active, and technology is viewed as part of the system with specific work for the system. To achieve this goal, AI applications were added to the system. Besides the robot described above, generative text AI was added to scan the EHR for changes to the patient and messages were started for the providers, including nurses. Employees learned to work with technology and trust the technology.

Each stage of the process that took several years was started with meetings with all employees and continued with employee input and education. It is important to note that there were as many philosophical changes as technology updates and changes. Both are suggested to add to the success of such a complex project. This system is fictional but combines several items from existing systems.

8   Summary

Responding to the challenge by the Institute of Medicine, the government enacted the HITECH Act requiring adoption of the EHR in care settings. At the time, little was understood about the risks to patient safety and the unanticipated deaths in the USA. Embedding technology into the health system revealed through data the risks to patient safety and successful interventions. Through Meaningful Use, medication-associated errors were reduced. It also revealed ongoing challenges such as hospital-acquired complications.

Contributing to the risks to patient safety is the design of the EHR not taking principles of end user technology interface. We stated that individuals have their own experiences and training that have them complete work using their processes. The current EHR lacks flexibility to support individual workflow and decision-making. Building on this was the burden of data entry by nurses. Here, we introduce cognitive load and impact of the environment on the burden of the nurses and risks to patient safety.

Technology is essential in healthcare. We have seen evidence of the decrease in medication errors. Since 2009, and moving forward, there remains the need for more advancements. We recommended a paradigm shift from technology system to communication system. We also recommended a review of nursing data entry to quantify the work and determine essential to nonessential. Finally, we recommended further advancements in technology in healthcare through artificial intelligence and sensors.

Perhaps the strongest sentence in this chapter is that with the implementation and adoption of technology in healthcare, i.e., errors are not inevitable, implying that unanticipated patient deaths are also not inevitable. Harnessing technology as a communication system and advancing innovation have the potential for increasing patient safety.

Key Points
- Health and technology systems are complex.
- Individuals with different experiences, training, and approaches to work provide complexities to the systems.
- Technology has revealed methods for reducing errors.
- There remain issues with the end users working with the technology.
- Advancing technology provides promise for further reducing errors and increasing patient safety.

References

1. Capra F. The web of life: the new scientific understanding of living systems. New York: Anchor Books; 1996.
2. von Bertalanffy L. General systems theory: foundations, development, and applications. Revised Edition. New York: George Braziller Publishers; 1968.
3. Meadows, D. Thinking in systems: a primer; 2008.
4. IOM (Institute of Medicine). Crossing the quality chasm: a new health system for the 21st century. Washington, DC: National Academy Press; 2001.
5. Miller JH, Page SE. Complex adaptive systems: An introduction to computational models of social life. Princeton University Press; 2007. January, 1. ISBN 9781400835522. OCLC 760073369
6. Jamshidi M, editor. System of systems engineering: Innovations for the 21st century. New York: John Wiley & Sons; 2009.
7. Samad T, Parisini T. Systems of systems. Computer Science Proceedings; 2011.
8. Agency for Healthcare Research and Quality. Rockville, MD: Defining Health Systems [updated January 2023]. Rockville, MD. Available from: https://www.ahrq.gov/chsp/defining-health-systems/index.html

9. Donabedian A. Quality of care. How can it be assessed? JAMA. 1988;260(12):1743–8.
10. Mitchell P. Quality health outcomes model. Image J Nurs Scholarship. 1998;30(1):43–6.
11. Laudon KC, Laudon JP. Management information systems. 13th ed. Upper Saddle River, NJ: Pearson; 2014.
12. Kohn LT, Corrigan JM, Donaldson MS. To err is human: building a safer health system. In: Institute of Medicine (US) Committee on Quality of Health Care in America. Washington, DC: National Academies Press (US); 2000.
13. Institute of Medicine (US). Committee on Quality of Health Care in America, Crossing the quality chasm: a new health system for the 21st century. Washington, DC: National Academies Press (US); 2001.
14. U.S. Department of Health & Human Services, Washington, DC.: HITECH Act enforcement interim final rule [Updated June 16, 2017]. Available from: https://www.hhs.gov/hipaa/for-professionals/special-topics/hitech-act-enforcement-interim-final-rule/index.html
15. Rogers E. Diffusion of innovations. New York: Free Press of Glencoe; 2003.
16. Adams DA, Nelson RR, Todd PA. Perceived usefulness, ease of use, and usage of information technology: a replication. MIS Quart. 1992;16(2):227–47.
17. Kobayashi M, Fussell SR, Xiao Y, Seagull J. Work coordination, workflow, and workarounds in a medical context. CHI late breaking results. New York: ACM Press; 2005. p. 1561–4.
18. Sum MT, Chebor MA. Documentation: historical perspectives, purposes, benefits and challenges as faced by nurses. Int J Human Soc Sci. 2013;3(16):236–40.
19. Blair W, Smith B. Nursing documentation: frameworks and barriers. Contemp Nurse. 2012;41(2):160–8.
20. Paul MM, Greene CM, Newton-Dame R, et al. The state of population health surveillance using electronic health records: a narrative review. Popul Health Manage. 2015;18(3):209–16.
21. Lee T. Nurses' perceptions of their documentation experiences in a computerized nursing care planning system. J Clin Nurs. 2006;15(11):1376–82.
22. Huryk LA. Factors influencing nurses' attitudes towards healthcare information technology. J Nurs Manage. 2010;18(5):606–12.
23. Wang N, Hailey D, Yu P. Quality of nursing documentation and approaches to its evaluation: a mixed-method systematic review. J Adv Nurs. 2011;67(9):1858–75.
24. Padden J. Documentation burden and cognitive burden: how much is too much information? Comput Inform Nurs. 2019;37(2):60–6.
25. Collins R. Clinician cognitive overload and its implications for nurse leaders. Nurse Leader. 2020;18(1):44–7. https://doi.org/10.1016/j.mnl.2019.11.007.
26. Haskins J. 20 Years of patient safety. AAMCNEWS. [Updated June 6, 2019] Available: https://www.aamc.org/news-insights/20-years-patient-safety
27. American Nurses Association. Principles for nursing documentation. MD: Silver Spring; 2010. Available from: http://www.nursingworld.org/~4af4f2/globalassets/docs/ana/ethics/principles-of-nursing-documentation.pdf
28. Gerbner G. Toward a general model of communication. Audio Vis Commun Rev. 1956;4(3):171–99.
29. Shannon CE. The mathematical theory of communication. In: Shannon CE, Weaver W, editors. The mathematical theory of communication. Chicago, IL: University of Illinois Press; 1967. p. 31–125.
30. Sengstack PP, Adrian B, Boyd DL, Davis A, Hook M, Hulett SL, Karp E, Kennedy R, Langford LH, Niblett TA. The six domains for Burden: a conceptual framework to address the burden of documentation in the electronic health record updated: June 23, 2020. Available from: https://www.ania.org/assets/documents/position/ehrBurdenPosition.pdf
31. Zhao Y, Rokhani FZ, Sazlina SG, Devaraj NK, Su J, Chew BH. Defining the concepts of a smart nursing home and its potential technology utilities that integrate medical services and are acceptable to stakeholders: a scoping review. BMC Geriatrics. 2022;22:787.
32. Chung J, Brakey HR, Reeder B, Myers O, Demiris G. Community-dwelling older adults' acceptance of smartwatches for health and location tracking. Int J Older People Nurs. 2023;18:e12490.

Part IV

Resilience, Healing and Moving Forward

Partnering for Patient Safety Through Patient Engagement

Stephanie Bennett and Armando Nahum

1 Introduction

Patients, families, and communities have essential, timely contributions to make in patient safety [1]. Patient engagement, sometimes referred to as patient participation or involvement, has increasingly become recognized as a pivotal consumer-oriented approach to achieving safe, high-valued care [1–3]. Sustainable improvement and the goals of zero harm require both the engagement and empowerment of patients, families, and caregivers. Throughout this chapter, we convey the importance of capacity building to empower patients. For the purposes of this chapter, family refers to broad use of the terms caregivers and care partners as defined by the patient. This chapter is designed to help you engage with patients and families on their journey to safer, high-quality healthcare and your leaders on the journey to zero harm.

2 Background: Why Learn More About Patient Engagement?

Researchers found the concepts of patient and family engagement (PFE) and patient- and family-centered care (PFCC) to be poorly understood and not well-defined [4, 5]. Still, PFE is being leveraged to decrease the risk of physical and

S. Bennett (✉)
Transformation and Patient Experience, Emory Healthcare and Emory University, Atlanta, GA, USA
e-mail: stephanie.bennett@emoryhealthcare.org

A. Nahum
Healthcare and Patient Partnership Institute (H2Pi), Smyrna, GA, USA
e-mail: anahum@h2pi.org

© The Author(s), under exclusive license to Springer Nature Switzerland AG 2024
C. A. Oster, J. S. Braaten (eds.), *The Nexus between Nursing and Patient Safety*, https://doi.org/10.1007/978-3-031-53158-3_15

psychological harm and improve the learning process when harm occurs [1]. Engagement requires care teams to work "with" patients and families, instead of doing "to" or "for" them. Notably, patients and families conceptualize themselves as experts in their experiences of health and well-being [6]. When invited to engage, patients "...bring insights from their experiences of care that cannot be substituted or replicated by clinicians, managers or researchers. This is especially so for those who have suffered harm" ([1], p. 40).

Box 1 Concepts Related Patient Participation in Care

Graffigna et al. [7] conceptualize patient engagement as a journey, whereby patients mature in their motivation and determination to participate actively in their care.

Leaders in healthcare systems require PFE during clinical encounters and in organizational councils and committees to approximate outcomes that matter to clinical teams and patients and families. Clinical teams and patients and families align around the goal of zero harm.

Patient and family engagement is explicitly demonstrated by applying the principles of patient- and family-centered care (PFCC) which include information sharing (transparency), collaboration, participation, and respect and dignity [8].

2.1 Continuously Learning on the Journey to Zero Harm

Park and Giap [4] conducted a systematic review on PFE and surmised that care team members need deeper understanding in partnering for safety and strategies to activate and reciprocate engagement. Consider this scenario:

Debra, a patient, presents to the ED with nausea/vomiting, pain, and jaundice. The work up is completed, and she needs to be admitted to the hospital. The nurse greets Debra with smiling eyes and comforting words as she prepares to start the IV and draw blood. Debra noticed the nurse didn't perform hand hygiene and don gloves. Exhaustedly, Debra managed to whisper a few words asking the nurse to don gloves. From that point on, Debra perceived that the patient–nurse partnership crumbled. The nurse started using harsh tones and abrupt communication. Most importantly, Debra recalls, "My call light went unanswered for hours. The nurse failed to return to check on me and give my pain medicine. I felt abandoned. I suffered alone (during COVID pandemic). It has been over a year and this horrible, gut-wrenching memory still lingers. I spoke up, but it wasn't well received." *This is my lived experience- Debra Smith, Patient Safety Advocate,*

Among patients and families, fear of offending care team members exists. This forms a barrier to engagement and patient safety [9–11]. One way to strengthen partnerships is to invite patients and families to participate in nurse residency and nursing professional development activities to help advance patient-centered knowledge, skills, and attitudes associated with safe, high-value care [8]. The inclusion of patients and families actually represents a pivotal change in how organizations learn "from" and "with" patients during the planning, implementation, and evaluation of care and organizational programs [8]. It introduces mutual learning and benefit as well as health outcomes prioritized by clinicians and those that matter most to patients [3, 12]. It requires a longer look at the safety culture, which is affected by the experiences of all who interact with the healthcare system. These experiences and perspectives include different observations about how the healthcare system operates and begs to be understood to deliver on the commitment of zero harm.

> **Quote Box:**
> Many patients and families will walk back through the very doors of the organizations where they were harmed, and they want to be a partner in improving the care that organization provides and in making sure patient safety is a priority. This is a gift that health care providers, leaders, and organizations should embrace.—Carole Hemmelgarn, Patient Safety Advocate

With hospitalized patients continuing to experience unnecessary harm at an alarming, estimated rate of over 400,000 per year [13], the engagement of patients and families is critical. The human impact of this overwhelming number of events includes:

- Patients who survived the harm.
- Families who became life-long caregivers of persons harmed.
- Families who lost a loved one to unsafe care.
- Care teams who suffered feelings of guilt.

More accurately, preventable harm takes its toll on the entire healthcare delivery ecosystem.

> **Quote Box:**
> Care team members involved in serious harm events also suffer long-term psychological harm. They often live with feelings of guilt and self-criticism [1].

2.2   Nursing Engagement with Patients

Given proper information and resources, patients and families can drive your organization's improvement engine forward and do so well beyond the capacity of siloed leaders and care teams within the organization [1]. Take the time to give patients and families information about how to take charge of their safety during the process of care. Invite them to participate in rounds and bedside shift report and show them how to use resources such as Speak Up® [14]. Educate staff to reciprocate PFE. Table 1 provides suggestions for planning how engagement will occur and specific examples of ways to engage [1, 3, 15]. Importantly, engagement needs to occur on different levels, such as:

Table 1 Strategies to plan for PFE in patient safety

Levels of engagement	Ways to engage and empower patients and families	Examples
Process of care	Educate to improve the self-management of their conditions and empower them for shared decision-making Invest in their knowledge, skills, and attitudes related to patient safety	Care decision, planning goals, bedside shift report, teach-back
Practice and organizational	Build the capacity of healthcare teams serving as champions in patient safety	Educational resources for professional development
Practice, organizational, community, and policy	Engage patients, families, and community organizations to cocreate policies, practices, and programs to make health care safer	Bring together the resources of community and healthcare organizations to promote safety Invite patients receiving care in community organizations to provide feedback about their care and to spread the word about safety campaigns
Practice, organizational, community, and policy	Learn from and with patients and care partners who experience unsafe care to improve understanding of the nature of harm and foster the development of more effective solutions	Patient and family advisor members participate in RCAs Patient and families who experience harm provide narrative to the RCA Team
Practice and organizational	Establish the principle and practice of information sharing with openness and transparency, such as disclosure of safety incident to patients and families	Patient and family advisor councils for quality and safety

From left to right, this table displays different levels of PFE, ways to engage, and practical examples [1, 3, 15]

- During the process of care (clinical encounters)
- At the practice and organizational level (hospital councils and committees)
- At the community level (partnered community organizations)
- At policy levels (local, state, national, and international)

2.3   Engagement and the Quadruple Aim

Ultimately, a safer culture for patients will usually also be safer for you and other staff [1]. The National Academy of Medicine [12] posits PFE as a driver of better health, better care, lower costs, and better work experience for those providing care, also known as the Quadruple Aim [16]. With this in mind, it is worth delineating that outcomes related to the experiences of those providing care matter. Clinician fatigue and burnout affect the organization's culture and the provision of respectful, dignifying care [12].

Engaging patients and families is of benefit to those who commit to quality and safety. Benefits include but are not limited to improved patient and family experiences [17–19] and reduced clinician burden [20–22]. These improvements bolster the financial state of the healthcare organization where care is delivered and promotes improved public health.

2.4 Engaging Patients and Families

The remainder of this chapter contains case studies designed to describe different levels of engagement and how nurses can preserve patient safety through the coproduction of outcomes during the care process and through involvement in organizational improvement activities.

The following case studies:

- Case Study 1: Portrays bedside shift report as an example of engaging during the process of care.
- Case Study 2: Describes organizational-level engagement in a quality and safety initiative with community and policy work.
- Case Study 3: Provides organizational-level work that is needed after a patient and family are harmed.
- Case Study 4: Allows you to explore tools and resources to develop or reinvigorate your organization's quality and safety-focused patient and family advisory council.

The case studies contain Donabedian's [23] three components, known as structure, process, and outcome. They illuminate different ways to measure improvement.

- Structural measures are important to ensure that the infrastructure needed to improve patient engagement and decrease the risk of harm is in place.
- Process measures are transactions between patients and providers throughout the delivery of healthcare.
- Outcome measures are critical regarding patient safety because they reflect the results of the care provided.

3 During the Process of Care: "I Desire to Partner with You in my Care"

Like you, patients are vested in their safety. Researchers found that approximately 91% of patients in a study believed they could help make their care safer [24, 25]. When you engage patients and families in shared decision-making and teach them how to use different patient safety strategies, you also build their confidence and capacity for self-management [4].

Quote Box:
We (patients and families) are the only constant in the 24-hour care provided while the patient is in your medical setting.—Carole Hemmelgarn, Patient Safety Advocate

Table 2 Patient-perceived barriers to engagement

My perspective about me	My perspective about my care team
− I lack knowledge about engagement or healthcare issues. − I feel too sick. − I prefer passive involvement and want to leave decision-making to care team. − I am ashamed of and embarrassed about topics such as sexual, bowel, or bladder issues. − I feel vulnerable. − There are limitations on independence and self-care when hooked up to machines or being labeled a fall risk.	− My doctor seems so busy. − My nurses seem task oriented. − Nurses control what's written on communication boards. So, it must just be for them. − I don't like rounds because there are too many people who show up in my room and they use too much medical jargon. − I lose a sense of control. It's hard to know when things will happen, such as tests and procedures, therapy, and getting result and the ability to talk them through.

Several factors hinder patient and family engagement, including their perceptions about their abilities and about the care team ([6]; [18]; [7]; [26]).

Table 3 Organizations with tools for patient engagement in safety

Name of organizations	Website
Institute For Patient- and Family-Centered Care	https://www.ipfcc.org/
World Health Organization	https://www.who.int/teams/integrated-health-services/patient-safety/policy/global-patient-safety-action-plan
Institute for Healthcare Improvement	https://www.ihi.org/resources/Pages/Publications/PartneringwithPatientsandFamiliesRecommendationsPromisingPractices.aspx
Nursing Alliance for Quality Care	https://www.nursingworld.org/practice-policy/naqc/?utm_term=&utm_campaign=&utm_source=adwords&utm_medium=ppc&hsa_src=x&hsa_ad=&hsa_tgt=&hsa_mt=&hsa_ver=3&hsa_acc=4209008328&hsa_kw=&hsa_grp=&hsa_cam=20144851679&hsa_net=adwords&gclid=Cj0KCQjwib2mBhDWARIsAPZUn_l6H1EfCFEXZlGhMQpI09Tpuu3pBHByIecpA9RN7MI41f5wkAV6tW4aAiFNEALw_wcB
Center for Consumer Engagement in Health Innovation	https://www.healthinnovation.org/
National Quality Forum	https://www.qualityforum.org/Topics/Person-_and_Family-Centered_Care.aspx
Society to Improve Diagnosis in Medicine	https://www.improvediagnosis.org/pfac-guides/

Even though patients desire to participate in their care and national and international patient advocacy organizations recommend such, barriers exist to achieving their involvement, as shown in Table 2. Patient-perceived barriers to engagement threaten the tenets of patient safety.

Address patient-perceived barriers by modeling engagement and using teachback and capacity-building strategies. Table 3 contains a list of patient-oriented groups that have developed useful tools for engagement, such as Ask Me Three® resources by the Institute for Healthcare Improvement [27, 28].

3.1 Bedside Shift Report: Effective Communication During Engagement

Effective communication is a high-value component of patient safety and quality care [1, 3]. Patients and families have the right to effective communication about their health and health care. Think about the structured ways, we share information during bedside shift report and interprofessional rounds, or even through communication boards. If information sharing is conducted in a manner that elicits participation, patients and families will gain an understanding of the nature of safe care and become the eyes and ears of the system. Therefore, introduce patients to different tools and techniques, so they understand why you use the tool, how it contributes to patient safety, and how they can participate.

3.1.1 Case Study 1: Bedside Shift Report—Patient Safety During the Process of Care

"Can you just tell me what's going on and why I need so many tests?"

Scenario

Meet Yanet Rodriguez, her off going nurse Rayshard King, and her oncoming nurse Johanna Silverman.

Yanet reports: "I was exhausted and in pain. During a conscious moment, I remember asking my nurse, Rayshard, what was wrong with me. Rayshard leaned in and rubbed my arm and said don't worry. You have the best doctor and team in this hospital. It was unsettling that he didn't answer my question. I didn't have the will to push the discussion further. Even though I probably slept the next day, I remember people doing things to me. I slowly started to feel better, and my daughter asked me what was going on and what they'd found. She could hear the uncertainty in my voice when I replied, "I don't know. I think it's something to do with my kidneys because they said I have the best kidney doctor at this hospital." She made me promise to start asking questions, but I didn't know where to start. Fortunately, during an evening shift, the oncoming nurse asked me what I wanted to get out of report and invited me to share my goals for the shift. Before I knew it, I told her that she was the first to ask. I proceeded to ask if she could tell me what was going on and why I needed so many tests. I told her that someone mentioned me having a history of diabetes. I told her that was wrong and asked her to check my chart."

After hearing the patient's concerns, Johanna explained the purpose of bedside shift report, spent a few minutes giving the patient an update, and agreed to share more during the course of the shift. She showed Yanet how to look at her information in the patient portal and how to share proxy access with her daughter. With each intervention, Johanna conducted teach-back.

A few weeks later, Johanna worked with her unit-based educator to investigate Yanet's report of not being included in BSR. They found variation in the way nurses conduct report on each shift. Some nurses performed a report outside the room, while others performed it in the room by reviewing real-time electronic health record (EHR) data but excluded the patient.

Yanet and the unit educator formed a workgroup to help plan a bedside shift report improvement project. Here are a few of her initial planning strategies:

- Gain an understanding of how patients experienced BSR to draft a plan for improving dialogue.
- Conduct a literature review to understand the latest evidence about incorporating safety checks into BSR.
- Work with her quality colleagues to plan how to measure improvement.

Discussion

Question   What are the examples of structure, process, and outcome measures for the bedside shift report project?

Answer   Table 4 provides examples of Yanet's starting point for structure, process, and outcomes measurements.

Question   Nurses spend the most time with patients at the bedside. Is it still essential to learn engagement strategies?

Answer   Yes. Nurses spend most of the time with patients and families at the bedside; however, their knowledge and understanding are severely limited by our "point-in-time" encounters. Preventing physical and psychological harm often requires understanding the entire journey and the larger context of factors affecting patients' health and well-being. For example, harm may occur when we do not understand the day-to-day symptom management, problem-solving, and even the issues patients face coordinating their care after leaving the hospital.

Question   What are the examples of patient-desired outcomes of bedside shift report?

Answer   According to Jerofke-Owen and Dahlman [6], patients reported that their motivation for participating in bedside shift report was to:
    - Decrease the risk of errors.
    - Understand their plan of care.
    - Stay informed about changes to the plan of care.

Have you asked patients what they would like to get out of BSR? What are their goals? It is worth asking so that they feel a sense of dignity and respect and to meet their information-sharing, collaboration, and participation needs.

Question   Are patients required to participate in bedside shift report?

Answer   No. Ask patients if they would like to participate and then respect their wishes.

Bedside shift report is a powerful relationship-building tool that supports patient safety and well-being [18, 29–31]. It is the perfect situation and a great invitation for the nurses and patients/families to lay the foundation for partnering during the rest of the shift. Bedside shift report is mutually beneficial for the patient, family, and the nurses involved. It also allows for the transfer of professional responsibility and accountability for patient care between nurses. Because communication occurs at the bedside, patients can request, confirm, or correct information in real time [30].

Table 4 Example measures for a bedside shift report initiative

Structure	Process	Outcome
Designated organizational leader, committee, or both with dedicated time focused on improving communication Error prevention integrated into BSR Patient and family advisory council with process-of-care, communication improvement on the agenda, and work plan Practice plan: Cocreated with patient and family advisory council • Policy and procedure • Standard performance • Keywords that resonant with patients	Percentage of patients verbalizing that they participated in bedside shift report Percentage of bedside shift report audits completed Number of root cause analyses completed per month for errors related to nurse communication	Patient safety: decrease in errors related to nurse communication HCAHPS: Nurse communication HCAHPS: Intent to recommend

Examples of structure, process, and outcome measures are listed based on the bedside shift report initiative

4 Patient and Family Engagement in Organizational Initiatives for Safety

4.1 Patient and Family Advisory Programs: Organizational Initiatives

There are several reasons to leverage a patient and family advisor's (PFA) unbiased lens and lived experiences in the realm of patient safety [8]:

- Patients and families consume care across all settings, while nurses and health system leadership often see care provided within a limited or narrow context. The observations and experiences of PFAs provide valuable information about areas of risk.
- PFAs have a sense of purpose toward improving outcomes for the next patient and family. They are laser-focused on driving change. As PFAs share their stories about medical errors, nurses can lean in to understand relevant system issues and the compounding effect of errors. Nurses can also partner to think through solutions to prevent them.
- PFAs can be a multiplier for your dissemination strategy. They are trusted community members with access to networks well beyond your reach. For example, they can share information about health maintenance and preventative strategies to improve health and well-being outcomes.

4.2   Precursors To Structuring Organizational Engagement

Before reading the case studies, consider a few tips about structuring PFE at the organizational level. Most organizations develop a framework or credo that represents their commitment to patient- and family-centered care, safety, and quality. Decisions and priorities stem from here and ground the work of care teams across different environments where patients interact to receive care. As you investigate, you may find that your organization espouses information about what patients should expect from care teams that differs from how care is delivered. If so, share your concerns with your leaders and ask them to partner with you to improve PFE. Earlier in this chapter, Table 1 described different ways organizations could engage patients in different initiatives. Precursors to deep engagement include [12]:

- Identifying progressive leaders who plan and develop initiatives with patients and families.
- Integrating patient and family engagement strategies into professional development.
- Leveraging national priorities and guidelines to gain traction.
- Having a plan for measurement.

4.2.1   Structuring Patient Engagement in the Safety Journey with Leaders

If you are interested in leading or supporting patient engagement in safety initiatives, there is enormous benefit in starting with your leadership team to situate engagement as a strategic priority [12, 32]. Leaders will direct zero-harm initiatives. They also provide resources and direct the accountability requirements of teams. In particular, you will need your leader's help when care team members are reluctant to move forward with different tactical strategies. Delays in the project may risk implementation efforts and the overall success and sustainability of the safety initiative [12]. During your initial steps, seek out leaders whose values, behaviors, decisions, and resource allocation indicate their commitment to PFE across the different levels of engagement.

4.2.2   Using Patient and Family Engagement Strategies

Be aware that there is an engagement continuum and that engagement practices must be "respectful of and responsive to individual preferences, needs, and values" [12]. We underscore the need for respectful, individualized approaches to engagement. Said differently, a "one size fits all" approach does not work. Patients have specific preferences regarding participating in their care [33]. There is a range of patient preferences, pinpointing the need for nurses to assess patients' preferences and tailor engagement efforts to the unique needs and circumstances of patients [6, 34]. Patients' gender, age, culture, severity of illness, and education levels have been associated with different engagement preferences [35, 36].

4.2.3 Leveraging National Priorities and Guidelines to Gain Traction

Did you know there are many patient advocacy organizations offering tools to help you and your leaders transform organizational structures and care team practices to approximate the quadruple aim? Many organizations, such as those listed in Table 3, have been advocating for patient and family engagement for decades and have developed toolkits and resources related to patient engagement in safety initiatives.

4.2.4 Having a Plan for Measurement

In terms of measurement, organizations need to commit to learning from the care they provide to improve their future state. If we ever hope to close existing gaps on quality and safety, we must have good cross-sectional and longitudinal data and data collection methods. With patient engagement in mind, Healthcare Consumer Assessment of Provider and Hospital Systems (HCAPHS) measures are collected nationally. HCAPHS includes a standard measure of patients' perception of care. Beyond HCAHPS, outcomes that are a priority for your organization and patients and families should be measured.

4.3 Case Study 2: Why PFE in Safety Is Important: It Takes a Village to Drive Toward Zero Harm: Sepsis Campaign

"I lost my son, and it was preventable. Now, I am leading safety initiatives to help others."

4.3.1 Scenario

This case study features the lived experiences of Armando Nahum, (Patient and Family Advisor, National Patient Safety Advocate) and Jeanne DeCosmo, RN, (Former Director of Clinical Quality) who led an organizational quality and safety initiative that included both community and policy work.

Armando: The Vice President of Quality and Safety at MedStar Health asked me to lead their new system-wide sepsis initiative from the patient's perspective. Our alliance was forged out of mutual respect, and it was based on shared goals. Additional partners were the Vice President of Clinical Care Transformation, and Jeanne DeCosmo, RN, who was the Director of Clinical Quality. Our team knew that executive leadership had to drive the project with us, or it would not survive the roadblocks that we would encounter. We also knew we needed to have the entire MedStar Health Leadership Team on board. I was nervous at first. I told the VP of Quality and Safety that I didn't know anything about sepsis. I told him that I wasn't clinically trained. He responded that I didn't need to be clinical. He needed a set of eyes from outside the clinical team.

Tip Box:
Patients may be reluctant to partner at first. Allay their concerns by highlighting their unique, valued vantage point.

Jeanne: I was thrilled to partner with Armando. My intent was to avoid influencing him in anyway. I wanted him to keep his objective lens. He learned what was important to question and where to engage us to go a layer deeper in our thinking.

> **Tip Box:**
> Bring PFAs in during planning and don't influence their understanding about the clinical aspect of things so they keep their objective lens.

Armando and Jeanne: As a team, we were persistent and determined to get the work done to drive mortality rates down. We worked as though lives depended on it, and it did. Keep in mind, this work was done during a time when sepsis was not an easy condition to identify. We knew that every patient presented with different signs and symptoms. Most importantly, we knew that patients' conditions would decline rapidly with sepsis.

Armando: I started asking questions to understand where sepsis comes from; learn how to identify it and drive change that would decrease the risk of sepsis. Thus, we began work in ED.

Armando and Jeanne: At the outset, it was a little jarring to experience the level of hesitancy from various leaders. Quite often, we perceived that things were not going well. For example, ED doctors and nurses didn't want to move the campaign forward for various reasons. Some reasons seemed legitimate, but they were not the solution to our zero-harm goal.

Armando: As a PFA, I learned that resilience was the key to pushing forward. I advocated for the sepsis awareness campaign and was told "no" very often. I pushed leaders to articulate why "no" was the answer. I asked why quite often. I said, let's talk about why we can't do it. Now, let's talk about why we must do it.

> **Tip Box:**
> It's imperative to bring PFAs at very beginning stages of the project. Share ALL your data and have meaningful conversations about each entity and the barriers they face. This is tough on leaders because it requires a high level of transparency. However, it needs to be done.

Armando and Jeanne: The team aimed to evaluate EHR documentation and the triage process, but we quickly found variability in the structure established across the organization. You probably recognize this as a common problem in healthcare systems in general across the US. For our project, we were dealing with:
- Different operational workflows for medical and nursing staff from 10 entities
- Different vendors for our EHRs

Variability in structure impacted how we could evaluate process data, such as the time from receiving the lactic acid result to administration of the antibiotic. We set out to review and revise the ED nurse triage forms. We thought through clinical and

Table 5 Example measures for driving a safety awareness campaign

Structure	Process	Outcome
Nursing and provider leadership: Vested in PFE, safety, and quality Dashboard of aggregate and hospital data Electronic health record reporting capability Patient and family advisory council	PFAC Data (a) Number of patient voices embedded (b) Number of PFAs on committees (c) Number of PFAs participating in the legislative session in MD Clinical data: Percentage completion of triage process documentation. For example: • Triage time • Lactate ordered and resulted • Lactate resulted • Antibiotic order time and administration time • Final diagnosis and disposition	Sepsis mortality outcome: System and hospital Number of patients diagnosed with sepsis Number of self-reported cases of sepsis Number of PFA stories

Examples of structure, process, and outcome measures listed are based on the sepsis awareness initiative described in this case study

4.4   Case Study 3: Harmed Twice

"We were harmed twice. Alyssa died due to medical errors. I was made vulnerable and intentionally excluded for over 3 years." Carole Hemmelgarn, Patient Safety Advocate

4.4.1   Scenario

Hi, I'm Carole, a founding member of the Patients for Patient Safety US organization. I sit on the quality and safety board in the hospital where my daughter died. I'm a patient advocate and I have shared my lived experiences across the US.

This case study contains a story that should never be told and that doesn't get easier to tell. Yet, it is a story that must be told for all to hear. Alyssa, my 9-year-old daughter, died. It was preventable. Our story is much greater than days, months, and years—yet it is punctuated by numbers, such as 3.7.28. I didn't experience an honest conversation for 3 years, 7 months, and 28 days, or 1,745,280 min.

Honestly, it does not matter the measurement of time you use, what's important is that my world stood still. There was zero communication. I was left with what felt like hundreds of questions, and ever more unknowns and "what ifs." A curtain is silence was intentionally hung to dangle between someone like me and someone like you.

What you don't understand is that those of us who are made vulnerable by the system of harm can only maneuver through the world in survival mode when we don't know the truth. You need to know that we lose the ability to actually live. We are frozen in time. Paralyzed. I lost Alyssa to medical errors; I lived this experience one day after the next.

You see, patients and families realize that you and other clinicians don't come to work with the intent to cause harm. Yet, when harm does occur and honest, transparent conversations aren't conducted, you inflict harm on us again. This is the 2nd preventable tragedy. What compounds the pain is when we are not told the truth about what has happened to our loved one and what kind of care they received.

I needed to learn what you experienced, saw, and believed happened with Alyssa's care.

I longed to have that difficult conversation to start my healing. I longed to enter into the organization's communication and resolution process.

> **Tip**
> Communication and resolution is an ongoing process. It ends when the patient or family says it ends, which can take days, weeks, months, and even years.

I've been a patient advocate for years. Although, patients and family will process the harm event differently, I've discovered five things that are needed for the healing process after medical harm occurs:

1. We need to know what happened.
    (a) It is simply about the truth, no more and no less. This means you need to tell us what we need and want to hear, not what you feel comfortable telling us, what you think we should hear, or what you want to share with us.
2. Tell us how you are going to fix the problem.
    (a) We need to know that what happened to our loved one is not going to happen to anyone else. If it does, we feel that our person's harm (injury or the loss of their life) was in vain.
3. Take responsibility.
    (a) Someone needs to take responsibility for the human and/or system error. Communication must remain empathic and remorseful so that patients and family feel you genuinely care.
4. Apologize.
    (a) Say, I'm sorry
5. Let us be part of the solution to fix the problems that led to the error.

To tell us what happened and how the organization is going to fix the problem, you must conduct an event or root cause analysis. The analysis is critical to the learning process for the organization and is the pathway to providing answers to the patients and family. To gain a 360-degree view of what happened, a narrative from the patient and/or family should be part of the root cause analysis discovery. We have valued perspectives on what happened. We are the only constant in the 24-hour-care provided while the patient is in your medical setting. No one should ever experience being harmed twice. Our story must be told to drive the goals of transparency that matter to patients and families and to elevate clinical interventions to zero harm. More of my story can be heard here

https://psmf.org/patient-safety/patient-stories/alyssa-hemmelgarn/.

Carole and other patient advocates worked with the AHRQ to develop CANDOR, a toolkit for the communication and resolution process. CANDOR stands for Communication and Optimal Resolution. A CANDOR event is defined as an event that involves unexpected harm (physical, emotional, or financial) to a patient. The toolkit contains resources that organizations and healthcare team members can use when harm occurs, and before the cause of the event is known. The AHRQ resources for CANDOR are found here:

https://www.ahrq.gov/patient-safety/settings/hospital/candor/index.html

4.4.2   Discussion

Question   Do patients and families who experienced harm typically participate in the Root Cause Analysis (RCA) process?

Answer   Participating in the RCA may or may not be their desire. Importantly though, there are risk management barriers to their participation. The answer is usually no. Thus, organizations should consider including their own patient and family advisors who have experienced harm. Victims of medical harm may feel comfort knowing that someone is representing their perspectives.

Question   What are the examples of structure, process, and outcome measures for organizational disclosure?

Answer   Most hospitals focus on developing processes to improve the reporting and monitoring of adverse events and to promote better care for patients through candid, caring communication in the wake of an adverse event. Table 6 includes measurable examples from CANDOR. The Patient and Family Partnership for Safety also provides a pathway to get measurable improvement. Patient and Family Partnership for Safety is the United States branch of the World Health Organization's international network of patient safety advocates.

Table 6   Examples of CANDOR-related measurements

Structure	Process	Outcome
Leadership structure for the patient-centered communication and resolution process Dashboard for transparency of harm data	Time of disclosure to unexpected patient harm events The number of checks completed to follow up on improvement of the root cause/contributing factor	Improved patient satisfaction scores Fewer medical liability claims Improved patient safety outcomes

Structure, process, and outcome measures are based on the CANDOR initiative [39]

Question   Are there different measures that are important for patients and families?

Answer   Yes. There are specific structure, process, and outcomes measures important to patients and families.

Structure measures:

- Patient and family advisory council with RCA on the agenda and work plan for improvement.
- Patient and family advisor on RCA teams to represent the voices of those suffering from harm.

Process measures:

- The number of patients or families who participate in the RCA process.
- The number of times the patient and/or family's narrative was included in the RCA process.
- The number of patients and family who experienced harm are invited to sit on quality and safety committees throughout the hospital.
- The number of times patients and families received communication throughout the RCA process.

Outcome measures

- Zero harm for anyone.
- Never repeat the same harm twice.

Question   Does the use of the communication and resolution process drive down medical liability claims?

Answer   Data indicate that less cases go to trial. Also, by not having the cost of an attorney and settling quicker, more money can go to the patient or family.

Table 7 CANDOR event reporting, investigation, and analysis team

Role	Responsibilities
CANDOR implementation team leader	The team leader role is usually occupied by an executive leader
	Leads the team in the CANDOR process
Nurse champion	Advances the goals of the process
	Teaches team members about the process
	Supports nurses with the implementation process
Direct patient care staff	Works to implement and sustain the process
Patient and family advisors liaison	Represents the voices of patients and families who have been harmed
	Participates in team meetings

Nurses may take on various roles when participating in communication and resolution process. Based on the Implementation Guide for the CANDOR Process [40]

Table 8 Harm-driven and resolution process additional resources

Organization	Content	Website
Patient safety movement	Global reach, unifying people for zero harm	https://psmf.org/
AHRQ— CANDOR Resources	Communication and resolution programs	https://www.ahrq.gov/patient-safety/settings/hospital/candor/index.html
Patients for Patient Safety US	Patient safety and communication and resolution programs	www.pfps.us
Collaborative for accountability and improvement	Communication and resolution programs	https://communicationandresolution.org/

To help you find more information about patient safety, this table lists the names of national patient safety organizations, the type of content offered, and the URL for the website. This is not an exhaustive list

Question   Based on CANDOR, what role do nurses play in the communication and resolution process?

Answer   Based on nurses' role in the organization, expertise, and skills, they can participate in the event analysis process. Table 7 provides examples of different ways nurses can engage.

Question   Where can I find more resources about harm-driven communication and the resolution process?

Answer   Table 8 lists several websites that provide additional resources.

---

5   Establish a PFA Program Using a Toolkit

5.1   Case Study 4: Start or Reinvigorate a Patient and Family Advisory Council (PFAC)

Nurses Designing a Project Team with Leadership and PFAs: Safety in Diagnostic Testing

5.1.1   Scenario

Anisa, the Director of Quality, notices an upward trend in the rates of errors in laboratory and diagnostic testing. Several incidents were traced back to preventable harm. A few included:

• An incidental finding on a CT scan with no follow-up. Later the patient was diagnosed with stage IV cancer.
• In the ED, critical laboratory results were missed during the change of shift. The patient was discharged home, requiring emergency medical treatment. The patient returned to the hospital via ambulance and was admitted to the ICU.

Anisa is interested in engaging patients and families to partner in laboratory and diagnostic safety but is not sure where to start. She's spoken with several patients and families who find it difficult to understand the results that display in their patient portal. She wonders if more can be done to teach patients and families how to review and follow up if they have questions. She consults the society to improve diagnosis in medicine and found a guide to develop a PFAC. After reviewing this information, she continued to search for a toolkit of resources that she could customize.

5.1.2 Establish a PFA Program Using a Toolkit

Anisa found customizable resources on a website at https://www.h2pi.org/pfac-tools, established by the Healthcare and Patient Partner Institute (H2Pi). Anisa intends to use the resources to develop a PFAC focused on quality and safety.

Anisa completed the steps shown in Fig. 1, the Road to Success diagram. The Road to Success is a road map indicating how to establish a Patient and Family Advisory Council for Quality and Safety (PFACQS®).

Step 1: Get Leadership Support.

Anisa garnered the support of the Director of Radiology, Chief Quality Officer and Chief Nursing Quality Officer to develop a PFACQS® to address trending errors in her department. She's aware that the goals of the Council need to align with the mission, vision, and values of her organization. View the following short videos to learn more about the role of leadership and to hear tips on identifying leaders.
- Leadership support: https://youtu.be/aQKzF0Qs1VQ
- Leadership on PFACQS: https://youtu.be/SbaYzhaChbk
- Identify different audiences: https://youtu.be/KI8m9uOruvw
- Understanding leadership expectations https://youtu.be/ShUEylHpLu0

Step 2: Form a PFACQS® Project Team.

Anisa worked to create a project team. This team focuses on planning and implementing the PFACQS®. This usually takes 6-to-9 months, but it may take less time depending on staff and PFA commitment to structuring the project and your desired go-live timeframe. The project team typically disbands after completing its goals. However, some team members will transition to serve as staff on the PFACQS® as part of their job function. With this in mind, as you start developing your project team, identify people who will staff the PFACQS® eight-to-nine months down the line. Click this link https://youtu.be/vSdYt5ZXYhw to learn why having administrative support is important when managing the project.

Step 3: Assess Opportunities

Anisa used the H2Pi Assessment Tool that was part of the toolkit. She worked with the project team to conduct an assessment to:
- Identify elements of effective patient and family engagement existing within her organization.
- Elucidate opportunities for improvement.
- Over time, the team will reassess their progress as the organization implements new, more effective structures and practices to engage PFAs.
- View the tool by accessing "Toolkit 1." Then, click the "Readme Files" folder and open the "H2Pi-Assessment Tool" document.

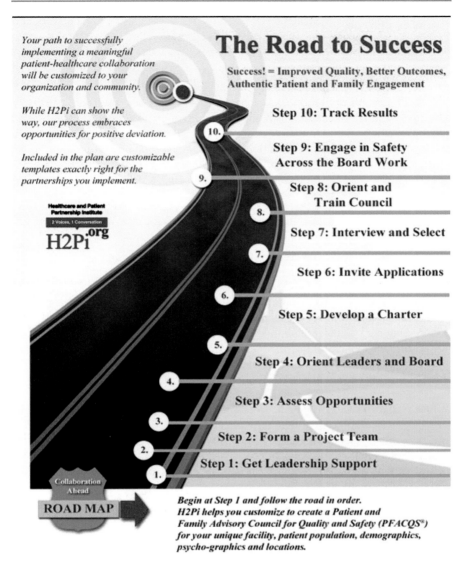

The Road to Success

Your path to successfully implementing a meaningful patient-healthcare collaboration will be customized to your organization and community.

While H2Pi can show the way, our process embraces opportunities for positive deviation.

Included in the plan are customizable templates exactly right for the partnerships you implement.

Healthcare and Patient Partnership Institute
2 Voices, 1 Conversation
H2Pi.org

Success! = Improved Quality, Better Outcomes, Authentic Patient and Family Engagement

Step 10: Track Results

Step 9: Engage in Safety Across the Board Work

Step 8: Orient and Train Council

Step 7: Interview and Select

Step 6: Invite Applications

Step 5: Develop a Charter

Step 4: Orient Leaders and Board

Step 3: Assess Opportunities

Step 2: Form a Project Team

Step 1: Get Leadership Support

Collaboration Ahead
ROAD MAP

Begin at Step 1 and follow the road in order. H2Pi helps you customize to create a Patient and Family Advisory Council for Quality and Safety (PFACQS®) for your unique facility, patient population, demographics, psycho-graphics and locations.

Fig. 1 Follow the steps in this roadmap to develop a safety and quality PFAC for your organization, department, or unit [41]Used with permission from H2Pi

Step 4: Orient Leaders and your Board of Directors

The PFACQS® becomes a strategic priority within the organization with board oversight. With this in mind, Anisa advocates for leadership and staff to embed the PFAC as part of its quality, safety, and operational improvement strategy and report outcomes to the Board of Directors.

Members of the project team helped orient new leaders to the work of the PFAC, letting them know:

- What PFAs do.
- How the PFACQS® aligns with the mission, vision and values of the organization.
- How staff and resources are needed to structure the program.
- How often they will receive a report on outcomes.
- Read tips on orienting leaders by accessing "Toolkit 1." Then, click the "Orientation" folder and open the "Internal Orientation" document.

Step 5: Develop a Charter

Develop a charter covering information, such as the mission and purpose, terms of service, and what to expect from patients, families, and staff.

View this video to gain more insight into developing a charter https://youtu.be/BHtkyMTO74A.

Read an example charter by accessing "Toolkit 1." Then, click the "ReadMe File" folder and open the "H2Pi-Charter" document.

Step 6: Invite Applications

Members of the project team created flyers to recruit patients, families, community leaders, and staff. Additional recruitment methods included:

- Asking help from various service lines.
- Looking for patients or families who provide solution-oriented, constructive criticism regarding their encounters.
- Asking the volunteer department to assist in recruiting.
- Use multiple recruitment methods so that the PFACQS® reflects the population served by your organization. View this video to learn more about the application process https://youtu.be/c4CuaOhGhFQ.

Step 7: Interview and Select

Anisa and the PFACQS® Project Team found that the application and interview processes took more time than they planned. As they interviewed and selected council members, they sought to achieve diversity in diagnosis, economic status, payor source, ethnicity, education, sexual identity, and geographic location, to name a few. View this video to hear perspectives on conducting interviews https://youtu.be/37zygnI1CJk.

View forms that you can customize and use to conduct interviews by accessing "Toolkit 1."

- Conducting interviews with staff: Click the "Associates" folder and open the "H2Pi-Associate-Review-Form" document.
- Conducting interviews with patients and families: Click the "External" folder and open the "H2Pi-External-Review-Form" document.

Step 8: Orient and Train Council

The PFACQS® Project Team developed orientation and training materials for PFAC members. They checked with their Legal and Human Resources department to determine onboarding and orientation requirements. Generally, there are policies describing what volunteers must do, such as HIPPA training.

Other information to cover includes:

(a) What to expect during the meeting.
(b) How to interact in a meeting.
(c) How to ask questions, especially when unfamiliar terminology is used.

(d) How to communicate in a manner that creates a safe environment for all attendees.

(e) How to manage conflict.

Read more about PFA orientation and training by accessing "Toolkit 1." Then, click the orientation folder and open the "Legal Checklist Volunteer Status.docx" document.

Step 9: Get Ready to Engage in Safety Work

After staff and PFAs were onboarded and oriented, an agenda was created for the PFACQS meetings. Agenda topics may arise from PFAs and staff who are part of the Council. Additionally, expect leaders to contribute topics that address trending quality and safety trends.

View this video to learn about activities for PFACQS® work https://youtu.be/WORQYbD1zTY.

Get ideas for agenda topics and learn about activities that should be organizational priorities by accessing "Toolkit 1." Then, click the "Orientation" folder and open the "Organizational Priorities for your PFACQS®" document.

Step 10: Track Results

Anisa engages the PFACQS® for suggestions on how to sustain the momentum of work performed by the Council, track results, and as appropriate, draw correlations to demonstrate how the PFACQS® connects with and helps advance the organization's mission, vision, and values.

As mentioned earlier, complete the PFACQS® self-assessment and show leaders the opportunities for improvement. Provide them with periodic reports to raise their awareness of the improvements achieved. In the beginning, sharing examples from other organizations or literature about the value of a PFACQS® in improving outcomes may also be helpful.

View the following video for ideas on building and sustaining PFACQS® Momentum https://youtu.be/WORQYbD1zTY.

For ideas on conceptualizing and articulating the value of PFACQS® access "Toolkit 1." Then, click the "Readme Files" folder and open the "Benefits of PFACQS" document. This document also provides ideas about project work that benefits the organization and that could be tracked and reported.

5.1.3 Discussion

Question   I really like the documents and videos. Can I use them within my organization?

Answer   You have permission to use the documents and videos to start your program. Keep the H2Pi logo on the document and work with your marketing team to include your organization's logo.

Question   What specifically will the PFACQS® Project Team do?

Answer   The PFACQS® Project Team will form, identify a lead or leads, get oriented to the tasks, perform a self-assessment of opportunities, organize one or more hospital orientation sessions for key audiences, guide recruiting efforts to populate the PFACQS®, interview candidates, and recommend candidates to be invited to serve as Founding Members of the PFACQS®.

Question   How big should the Project Team be?
Answer   A project team should consist of at least 6–10 active members. If you
             have less than six, the work can start to feel onerous especially when
             you start scheduling PFACQS® candidate interviews. Some organiza-
             tions add additional members to be inclusive, get their input and per-
             spective and get their departments engaged in thinking about how to
             partner with the PFAs when the council is established. Teams may have
             as many as 20 members.
Question   How much work is involved for members of the PFACQS® Project Team?
Answer   The project team has three time-sensitive jobs:
             1. In the first month of activity, complete the self-assessment tool. A
                 single team member may complete the assessment, but it is best to
                 divvy the work up among several people.
             2. Across the 2nd and 4th months, disseminate invitations. The dis-
                 semination step typically involves connecting with patients who
                 completed a patient satisfaction survey in the last 2–3 years as well
                 as internal distribution to organizational staff.
             3. During months 5 through 7, interview candidates for the PFACQS®.
                 One organization conducted 20 interviews per hospital PFACQS®,
                 with three interviewers from the Project Team per candidate. If pos-
                 sible, create a pool of six to ten interviewers to ease the burden of
                 scheduling.
Question   Who should be on the Project Team?
Answer   Include a person from your patient safety or quality improvement areas,
             someone familiar with outreach to patients and families (typically com-
             munications department function, sometimes community relations or
             patient experience), and someone with responsibility for internal com-
             munications (typically human resources, sometimes communications).
             To create internal momentum, seek to partner with a physician and
             nurse leader who has the bandwidth to participate. When a CNO or
             CMO is involved, the teams generally have more stature and are better
             attended. If you know of a person in your community who is passionate
             about patient and family engagement, it really adds value to bring the
             dimension of personal commitment into the team. For example, in one
             organization a board member joined the team. Finally, if you know that
             certain staff have concerns about discussing hospital performance
             issues with "outside" audiences, meet with them to discuss the role and
             training of PFAs. Cautious audiences typically are medical staff or peo-
             ple from the communications, legal and risk departments.
Question   When is the PFACQS® project team's job done?
Answer   The last event is usually launching the PFACQS® itself. During this
             meeting, typically a luncheon or dinner is served. Senior management
             welcomes the PFACQS® members and thanks the project team for its
             work in building a new hospital or system-wide resource. Again, some
             members of the PFACQS® project team may transition to being staff as
             part of their job function.

6   Summary

The journey to zero harm requires using structured methods, such as those provided in this chapter, to learn "from" and "with" patients when planning initiatives related to practice, programs, and policy. For decades, national attention has been given to the need for patient and family engagement in patient safety. Even though this call to action is not new, there is a sense of urgency in simultaneously approximating zero harm and the quadruple aim. The return on investment of patient and family engagement stands to yield improved care experiences and decreased clinician burden, which in turn lowers the cost of care, decreases medical liability costs, and promotes improved public health. This is a win-win. As a nurse, your specific call to action is to collaborate with leaders to plan how care teams will consistently engage with patients and families during the care process and at different levels of your organization's initiatives.

Key Points
- There is room for improvement in today's healthcare culture and within hospital organizational structures to prevent harm and respond to and learn from harmful events after they occur.
- The goal of zero harm requires different ways of thinking about and implementing engagement strategies to achieve outcomes that matter to the organization as well as patients and families.
- Ask patients and families how they would like to engage with you during the process of care. Often, you will need to build their capacity for engagement.
- Engagement across different organizational initiatives invites patients and families to partner and share insights about hidden safety-related risks existing within the healthcare system.
- When harm occurs, organizations should invite patients and families to engage in communication and resolution to decrease the likelihood of harm happening twice.
- Patient and family engagement in patient safety will not occur by happenstance. Thus, leader buy-in and partnership are needed to scale and spread engagement initiatives.

References

1. World Health Organization. Global patient safety action plan; 2021. https://www.who.int/teams/integrated-health-services/patient-safety/policy/global-patient-safety-action-plan. Accessed 1 Mar 2023.
2. Agency for Healthcare Research and Quality. AHRQ's making healthcare safer reports: shaping patient safety efforts in the 21st century; 2020. https://www.ahrq.gov/research/findings/making-healthcare-safer/index.html. Accessed 1 Mar 2023.
3. Institute of Medicine. Best care at lower cost: The path to continuously learning health care in America. The National Academies Press; 2013. https://doi.org/10.17226/13444.
4. Park M, Giap TTT. Patient and family engagement as a potential approach for improving patient safety: a systematic review. J Adv Nurs. 2019;76:62–80. https://doi.org/10.1111/jan.14227.

5. Santana MJ, Manalili K, Jolley RJ, Zelinsky S, Quan H, Lu M. How to practice person-centred care: a conceptual framework. Health Expect. 2018;21:429–40. https://doi.org/10.1111/hex.12640.
6. Jerofke-Owen T, Dahlman J. Patients' perspectives on engaging in their healthcare while hospitalised. J Clin Nurs. 2019;28:340–50. https://doi.org/10.1111/jocn.14639.
7. Graffigna G, Barello S, Bonanomi A, et al. Factors affecting patients' online health information-seeking behaviours: the role of the Patient Health Engagement (PHE) model. Patient Educ Couns. 2017;100:1918–27. https://doi.org/10.1016/j.pec.2017.05.033.
8. Minniti M, Abraham M. Essential allies patient, resident, and family advisors: a guide for staff liaisons. Maryland: Institute for Patient- and Family-Centered Care; 2013.
9. Huisman-de Waal GJ, Feo R, Vermeulen H, et al. Students' perspectives on basic nursing care education. J Clin Nurs. 2018;27:2450–9. https://doi.org/10.1111/jocn.14278.
10. Seale, et al. Lifting the curtains of silence: patient perceptions towards needs and responsibilities in contributing to the prevention of healthcare-associated infections and antimicrobial resistance. Am J Infect Control. 2022:1–7. https://doi.org/10.1016/j.ajic.2022.11.013.
11. van Belle E, Giesen J, Conroy T, et al. Exploring person-centred fundamental nursing care in hospital wards: a multi-site ethnography. J Clin Nurs. 2020;29:1933–44. https://doi.org/10.1111/jocn.15024.
12. Frampton SB, Guastello S, Hoy LM, et al. Harnessing evidence and experience to change culture: a guiding framework for patient and family engaged care. NAM Perspect. 2017; https://doi.org/10.31478/201701f.
13. James JT. A new, evidence-based estimate of patient harms associated with hospital care. J Patient Safety. 2013;9:122–8. https://doi.org/10.1097/PTS.0b013e3182948a69.
14. The Joint Commission. Speak up campaigns; 2023. https://www.jointcommission.org/resources/for-consumers/speak-up-campaigns/. Accessed 1 Mar 2023.
15. Carman KL, Dardess P, Maurer M, et al. Patient and family engagement: a framework for understanding the elements and developing interventions and policies. Health Affairs. 2013;32:223–31. https://doi.org/10.1377/hlthaff.2012.1133.
16. Bodenheimer T, Sinsky C. From triple to quadruple aim: care of the patient requires care of the provider. Ann Fam Med. 2014;12:573–6. https://doi.org/10.1370/afm.1713.
17. Kuntz JL, Safford MM, Singh JA. Patient-centered interventions to improve medication management and adherence: a qualitative review of research findings. Patient Educ Couns. 2014;97:310–26. https://doi.org/10.1016/j.pec.2014.08.021.
18. Tobiano G, Bucknall T, Sladdin I. Patient participation in nursing bedside handover: a systematic mixed-methods review. Int J Nurs Stud. 2018;77:243–58. https://doi.org/10.1016/j.ijnurstu.2017.10.014.
19. Tzeng H, Yin C. Engaging as an innovative approach to engage patients in their own fall prevention care. Patient Prefer Adher. 2014;8:693–700. https://doi.org/10.2147/PPA.S62746.
20. Lown BA, Shin A, Jones RN. Can organizational leaders sustain compassionate, patient-centered care and mitigate burnout? J Healthcare Manag. 2019;64:398–412. https://doi.org/10.1097/JHM-D-18-00023.
21. McClelland LE, Vogus TJ. Compassion practices and HCAHPS: does rewarding and supporting workplace compassion influence patient perceptions? Health Serv Res. 2014;49(5):1670–83. https://doi.org/10.1111/1475-6773.12186.
22. McClelland LE, Gabriel AS, DePuccio MJ. Compassion practices, nurse well-being, and ambulatory patient experience ratings. Medical Care. 2018;56:4–10. https://doi.org/10.1097/MLR.0000000000000834.
23. Donabedian A. Evaluating the quality of medical care. Milbank Q. 2005;83:691–729. https://doi.org/10.1111/j.1468-0009.2005.00397.x.
24. Schwappach DLB, Frank O, Buschmann U, et al. Effects of an educational patient safety campaign on patients' safety behaviours and adverse events. J Eval Clin Pract. 2013;19:285–91.
25. Waterman AD, Gallagher TH, Garbutt J, et al. Brief report: hospitalized patients' attitudes about and participation in error prevention. J Gen Intern Med. 2006;21:367–70.

26. Graffigna G, Barello S. Spotlight on the Patient Health Engagement Model (PHE model): a psychosocial theory to understand people's meaningful engagement in their own health care. Patient Prefer Adher. 2018;12:1261–71. https://doi.org/10.2147/PPA.S145646.
27. Institute for Healthcare Improvement (2023a) Partnering with patients and families to design a patient- and family-centered health care system: recommendations and promising practices. https://www.ihi.org/resources/Pages/Publications/PartneringwithPatientsandFamiliesRecommendationsPromisingPractices.aspx. Accessed 1 Mar 2023.
28. Institute for Healthcare Improvement. Ask me 3: Good questions for your good health; 2023b. https://www.ihi.org/resources/Pages/Tools/Ask-Me-3-Good-Questions-for-Your-Good-Health.aspx. Accessed 1 Mar 2023.
29. Baldwin KM, Spears MJ. Improving the patient experience and decreasing patient anxiety with nursing bedside report. Clin Nurs Specialist. 2019;33:82–9. https://doi.org/10.1097/NUR.0000000000000428.
30. Friesen MA, Herbst A, Turner JW, et al. Developing a patient-centered ISHAPED handoff with patient/family and parent advisory councils. J Nurs Care Qual. 2013;28:208–16. https://doi.org/10.1097/NCQ.0b013e31828b8c9c.
31. Sand-Jecklin K, Sherman J. A quantitative assessment of patient and nurse outcomes of bedside nursing report implementation. J Clin Nurs. 2014;23:2854–63. https://doi.org/10.1111/jocn.12575.
32. Center for Consumer Engagement in Health Innovation. Person-centered engagement at the organization level; 2022. https://www.healthinnovation.org/change-package/planning/role-of-leadership. Accessed 1 Mar 2023.
33. Florin J, Ehrenberg A, Ehnfors M. Patient participation in clinical decision-making in nursing: a comparative study of nurses' and patients' perceptions. J Clin Nurs. 2006;15:1498–508. https://doi.org/10.1111/j.1365-2702.2005.01464.x.
34. Higgins T, Larson E, Schnall R. Unraveling the meaning of patient engagement: a concept analysis. Patient Educ Couns. 2017;100:30–6. https://doi.org/10.1016/j.pec.2016.09.002.
35. Aasen EM. A comparison of the discursive practices of perception of patient participation in haemodialysis units. Nur Ethics. 2015;22:341–51. https://doi.org/10.1177/0969733014533240.
36. Hawley ST, Morris AM. Culture challenges to engaging patients in shared decision making. Patient Educ Couns. 2017;100:18–24. https://doi.org/10.1016/j.pec.2016.07.008.
37. Martin JH, Armando N, Roger L, et al. Jt Comm J Qual Patient Saf. 2020;46:158–66. https://doi.org/10.1016/j.jcjq.2019.12.001.
38. Meena S, Armando N, Jeanne D. How to effectively engage patients and families in quality improvement: a deep, transparent partnership. Int J Qual Health Care. 2021;33 https://doi.org/10.1093/intqhc/mzab112.
39. Agency for Healthcare Research and Quality. Communication and optimal resolution; 2022. https://www.ahrq.gov/patient-safety/settings/hospital/candor/index.html. Accessed 1 Mar 2023.
40. Agency for Healthcare Research and Quality. Implementation Guide for the CANDOR Process: Appendix B; 2022. https://www.ahrq.gov/research/findings/making-healthcare-safer/index.html Accessed 1 Mar 2023.
41. Healthcare and Patient Partnership Institute. H2Pi road to success; 2023. https://www.h2pi.org/roadmap. Accessed 1 Mar 2023.

Healing and Learning: A Restorative Just Culture

Marian Savage and Marissa B. Jamarik

1 Background: What Is a Just Culture and Why Is It Important?

The Institute of Medicine (IOM) report *"To Err Is Human: Building a Safer Health System"* still resonates across healthcare as one of the most influential documents that changed the course of patient safety. The report exposed how medical errors arise from "faulty systems, processes, and conditions that lead people to make mistakes or fail to prevent them" and not the individuals themselves that are reckless working within those systems [1]. The Institute of Medicine's landmark report revealed that up to 98,000 people die every year because of medical errors and in many ways forced healthcare to evaluate and re-evaluate safety [2]. The document gave rise to the development of what we coin today as "just culture" to help cultivate and guide organizations to adopt processes that instead offer opportunities to evaluate errors or "almost" errors in a holistic manner. It also evaluates individual choices

M. Savage (✉)
Quality & Patient Experience, Roper St. Francis Healthcare, Charleston, SC, USA
e-mail: Marian.Savage@rsfh.com

M. B. Jamarik
Roper St. Francis Healthcare, Charleston, SC, USA
e-mail: Rissa.Jamarik@rsfh.com

© The Author(s), under exclusive license to Springer Nature Switzerland AG 2024
C. A. Oster, J. S. Braaten (eds.), *The Nexus between Nursing and Patient Safety*,
https://doi.org/10.1007/978-3-031-53158-3_16

and lack of infrastructure and supports learning versus punishment. Learning from errors allows for organizations to gain insight and improve safety, reliability, and resilience [3].

> A general definition of a "just culture" is when an organization is motivated by patient safety and strives to improve through a process of shared or balanced accountability between the system for structural design and individuals for their choices [4].
> The model is a guide for healthcare organizations that includes human factors, error prevention, and steps to mitigate issues before they become critical. The priorities are to create a fair environment that promotes learning, safe systems, and safe behavioral choices [5].

Human error is now regarded as an expected event that requires organizations to put in place exceptionally reliable processes that limit their occurrence, recognize them before they occur, and manage those involved with support and education [5]. Frequently, when framing up errors within an organization, you will hear references to the "intent" of the individual who made the error. Most often, it denotes that by nature of the profession, individuals do not come to work with the intention of harming others as a goal. Organizational codes such as the Code of Ethics for Nurses [6] and the American Medical Association's Code of Medical Ethics Opinion 8.6 [7] speak to the responsibility of these professional roles to support safety as well as acknowledge personal accountability. Restorative just culture supports this professional good intent while creating the framework for healthcare professionals to be able to live their mission to heal and protect by using an error as a true learning event.

1.1 Retributive Versus Restorative Justice

To understand the types of responses to safety events, it is important to understand retributive versus restorative justice. Retributive justice focuses on punishment and finding someone to "pay," while restorative justice focuses on healing and making those who are hurt whole. In other words, retributive justice causes more hurt after the initial insult, while restorative justice attempts to heal.

Organizationally, retributive culture has dominated our history in not only healthcare but also many industries, with a very top-down approach to assess the severity of errors and assign consequences based on the level of harm [8–10]. Kaur et al. [11] surmise that retributive justice is linked less to justice than to the organizational power of an individual or individuals. Clearly, the "blaming" approach to events contributed to lost trust, a lack of willingness to come forward, and an overall sense of power versus promotion of justice [11]. Although we feel that we have come a very long way from this retributive culture, current Patient Safety Culture surveys still find the question regarding non-blaming culture as one of the least positive responses. In other words, we still do not have the just culture that we desire [12].

Restorative just culture, in contrast, takes a cross-organizational approach to evaluate the causal effects of the error and focuses on repairing the damage and restoring the well-being of those involved [3]. However, the most beneficial attribute of restorative just culture remains in its promotion of fostering a culture where employees feel free to speak up, voice overall concerns, and be actively engaged in preventing future errors moving safety from a reactive to a proactive model [13]. In many ways, restorative just culture establishes that despite their best efforts, healthcare clinicians will inevitably make mistakes of omission, commission, human nature, and imperfect work environments [4]. However, how an organization responds to this determines its overall success in preventing patient harm. Table 1 summarizes the differences between a retributive and a restorative just culture.

Patient safety experts have begun to distinguish between what it means to have a just culture that heals and a just culture that causes more hurt. Sidney Dekker [14] developed a checklist noted in Fig. 1 that probes all parties involved in a situation and seeks to resolve while repairing harm. Questions that should be asked include: Who was harmed? What do they need to heal? Are we ready to forgive?

Table 1 Comparison: retributive versus restorative just culture

Retributive culture	Restorative just culture
• Victimization of caregiver	• Understanding of underlying processes
• Decrease in reporting events	• Increase in reporting of events
• Psychological stress	• Psychological support
• Increase in nursing turnover	• Nursing retention
• Focus on blame	• Focus on healing

RESTORATIVE JUST CULTURE CHECKLIST

Restorative Just Culture aims to repair trust and relationships damaged after an incident. It allows all parties to discuss how they have been affected, and collaboratively decide what should be done to repair the harm.

WHO IS HURT?

ACKNOWLEDGED:
NO   **YES**

Have you acknowledged how the following parties have been hurt:
First victim(s) – patients, passengers, colleagues, consumers, clients
Second victim(s) – the practitioner(s) involved in the incident
Organization(s) – may have suffered reputational or other harm
Community – who witnessed or were affected by the incident
Others – please specify:..

WHAT DO THEY NEED?

EXPLORED:
NO   **YES**

Have you collaboratively explored the needs arising from harms done:
First victim(s) – information, access, restitution, reassurance of prevention
Second victim(s) – psychological first aid, compassion, reinstatement
Organization(s) – information, leverage for change, reputational repair
Community – information about incident and aftermath, reassurance
Others – please specify:..

WHOSE OBLIGATION IS IT TO MEET THE NEED?

IDENTIFIED:
NO   **YES**

Have you explored the needs arising from the harms above:
First victim(s) – tell their story and willing to participate in restorative process
Second victim(s) – willing to tell truth, express remorse, contribute to learning
Organization(s) – willing to participate, offered help, explored systemic fixes
Community – willing to participate in restorative process and forgiveness
Others – please specify:..

READY TO FORGIVE?

NO   **YES**

Forgiveness is not a simple act, but a process between people:
Confession – telling the truth of what happened and disclosing own role in it
Remorse – expressing regret for harms caused and how to put things right
Forgiveness – moving beyond event, reinvesting in trust and future together

ACHIEVED GOALS OF RESTORATIVE JUSTICE?

ACHIEVED:
NO   **YES**

Your response is restorative if you have:
Moral engagement – engaged parties in considering the right thing to do now
Emotional healing – helped cope with guilt, humiliation; offered empathy
Reintegrating practitioner – done what is needed to get person back in job
Organizational learning – explored and addressed systemic causes of harm

Public Domain. By Professor Sidney Dekker—Griffith University, Delft University and Art of Work. **sidneydekker.com**

Fig. 1 Restorative just culture [14]

BACKGROUND OF RESTORATIVE JUSTICE

Restorative Just Culture asks:
- **Who is hurt?**
- **What do they need?**
- **Whose obligation is that?**

Accountability is *forward-looking*. Together, you explore what needs to be done and who should do it

An **account** is something you tell and learn from

Retributive Just Culture asks:
- What rule is broken?
- How bad is the breach?
- What should consequences be?

Accountability is *backward-looking*, finding the person to blame and imposing proportional sanctions

An **account** is something you settle or pay

WHY AVOID RETRIBUTIVE JUST CULTURE?

A retributive just culture can turn into a blunt HR or managerial instrument to get rid of people.
It plays out between 'offender' and employer—excluding voices of first victims, colleagues, community.
A retributive just culture is linked with hiding incidents and an unwillingness to report and learn.
The more powerful people are in an organization, the more 'just' they find their retributive just culture.
A retributive response doesn't identify systemic contributions to the incident, thus inviting repetition.

GUIDANCE FOR USE OF *RESTORATIVE* JUST CULTURE CHECKLIST

On the checklist, mark where you think you are, like so: or so:
Together, the marks reveal what you still need to do.

HURTS, NEEDS AND OBLIGATIONS

An incident causes (potential) hurts or harms. This creates needs in the parties harmed.
These needs produce obligations for the (other) parties involved.
Restorative justice allows parties to discuss their hurts, their needs and the resulting obligations *together*.
Incidents don't just harm their (first) victim(s). They also (potentially) harm the second victim, supervisors, the organization, colleagues, bystanders, families, regulatory relationships and the surrounding community. All these parties have different needs arising from the harms caused to them.
The checklist allows you to trace the harmed parties, their needs, and the obligations on them/others.

FORGIVENESS

Forgiveness is not a simple act of one person to another. Forgiveness is a relational process that involves truth-telling, repentance and the repair of trust. It takes time. Trust is easy to break and hard to fix. Some first victims may be unwilling or unable to forgive. Second victims can also have difficulty forgiving themselves. Parties need to have patience and compassion, and may end up going separate ways.

GOALS OF RESTORATIVE JUSTICE

- *Moral engagement* can mean accepting appropriate responsibility for what happened, recognizing the seriousness of harms caused, and humanizing the people involved. Incidents can overwhelm an organization (e.g. a legal, reputational, financial, managerial issue). It is easy to forget that it is also a moral issue: What is the right thing to do?
- *Emotional healing* aims to deal with feelings such as grief, resentment, humiliation, guilt and shame. It is a basis for repairing trust and relationships.
- *Reintegrating* the practitioner expresses the trust and confidence that the incident is about more than just the individual. Expensive lessons can disappear from the organization if the practitioner is not helped back into the job, and letting them go tends to obstruct the three other goals. If you fire someone, what have you fixed?
- Restorative justice is better geared toward *addressing the causes* of harm because it goes beyond the individual practitioner and invites a range of stories and voices. Forward-looking accountability is about avoiding blame, and instead fixing things.

Public Domain. By Professor Sidney Dekker—Griffith University, Delft University and Art of Work. **sidneydekker.com**

Fig. 1 (continued)

2   Components of Highly Reliable Organizations

Error-prone processes are plentiful within healthcare. Multiple processes including medication administration, surgical procedures, and specimen retrieval are complex and require multiple steps. The addition of electronic systems in the process has reduced the probability of error, but the possibility of human error remains. Additionally, the emergence of technology may lead to complacency of the staff performing the task [15]. This is evident in the reliance and overreliance of technology that may create drift from fundamental safety checks such as the five rights to medication administration. Medication scanning is an excellent tool to prevent errors but does not remove the ultimate accountability of the last check to remain with the bedside clinician.

Highly reliable organizations focus on processes and overall safety. The organizational design must focus on common goals with strategic oversight while supplying the structure and resources to evaluate potential issues. High reliability includes managerial oversight and structure within policies, procedures, and processes. This much-needed structure allows for collaboration, which leads to action. Organizations that provide an open, collaborative culture foster an inclusive environment that allows for learning from errors, instead of blame. One common aspect of highly reliable organizations includes involving frontline staff in the decision-making process. Frontline staff are the ones performing the most complex tasks within healthcare, so their input in decision-making is invaluable. Without this type of input, organizations design processes and policies that do not match everyday practice. In addition, this form of shared decision-making not only optimizes the process redesign but also engages the front line as true stakeholders of the improvement process, which will support the overall success of implementation and its ultimate sustainability.

3   Focusing on Multiple Victims

When errors occur within healthcare, many times they reach a patient. The level of harm to the patient can vary from no reaction to patient death. Organizations that engage in retributive culture tend to blame the nurse, if applicable, for the error while consoling the patient and loved ones. When a patient is the victim of a medical error, it is always important to provide support and empathy to them, but many times there is also a second victim that goes unnoticed. In healthcare, understandably areas where fast-paced care is delivered with high acuity and trauma yield the highest rates of reported distress. This distress contributes to second victim syndrome and can lead to post-traumatic stress disorder (PTSD) if not addressed adequately. As recent as July of 2022, high levels of distress were reported to be 27% of emergency room nurses and 22% of ICU nurses [16].

When errors within healthcare occur, usually a person is the last step in the process. Restorative just culture understands that patients and their loved ones need comfort and support, but additionally the nurse may need reassurance and compassion. It is extremely rare for a nurse to purposely want to cause harm to any patient, so when an error occurs, the effects can be overwhelming. Highly reliable organizations provide a safe space where the nurse can speak freely about what occurred during the error. This type of atmosphere is important to understand the true root cause of the error. Without this direct information, organizations would be left to guess what led to the error. Using a consultative approach, asking non-accusatory questions allows the nurse to feel safe and free to speak about the error. The nurse may need additional support outside of the organization, particularly if the error caused extreme harm to a patient. According to the Joint Commission, second victims experience a range of emotions including sleep disturbances, fear, guilt, and anxiety. One study by Ullstrom and colleagues [17] determined that one-third of second victims had not received adequate support from their organizations and continued to struggle with job satisfaction after an adverse event.

4 Outcome Bias and Severity of Judgment: No Harm, No Foul?

Overcoming outcome bias is a skill that requires practice and reinforcement within the restorative just culture model. Outcome bias is often the prompt for individuals to focus on blaming healthcare providers for the error by focusing on the outcome of the error versus the systemic or process failures leading to the error. When an error occurs, individuals tend to focus on the outcome of the error, rather than the error itself. This type of focus might be described as outcome bias and can lead to a retributive culture.

Take for example a person that has multiple drinks in a bar and decides to drive home. Many different outcomes can arise from this poor choice. The driver could make it home with no incident, the driver could hit a tree and injure themselves, or the driver could crash into a vehicle and injure the driver and passengers. The act that caused the accident (drinking and driving) did not change, though the punishments for the act change dramatically in current culture. In some sense, the driver is rewarded for arriving safely at home without an incident. The driver may feel an incorrect sense of safety because they did not understand how much alcohol they consumed. The driver that hit a tree may encounter some damage to their vehicle but may or may not have any police involvement with the incident. The driver may or may not think about having a drink and driving in the future. When a driver hits another car and injures others, the consequences are very severe. There may be police intervention, and the judicial system might be involved. The punishment for this type of crime might be drastic, but the initial act of deciding to drive while drinking has not changed. It is common in our culture to use the sentiment of "let the punishment fit the crime," but does that same sentiment seek to understand why the crime occurred?

Medication errors in nursing may follow a similar pattern in organizations that use a retributive approach to error management. Most organizations use incident reporting systems for individuals to report unusual events. Nurses frequently report medication errors of overdosing, timing, and administering medications that cause an allergic reaction. When a medication error occurs, one of the three outcomes can happen to the patient. Errors may have no effect on the patient, patients may suffer from a minor reaction and need extended monitoring, or, in extreme cases, the patient may die from the error. Organizations typically do not terminate a nurse when a single medication error is made. But there are instances when this has occurred. The recent case of RaDonda Vaught proved that over a single medication error, the nurse can be terminated and criminally charged by the State of Tennessee [18]. In 2017, Vaught administered a dose of medication to a patient during a radiology procedure. The order was for a sedative, but mistakenly Vaught administered a paralytic drug. The patient subsequently died after the medication error.

The outrage and criminal charges arose because the patient died from the medication that Vaught administered. It is unknown if the organization used restorative just culture to understand all the components of medication errors. Restorative just culture practices would have examined previous medication errors within the organization and attempted to put barriers in place to prevent future ones. Also, support would be provided to the nurse since the patient's outcome was tragic.

Outcome bias occurs in healthcare when the punishment for an error is more severe based on the outcome to the patient. Outcome bias occurs when we want to attribute blame and find a quick solution to the problem [19]. Without a deep analysis of the causes of the error, along with the use of a restorative just culture structure, individuals may be blamed for an error that their colleagues are not. Successful restorative just culture implementation requires training and ongoing practice. Familiarity with the algorithm and how to navigate it should be exercised routinely. Case studies are an excellent and practical way to train teams on how to best utilize and implement restorative just culture. Literature suggests that initial training is imperative in establishing just culture within an organization but that sustainability of restorative just culture requires ongoing refinement and learning.

5   Case Studies

Sally, a registered nurse (RN) works as a nurse in an elementary school in a rural area. She has been a nurse for 7 years and has been working at the school for the past 18 months. She has an excellent rapport with the other teachers and received a great review after her first year of employment. Previously, Sally worked as a nurse in a pediatric patient clinic.

One day, a well-known diabetic student became dizzy and collapsed. The student had just told their teacher that they did not feel well and that they needed to see the school nurse. The teacher carried the student into the nurse's area and placed them on a bed. Sally was aware that the student had type 1 diabetes, so she took the student's blood sugar while asking a colleague to call 911 and the guardians. The student's blood sugar was 24. The student's parents provided emergent glucagon injectors to the school nurse in case the student's blood sugar dropped to a dangerous level. Sally administered the glucagon injection to the student. Sally did not recheck the student's blood glucose before the emergency team arrived. The paramedics took the student to the hospital where the blood sugar remained low, and the student was found to have an insulin pump that was still running. Once the pump was removed, the hospital gave dextrose fluids and glucagon to raise the blood sugar, and the student spent a few days in the hospital, eventually recovering.

The student's parents were outraged that such an incident would happen and stated that Sally did not know how to handle emergency situations. They told the principal of the school that they were extremely disappointed in the care that their child had received and that the child could have died under the care of the school. The principal made the decision to terminate Sally effective immediately. Sally was never provided with a forum to discuss what happened from her perspective or given any psychological support. The school hired a new nurse and did not provide any additional training to the new nurse.

Did Sally have adequate training as a school nurse?
Did the principal have justification for terminating Sally?
Did the school do anything to prevent a similar event from happening in the future?

Mark, RN, works in the emergency department of a large teaching hospital. He has been a registered nurse for 2 years. He completed the nurse residency program that his hospital provided 1 year prior. The emergency department had recently hired multiple new graduates due to staffing shortages. Mark was working a night shift and had an order to give his patient 0.5 mg of hydromorphone IV for a bone fracture. The patient was in room 4, and when Mark went to give the medication, he realized that the bar code scanner was broken in the room. Mark checked the patient's name on the armband and checked the order in the computer and then administered the hydromorphone.

About 15 min after Mark administered the medication, the patient's wife rushed to the nursing station to ask for help. The patient was unresponsive, and an overhead announcement was called for assistance. The physician arrived and asked what medications that patient received, and Mark stated that he had just been given hydromorphone. An order was given to administer naloxone. The patient started to regain consciousness and was admitted overnight for continued observation.

The patient's wife complained to the emergency room manager that Mark overdosed her husband on medication and was angry that the event occurred. The nursing manager apologized to the wife and assured them that she would review the events that led up to the overdose.

The emergency department manager met with Mark and asked for his recollection of what occurred. Mark remembered pulling the hydromorphone from the medication administration cabinet and checking the patient's name and order. The manager obtained the report of the medications that Mark pulled from the medication administration cabinet and noticed that he pulled a 4 mg syringe of hydromorphone. When the manager asked if he scanned the medication, he stated that he did not because the scanner was not working. When asked if he used the entire syringe, Mark stated that he did, thinking he pulled a 0.5 mg syringe. The manager discussed the issue with pharmacy and determined that there was a shortage of the 0.5 mg syringes usually stocked in the emergency department. The pharmacy had back-filled the stock with 4 mg syringes until the shortage subsided. The manager discussed the importance of timely reporting of equipment failures and the safety aspects of bar code scanning. The emergency room manager asked Mark to present the medication error at the next staff meeting along with the safety steps that may have prevented the error.

Did Mark have adequate training as an emergency department nurse?
How did the emergency department manager investigate the medication error?
What system issues led to the medication error?

5.1   Discussion of Case Studies

Using restorative just culture, many contributing factors should be discussed. The main components that should always be evaluated include people, process, and environment. The first step in the evaluation is interviewing the nurses involved in the errors. In the first case study, the nurse was not given a chance to provide information about why she made certain decisions, so we are unclear about what exactly led to the error. Is it possible that the ambulance came faster than she would have been able to take another blood sugar? Was the nurse assessing other vital signs on the student? Were other colleagues present to help her in an emergency? Onboarding and training would be another area to explore. Was the nurse properly onboarded with resources for emergencies? Had she ever been exposed to emergencies in her previous role? What emergency equipment and supplies did the school have? Next, the investigation would seek to understand what the nurse knew about the insulin pump. Was she trained by the parents in how to stop the pump? Was she given a chance to practice those skills? All these questions and more should have been discussed before a decision was made to remove the nurse from her position.

In the second case study, the nurse provided details of why they gave the incorrect dose of medication to a patient. Mark had been through the nursing residency program and was aware of the five rights of medication administration. The organization provided an orientation process, and this was not the first time that he had given medications to patients. Did the switch-in process by the pharmacy contribute to the error? Is it possible that the emergency department was terribly busy that day and Mark had just been asked to take on an additional patient because of staffing shortages? How were the medication shortages communicated to the nursing staff? Was there a warning on the electronic medication cabinet? How often do shortages occur? Why were the scanners nonfunctional? Is there a process to remove broken equipment and obtain functional equipment?

It is clear from both case studies that neither nurse intended to cause harm to their patients. Using restorative culture takes time and investigation to understand all the components of the error. Additionally, there needs to be time spent with the nurses to understand how they are feeling and processing the error. A strong restorative just culture allows nurses to grieve the error and impact on the patient.

6 Barriers to Implementing a Restorative Culture

Despite best efforts to foster restorative just culture in healthcare, the reality check is that in some regards, the pendulum has swung in a way that overlooks the goal of both understanding the contributing factors and how to mitigate them. Restorative just culture is not blame free; it considers the intention and frequency of errors as well as individual accountability [5]. The Agency for Quality Healthcare and Research [20] defines restorative just culture as one which "focuses on identifying and addressing systems issues that lead individuals to engage in unsafe behaviors, while maintaining individual accountability by establishing zero tolerance for reckless behavior." Within the restorative just culture framework, medical errors fall into three categories: simple human error, risky behaviors, and recklessness. The restorative just culture framework guides the end users to address these mistakes through consolation, coaching, and in some instances punishment [5]. However, the initial intent of restorative just culture was to balance the accountability of both the system and the individual while allowing fair treatment when addressing adverse events [21]. Many factors have contributed to this: workforce shortages, staff burnout from a global pandemic, and an ardent desire for healthcare to deliver safe care in an environment that puts safety first. The first step is to acknowledge that restorative just culture is still fundamentally the path to the highest, most transparent culture in safety and quality. However, healthcare may also need to accept that it too may have an unconscious bias due to extraneous pressures. Organizations may need to pause and reevaluate how restorative just culture fundamentals should be re-engaged.

Understanding the complexities of errors in systems is important. When a single person is blamed for an error, many underlying issues remain unknown. When an error happens in healthcare, there is usually one or more people involved. It becomes easy to "blame" the person for the error and simply close an investigation since blaming an individual is often the easiest path forward. Spending time investigating the reasons that the incident occurred, all of the system issues involved take dedicated resources and time. When individuals are blamed for errors, their psychological safety is impaired. This psychological danger can lead to increased organizational turnover, underreporting of events, and fear within cultures [22]. When these factors are prevalent within an institution, it is unlikely that the root cause of the event has been determined. For example, when a patient receives the incorrect medication, it is easier for an organization to say that the nurse administering the medication did not follow the five rights of medication administration and put the nurse through some type of disciplinary process. The issue is thought to be resolved, and the management may be satisfied that the situation is over. In actuality, the system issues that allowed the medication error to occur may not be understood.

To determine the root cause of any event, a thorough investigation and extensive time must be spent to understand the causes of the failure. While there are many different tools available to understand the root causes, taking the time to use the tools effectively presents a challenge for the organization. Take for example the five whys approach endorsed by the Institute of Healthcare Improvement [23]. The tool states to ask five different "why" questions until you reach the root cause of the problem. Let us explore an easy example of using the five whys method. Let us review a medication administration error.

A patient received the incorrect medication.

Why? The nurse gave the incorrect medication to a patient.

Why? The nurse thought it was the correct medication.

Why? The nurse picked the incorrect medication from the patient's drawer that comes up from pharmacy daily.

Why? Most of the medications on the unit were stocked in the electronic medication cabinet, but a few were brought up from pharmacy each day intermixed with other medications. There were two medications that had similar names in the drawer.

Why? The hospital ran out of drawer space in their electronic medication cabinet so infrequently used medications were sent up from pharmacy to be administered by the nurse.

Determining that an error may have occurred because there was a system failure takes investigation. As you can see, taking the time to interview participants of a medication error takes purposeful probing. Multiple persons and departments may need to be interviewed to understand what the root cause is. In the example above, the root cause might be the lack of medication oversight and financial constraints. While the nurse did not use the five rights of medication administration, deeper underlying systemic issues placed the nurse in a dangerous scenario.

Given the staffing shortages within nursing, it becomes much more difficult to spend the needed time to investigate errors. Even more importantly is the time spent to remedy system failures. Highly reliable organizations may need to dedicate multiple individuals and provide time for teams to meet and discuss events. Organizations with a strong safety component can provide resources to help with investigations and determine root cause failures.

A literature review by Thiesse-Yount [24] identified perceived barriers to error reporting that included:

- Inadequate staffing levels affecting environmental conditions and negative outcomes.
- Management support of patient safety rates as low [25].
- Lack of trust [26].
- Lack of feedback on events, no solutions or changes based on events, and skepticism on the value of reporting [27].
- Fear of rude or confrontational behaviors from peers [28].

- Reliance on oral reporting versus written [29].
- Lack of reporting unless there was perceived harm experienced by the patient [29].

7   The Way Forward

Post-pandemic, organizations need to regrind the principles of restorative just culture. The process should be viewed by organizations as a dynamic, ongoing process that requires structure, focus, and constant re-evaluation. Tasker, Jones, and Brake [30] conducted a qualitative study to examine the barriers to effective restorative just culture as well as how clinicians and managers were aligned to the principles of restorative just culture. Several themes arose from their study that included familiarity with restorative just culture process and meaning to the frontline staff. In addition, they found that there were varying definitions of restorative just culture among the team leading to further confusion on the concepts of restorative just culture. Another significant finding was that lessons identified through investigations failed to drive any improvement in the organization. Consistently, this was driven by a lack of communication of the findings and the subsequent perception that "nothing had happened." A final compelling note from Tasker et al. [30] was the data that demonstrated that those performing the investigations lacked formal training. This suggests that organizations need ongoing emphasis of restorative just culture training to ensure that the process is clear to all as well as accountability for using the tools. In addition, Tasker et al. demonstrate the need for ongoing evaluation of the restorative just culture process for true sustainability.

Restorative just culture remains a viable and desirable model for addressing error prevention and remediation. The success of restorative just culture is highly dependent on the organizational culture for success [31]. Trust remains a constant trait in organizations that enculturate restorative just culture and high reliability. This is inherently driven by leadership and is evidenced by the ability of the entire workforce, top-down, to be able to articulate fair treatment, absence of blame, and a focus on systemic factors impacting errors [31]. Trust is foundationally important to just culture to promote and ensure event reporting [32]. Organizational self-assessment and current state reflection are an imperative to refresh the concepts of restorative just culture and help catapult high reliability and a true safety culture forward.

Just culture and restorative just culture are a journey work, not a quick solution. Ongoing research and evidence are needed to help healthcare organizations refine, enculturate, and sustain its principles. Across the world, healthcare is realigning safety priorities and regaining focus on fundamentals. Restorative just culture needs to be a priority in this process to ensure that healthcare professionals are acknowledged and supported when an error occurs and most importantly that our patients remain the focus of safety culture by ongoing learning and improvements.

In summary, retributive just culture persists in some organizations; however, its far-reaching implications are better understood. Restorative just culture continues to be the path forward; however, it too has its challenges as far as the ability to implement and sustain.

Key Points

- Retributive culture focuses on punishment and individual. Restorative culture focuses on process and system.
- Retributive culture is easier to implement and less complex than restorative culture that requires time, resources, and sustainability.
- Second victim syndrome has the potential to exist even in restorative culture and requires organization to have a high focus on well-being.
- Restorative culture is not just an algorithm of how to treat an error, but a culture of inquiry, understanding, learning, and evaluation.

References

1. Institute of Medicine. Report brief: to err is human: building a safer health system. https://www.nap.edu/resource/9728/To-Err-is-Human-1999-report-brief.pdf. Published November 1999.
2. Kohn LT, Corrigan J, Donaldson MS. To err is human: building a safer health system. Washington, DC: National Academy Press; 2000.
3. Baarle E, Harman L, Rooijakkers S, Wallenburg I, Weenink J, Bal R, Widdershoven G. Fostering a restorative just culture in healthcare organizations: experiences in practice. BMC Health Serv Res. 22(1):1035. https://doi.org/10.1186/s12913-022-08418-z.
4. Boyson PG II. Restorative just culture: a foundation for balanced accountability and patient safety. Oschner J. 2013;13(3):400–6.
5. Eng DM, Schweikart SJ. Why Accountability sharing in healthcare organizations cultures means patients are probably safer. AMA J Ethics. 2020;22(9):E779–83. https://doi.org/10.1001/amajethics.2020.779.
6. American Nurses Association. Code of ethics for nurses with interpretive statements. https://www.nursingoworld.org/practice-policy/nursing-excellence/ethics/code-of-ethics-for-nurses/. Published 2015. Accessed November 6, 2023.
7. American Medical Association. Opinion 8.6 promoting patient safety. Code of medical ethics. https://www.ama-assn.org/delivering-care/ethics/promoting-patient-safety. Published November 14, 2015. Accessed November 6, 2023.
8. Marx D. Patient safety and the "just culture": a primer for health care executives. New York: Columbia University; 2001.
9. Reason JT. Managing the risks of organizational accidents. Aldershot, UK: Ashgate Publishing Co; 1997.
10. Wachter RM, Pronovost PJ. Balancing "no Blame" with accountability in patient safety. N Engl J Med. 2009;361:1401–6.
11. Kaur M, de Boer R, Oates A, Rafferty J, Dekker S. Restorative just culture: a study of the practical and economic effects of implementing restorative justice in an NHS Trust. MATEC Web of Conferences. 2019;273:01007. https://doi.org/10.1051/matecconf/201927301007.
12. Hare R, Tapia A, Tyler ER, Fan L, et al. Rockville, MD: Agency for Healthcare Research and Quality; October 2022. AHRQ Publication No. 22(23)-0066.
13. Hollnagel E. Safety-I and safety-II: the past and future of safety management. London: CRC Press; 2018.
14. Dekker S. RestorativeJustCultureChecklist_MD (safetydifferently.com); 2018.

15. Carroll JS, Rudolph JW. Design of high reliability organizations in health care. Qual Saf Health Care. 2006;15(Suppl 1):i4–9. https://doi.org/10.1136/qshc.2005.015867.
16. Guttormson JL, Calkins K, McAndrew N, Fitzgerald J, Losurdo H, Loonsfoot D. Critical care nurse burnout, moral distress, and mental health during the COVID-19 pandemic: a United States survey. Heart Lung. 2022;55:127–33. https://doi.org/10.1016/j.hrtlng.2022.04.015.
17. Ullström S, Andreen Sachs M, Hansson J, Ovretveit J, Brommels M. Suffering in silence: a qualitative study of second victims of adverse events. BMJ Qual Saf. 2014;23(4):325–31. https://doi.org/10.1136/bmjqs-2013-002035.
18. Harrington L. The RaDonda vaught case: a critical conversation on nursing practice and technology. AACN Adv Crit Care. 2023;34(1):11–5.
19. Berlin L. Outcome bias. Am J Roentgenol. 2004;183:557–60. https://doi.org/10.2214/ajr.183.3.1830557.
20. Agency for Healthcare Research and Quality (AHRQ). 2012. Patient safety primers, safety culture. https://psnet.ahrq.gov/primer/culture-safety
21. Barkall NP, Snyder SS. Restorative just culture in healthcare: an integrative review. Nurs Forum. 2020.
22. Okpala P. Nurses' perspectives on the impact of management approaches on the blame culture in health-care organizations. Int J Healthc Manag. 2020;13(Suppl. 1):199–205. https://doi.org/10.1080/20479700.2018.1492771.
23. 5 Whys: finding the root cause | IHI—Institute for Healthcare Improvement. https://www.ihi.org/resources/tools/5-whysfinding-root-cause
24. Thiesse-Yount R. Cultivating a just culture: identifying barriers to reporting safety events. Radiol Manage. 2022;44(6):10–36.
25. Danielsson M, Nilsen P, Rutberg H, Årestedt K. A national study of patient safety culture in hospitals in Sweden. J Patient Saf. 2019;15(4):328–33. https://doi.org/10.1097/PTS.0000000000000369.
26. Deyo-Svendsen ME, Palmer KB, Albright JK, Phillips MR, Schilling KA, Cabrera Svendsen ME. Provider approachability: an all-staff survey approach to creating a culture of safety. J Patient Saf. 2019;15(4):64–9.
27. Miller N, Bhowmik S, Ezinwa M, Yang T, Schrock S, Bitzel D, McGuire MJ. The relationship between safety culture and voluntary event reporting in a large regional ambulatory care group. J Patient Saf. 2019;15(4):e48–51. https://doi.org/10.1097/PTS.0000000000000337.
28. Morrow KJ, Gustavson AM, Jones J. Speaking up behaviours (safety voices) of healthcare workers: a metasynthesis of qualitative research studies. Int J Nurs Stud. 2016;64:42–51. https://doi.org/10.1016/j.ijnurstu.2016.09.014.
29. Yung HP, Yu S, Chu C, Hou IC, Tang FI. Nurses' attitudes and perceived barriers to the reporting of medication administration errors. J Nurs Manag. 2016;24(5):580–8. https://doi.org/10.1111/jonm.12360.
30. Tasker A, Jones J, Brake S. How effectively has a Just Culture been adopted? A qualitative study to analyse the attitudes and behaviours of clinicians and managers to clinical incident management within an NHS Hospital Trust and identify enablers and barriers to achieving a Just Culture. BMJ Open Qual. 2023;12(1):e002049. https://doi.org/10.1136/bmjoq-2022-002049.
31. Neiswender K, Figueroa-Altmann A, Granahan K, Barkman D. Rooting an error review process in just culture: lessons learned. Patient SayJcom. 2022;4(3) https://doi.org/10.33940/2002.9.5.
32. Dekker S. Just culture: balancing safety and accountability. United Kingdom: Ashgate; 2007.

The Nexus of Nursing and Patient Safety: Keeping Patients Safe

Cynthia A. Oster and Jane S. Braaten

1 Introduction

"First, do no harm" or nonmaleficence is a well-known principle in nursing ethics and means selecting interventions and care that will cause the least amount of harm to achieve a beneficial outcome [1]. The principle of nonmaleficence ensures the safety of the patient in care delivery. Patient harm during the provision of healthcare is one of the top ten contributors to disability and death in the world according to the World Health Organization [2]. The purpose of this chapter is to describe and explore the connection between nursing practice and patient safety including a discussion of synergistic factors to create safe outcomes.

2 Background

Patient safety is a priority for healthcare organizations. Nurses play a pivotal role in patient safety within health systems throughout the world. The nursing profession is committed to providing safe quality healthcare directed at achieving optimal patient outcomes [3]. The role of nursing and the nurse is central to the provision of safe quality patient care. Nursing is expected to provide high-quality safe care to each patient every time. The delivery of quality healthcare and patient safety are indistinguishable from each other according to the IOM [4]. Patient safety is

C. A. Oster (✉)
Nursing and Professional Development, CommonSpirit Health – Mountain Region, Centennial, CO, USA
e-mail: oster.cynthia.a@gmail.com

J. S. Braaten
Quality and Patient Safety, AdventHealth Parker, Parker, CO, USA
e-mail: jane.braaten@adventhealth.com

"prevention of harm to patients" [4]. Quality is defined as "the degree to which health services for individuals and populations increase the likelihood of desired health outcomes and are consistent with current knowledge" [5]. Quality is further defined as safe, effective, patient-centered, timely, efficient, and equitable. In essence, quality care cannot exist without safe care.

The profession of nursing's interest in quality care and safe care can be traced to Florence Nightingale. She established nursing as a profession and defined what it meant to be a nurse [6]. Nightingale established standards of nursing practice and expectations of professionalism during her years of service during the Crimean War. As a data scientist, she showed the value of quality safe patient care: survival rates increased from 50% to nearly 80% under the care of Nightingale and her nurses [7]. She revolutionized nursing care practices and improved clinical outcomes through attention to rigorous infection prevention, hygiene and cleanliness, nutrition and hydration, and compassionate care [8]. In addition, her contributions to quality and safety go beyond nursing into other dimensions of today's healthcare system including crafting the modern hospital administrative structure, architecture, aesthetics, supply chain management, and financial management; establishing medical records; originating hospital epidemiology; starting medical triage; and initiating patient education and empowerment—the precursor to patient-centered care [9]. Furthermore, Nightingale advocated for positive culture in hospitals by reducing institutional tolerance for toxic emotional negativity like gossip, complaining, and mistrust [9].

The contemporary role of the nurse and the nursing profession in promoting patient safety has notably evolved during the last century [10]. Focus on asepsis safety measures and the germ theory in the early 1900s gave way to medication error prevention and development of written standardized care procedures during the 1930s. Nurses were active inventors of safety equipment and protocols during the 1940s. World War II nurses recognized that close observation of patients in "shock wards" improved survival of surgical and obstetrical patients with patients assigned to various levels of care based on acuity during the 1950s. Medication and nursing procedure safety were the primary emphasis for the next 40 years. Since 2000, the focus has shifted away from solely the actions of individuals to include systemic factors that affect patient safety. The development of a professional identity has empowered nurses to spotlight safety concerns and propose solutions to those concerns.

An important factor for quality and safety in patient care is an environment in which quality and safety are prioritized and embedded into the culture [11]. The nursing profession has championed the very culture of safety proposed by the IOM report *To Err Is Human* [12] that encouraged research to focus on systemic solutions rather than individual performance solutions to errors. Nursing practice plays a critical role in safeguarding patients and families. Nurses ensure patient safety by monitoring patients for clinical deterioration, detecting near errors and near misses, understanding care processes and weaknesses inherent in systems, identifying and communicating changes in patient condition, as well as performing other tasks such as detecting diagnostic and treatment errors and administering medications [13]. The practice of nursing requires nurses to regularly interact with other healthcare team members (i.e., physicians, pharmacists, surgeons, physical therapists). This frequent and repeated interprofessional interaction allows nurses to influence patient safety across the entire continuum of care.

Building a safe and healthy nursing practice work environment is essential to reducing adverse events and contributes to a culture of safety [14–16]. For hospitals with improved clinical work environments, nurses report a favorable grade on inpatient safety, while nurses practicing in hospitals with deteriorated clinical work environments report a less favorable grade on patient safety [17]. Building a culture of safety does not just happen; it requires teamwork, evidence-based practice, communication, ongoing education, a just culture, leadership, and patient-centered care [18].

Practice, research, and theory are cornerstones to the disciplines of patient safety science and nursing science (Fig. 1). The relationships among these three cornerstones are reciprocal and cyclical [19]. Practice generates research questions and knowledge; research guides practice and builds knowledge through theory development, while theory guides research and improves practice.

Effective patient safety and nursing practice require the application of knowledge, skills, and care to patients in an effective, efficient, and considerate approach. The knowledge used in making practice decisions is grounded in research findings. "In any discipline, science is the result of the relationship between the process of inquiry (research) and the product of knowledge (theory)" [19]. Research guides practice and builds knowledge through theory generation. Theory improves practice. Practice is the basis for the development of theory, and theory is validated in practice. Nurses must appreciate the value of evidence in practice, be able to understand and appraise research, apply relevant theory and research findings to their work, and identify areas for further investigation [20].

As nursing has evolved into a practice that prioritizes patient safety, it is interesting that overall patient safety improvements have occurred at a much slower rate than expected [21, 22]. The reasons are varied: lack of priority due to other urgent factors, lack of real system fixes, lack of real application of safety science such as human factors into healthcare safety, lack of standard measurement, and lack of involving those most knowledgeable about process within process improvement strategies, including the patient [23]. The goal is zero harm [24]. The integration of

Fig. 1 The relationship of practice, research, and theory

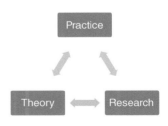

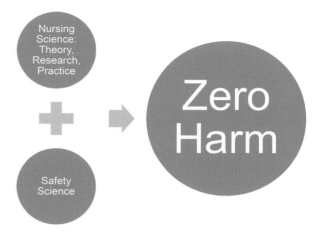

Fig. 2 Safety science and nursing science: nursing theory, nursing research, and nursing practice achieve zero harm

safety science and nursing science as applied to the nursing theory, research, and practice cycle can make zero harm a reality (Fig. 2). Nursing leaders, administrators, and clinicians can and must work tirelessly to apply safety science, nursing theory, nursing research, and nursing practice to achieve zero preventable harm and zero injury to patients and families served in healthcare systems.

3   The Nexus of Nursing and Patient Safety

Reflect on a healthcare world where:

- Hospital-acquired pressure injuries never occur due to meticulous attention to relieving pressure and programs dedicated to mobility for identified high-risk patients.
- Indwelling urinary catheter-acquired infections are a thing of the past as protocols allow nurses to remove catheters or use alternatives.
- Medication errors are caught and corrected due to redundancies and checkpoints prior to administration.
- Procedural staff speak up and stop the line when a count is not completed prior to closing the surgical site. The team prevents a retained object, and this is celebrated at the daily safety huddle.
- A nursing aide stops a nurse from entering a patient room without performing hand hygiene. The nurse says, "Thanks for the reminder."
- Ventilator-associated pneumonias do not occur due to nursing, respiratory, and physicians collaborating on care protocols.
- New technology is simulated at the front line to identify failure modes with the end users in human conditions (fatigue, distraction, interruptions).

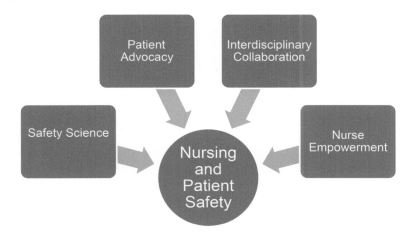

Fig. 3 The nexus of nursing and patient safety

- Clinical patient changes are discussed as a team with all team members' input encouraged. Expertise is valued at all levels.
- Patients are encouraged to ask questions before taking any new medication.

These are examples of the impact that is occurring as nursing integrates safety science principles into practice with the interprofessional team. This is the nexus of nursing and patient safety.

Nexus is a connection or link between things, persons, groups, or events [25] and is a central or most important point of interaction [26]. The nexus—the central or most important point of interaction—where patient safety connects or meets nursing keeps patients safe. Nursing and patient safety are interdependent, as nursing is a necessary element of patient safety. Figure 3 depicts the centrality of nursing and patient safety and the important components that optimize the nexus: safety science integrated into key nursing functions including patient, advocacy, collaboration, and empowerment. These factors combine to create a synergy of nursing theory, research, and practice integral to safety outcomes.

4   Nursing and Patient Safety: Synergistic Factors

Nursing, the largest healthcare profession in the United States, is the structural backbone of the healthcare system and is the primary provider of hospital patient care and long-term care [27]. Nursing and patient safety blend to create a synergy that positions nursing and patient safety as a powerful combined presence. However, this synergy must be intentionally designed and sustained. Synergy will come through focus on environments that support nurses as leaders of patient safety and integrating key elements of safety science into the entirety of nursing practice. Furthermore, nurses themselves need to believe that as the prime discipline that advocates for patients, they are the leaders of patient safety. Where patient safety and nursing connect with that synergy keeps patients safe. Synergistic and necessary factors as seen in Fig. 3 are subsequently discussed.

4.1   Safety Science

Nursing has distinct disciplinary knowledge that is strengthened by research, theory, and application of current safety science principles to practice. Application of safety science principles to the practice of nursing provides an additional resistant barrier to patient harm. Recommendations for strengthening nursing practice that integrate current safety science principles to keep patients safe are discussed next.

Nurse's voice as a strong barrier to harm. The Swiss cheese model (SCM) creates a view of safety that adds value [28]. The SCM describes a system of either strong or weak barriers that allow or stop an error from making its way through a system to cause harm to a patient. Nurses are a strong barrier to harm. Errors will always occur in a healthcare system; however, nurses are often the ones who find and correct errors to stop them from causing harm. The nexus of nursing and patient safety to keep patients safe is to realize that one of the strongest barriers to patient harm is the power of the nurse's voice when speaking up with concerns about safety. Not all professions are in the position to witness or recognize high-risk conditions. Nurses create safety at the front line by using their knowledge, skills, clinical expertise, and voice to:

- Recognize high-risk situations arising in daily patient care such as medication inconsistencies particularly dosage errors and circumstances placing patients at risk for hospital-acquired injuries such as indwelling urinary or intravenous catheters remaining in place when not necessary.
- Express concerns by asking questions, escalating issues, and stopping the line for safety when needed.
- Create structures that support speaking up behaviors with a culture that values all contributions on behalf of patient safety.
- Provide positive recognition and support for errors that are found and corrected at the front line.

Human factors and nursing. Nursing is ideally situated to adopt and adapt human factors science to keep patients safe. Human factors engineering is the application of human factors science and practice of designing work systems to fit the needs limitations and capabilities of humans [29]. The goals of human factors engineering are to improve safety by minimizing the prevalence of hazards, accidents, and injuries; improve performance by increasing the efficiency of workers performing tasks having physical, cognitive, or social demands; and improve satisfaction of humans in the work system. Human factors engineering considers human interaction with interactive systems that involve people, tools and technology, and work environments. Human factors engineers know that human beings and technology interact to create outcomes [30].

Healthcare systems of today are filled with new technology, and the quest for better technology is ever present [31]. Busy nurses rely on equipment to carry out potentially lifesaving interventions under the assumption that technology will improve outcomes. Nurses must participate in usability testing or the testing of new systems and equipment under real-world conditions in order to identify potential problems or unintended consequences of the new technology. Frontline safety threats related to new equipment are often undetected until after technology implementation. For example, infusion pumps are often upgraded with new software programs. Errors can occur with new infusion pump programming that might not be anticipated without usability testing or guidance of the end users (nurses). Proactive questions need to be addressed such as how does the pump perform in low lighting, in rushed situations, and in situations when medications have like names. Nurses can assure that human factors are always considered to create better outcomes by:

- Participating as an expert in the purchase decision and integration of new technology in a system.
- Using a structured system such as a failure mode and effects analysis (FMEA) to assess how technology coupled with real situations in the context of actual care can fail [32].
- Recognizing and identifying critical safety tasks that may be prone to rushing, distractions, interruptions, and shortcuts.
- Validating and using practice tools that make it more difficult for humans to make errors such as forced functions, checklists, and visual cues.

High reliability: Anticipation of error. High-reliability science is the study of organizations that operate under hazardous conditions while maintaining safety [33]. High-reliability science focuses on how harm can be avoided by anticipating errors and remaining observant to changing conditions in order to problem solve and change course prior to a bad outcome [34]. Nurses are constantly interacting with and vigilantly monitoring patients across the care continuum. Thus, nurses are ideally positioned to observe red flags or warning signs that something could go wrong and thereby coordinate resources to prevent harm. High reliability depends on team collaboration and making sense of vague changes. Nurses integrate high-reliability science into their practice every day by:

- Monitoring for slight changes in clinical conditions and escalating concern to the interdisciplinary team for early treatment.
- Anticipating complications and being prepared for their occurrence.
- Being empowered and encouraged to speak up with concerns in the moment and to escalate when speaking-up behaviors are not encouraged.

Safety II: Shining a light on the positive results of everyday nursing work. Safety II principles suggest that larger safety learning does not rely only on investigating events that do not go right [35]. The opportunity for learning exists within looking at everyday events and how those at the front line adapt to varying conditions to create success or avoid errors [36]. Nurses have the greatest opportunity to impact safety in this space sometimes without even realizing it. For example, a recent study sought to dispel the myth that nurses have limited impact on antimicrobial stewardship efforts. The researchers analyzed the literature and found that nurses influence antimicrobial stewardship by the nature of what they do every day at the front line including administering, monitoring for adverse effects, escalation of timing and dosage issues, and educating patients. Notably, these tasks spring from the lens of the nurse as a highly educated patient advocate. Also notable is that this work has not been recognized widely [37].

Nurses are constantly adapting to manage policies that break down or are faulty at the front line, to emergent or unexpected conditions for which there are no protocols or guidelines, and to varying conditions in the workforce and work environment such as pressure to work faster, staff shortages, new staff, or surges of patients. In other words, nursing is always adapting, using their knowledge and expertise, collaboration, and patient advocacy skills to organize optimal care. These issues are the everyday experience of a nurse working in healthcare today, and most of the time, nurses use their resources to adapt for a successful outcome. Davina Allen [38], in *The Invisible Work of Nurses*, discusses how the everyday work of nursing becomes integrated into the production cycle and metrics of the organization and can become an assumed or invisible process unless intentionally called out. As in the example of the myth of nurses and their impact on antimicrobial stewardship [37], nursing's meticulous organizing work can be overlooked because no failure occurs. Focusing on how nurses create safety everyday will shed light on how success in patient safety occurs. Nurses can create this focus on the positive results of everyday work by:

- Analyzing near misses and close calls to understand what adaptions were made that avoided harm.
- Researching everyday nursing practice in interactions with patients and colleagues to create theory and make visible how nurses create safety every day.
- Using interdisciplinary collaboration to review successful critical events such as code blues and massive hemorrhage events to analyze what conditions supported the success.
- Highlighting the supporting conditions that hardwire safe practices into care.

Practice, research, and theory are the foundation of patient safety science and nursing science. In any discipline, science is the result of the relationship between the process of inquiry (research) and the product of knowledge (theory). Evidence-based practice is the stimulus for research, thereby refining the scientific basis for practice. Incorporating safety science as previously discussed into nursing theory and research can further distinguish nursing science as a science committed to the practice of patient safety.

4.2   Interprofessional Collaboration

Interprofessional collaboration is a key factor that is evident in successful healthcare outcomes [39]. Nurses constantly serve as connectors and collaborators within the healthcare team. The knowledge base and inquiry focus of nursing strengthen the whole team. Furthermore, it is the collaborative nature of nursing and the focus on inclusiveness that allow all team voices to be heard while advocating for the patient. For example, nurses are often the conduit of patient concerns to the interdisciplinary team. Nurses are also commonly the ones that bring up environmental factors and social determinants that affect discharge. This unique focus of nursing is supported by a commitment to teamwork science, strong communication, and leadership skills. Threats to true interprofessional collaboration include hierarchy and power distance [40, 41]. Nurses use safety science to support interdisciplinary collaboration by:

- Recognizing that expertise is not within only the leader of the team; expertise can be found within all team members [34].
- Allowing all voices to be heard, including the patient.
- Recognizing that power distance in teams can occur innocuously and researching best practice to decrease this safety risk [40].

4.3   Patient Advocate

Nurses spend the most time one on one with patients and create connections that transcend the patient care encounter [38]. This connection and focus on protection and advocacy for the patient and family distinguish nursing as a point of synergy for patient safety. Patient safety suffers when patients are not involved in their safety. Often, the nurse is a direct conduit from the patient to the interprofessional team. Nurses as advocates promote this involvement by:

- Educating patients on their condition, medications, and procedures.
- Assisting patients with asking questions regarding safety.
- Identifying social determinants that may be affecting patient care such as access to resources, transportation, and food or home insecurity.
- Recognizing bias and the impact that it has on patient safety.
- Assuring that patient needs and desires are strongly present in decision-making.

4.4   Empowerment

A key to assuring the synergy of nursing and safety to create the nexus we are describing is the concept of empowerment. An empowered nursing workforce is imperative in order to truly realize the power of nursing to impact patient safety. We still have instances where nurses do not speak up, do not consult on new processes that affect safety, and do not have an equal voice with other disciplines [41, 42]. Furthermore, nurses often struggle to see themselves as leaders, which is a key factor in fully realizing nursing's impact [43].

Empowerment has been described extensively in the literature and refers to structural empowerment (support, resources) and psychological empowerment [44]. Empowered nurses access resources, information, and support needed to provide patient care. They also tend to speak up about safety concerns to escalate issues for timely resolution. Empowerment is one of the key elements of a positive work environment that enable safe, high-quality care to be delivered, despite challenges [45].

Nurses have so much to offer, and there is no argument that their contribution to patient safety is critical. However, the issue of true empowerment continues to be a barrier. Perhaps, empowerment is not all that we need. López-Deflory, Perron, and Miró-Bonet [42] discuss nurse empowerment versus nurse agency. Empowerment is given or granted by someone else. For example, leadership practices psychological safety, so nurses can speak up; just culture is practiced by human resources, so blaming does not occur for honest mistakes; nurses are required to be on practice councils. In comparison, agency enacts a realization that hierarchy and oppression can exist, and nurses, as opposed to being given authority, realize that they have the authority to exercise control over their practice, themselves, and patients. The difference is subtle; however, what is important is how nurses see themselves as leaders of patient safety.

In summary, empowerment and also agency are essential components that promote nurses creating safety at the front line of care. Empowered nurses with agency in the work environment:

- Recognize themselves as leaders no matter what position they hold.
- Identify power differentials and the effect they can have on patient safety.
- Feel responsible to speak up with concerns for patient safety and know that their concerns will be addressed.
- Feel comfortable escalating safety concerns to leadership.
- Create a work environment where all staff, no matter their status, can freely raise concerns on behalf of patient safety.

The vision for nursing to lead patient safety for the future is clear and inevitable as nurses evolve to adapt nursing theory, research, and practice to global healthcare needs. Essential for this evolution is a type of revolution. Nurses need to intentionally identify and dissolve the limits and assumptions placed by organizations and themselves to fully evolve to be safety leaders. Integral to this change is making the everyday work that nurses do to assure patient safety visible. This involves integrating safety science into nursing science, fully utilizing nursing skills of advocacy for patients and those who are not heard, optimizing interprofessional collaboration and communication, and realizing the reality that nurses are all change agents and leaders dedicated to improving healthcare for ourselves, our patients, and our communities.

5   Summary

Nurses are the reliable safety sentinels that often prevent errors from reaching patients in our healthcare systems. The most critical contribution of nursing to patient safety is the nurse's ability to collaborate, coordinate, and integrate the multiple aspects of care across care settings [46]. The bottom line is that nurses have the knowledge, expertise, communication, and collaboration skills to be leaders of patient safety. The synergy of nursing and patient safety is contingent on integrating current safety science into nursing science, interprofessional collaboration, connection with the patient, and recognition of the power of nursing. Empowerment from the inside and outside creates the visibility and sustainability for the future of patient safety and nursing. This integration enhances the power of nursing theory, research, and practice in the realm of patient safety. The nexus—the central or most important point of interaction—where patient safety connects or meets nursing is what keeps patients safe.

Key Points

- The nexus—the central or most important point of interaction—where patient safety connects or meets nursing keeps patients safe.
- Nursing and patient safety blend to create a synergy that positions nursing and patient safety as a powerful combined presence.
- Nurses are a strong barrier to harm. The best nurse is not one who never makes a mistake, but one who finds mistakes and stops them from causing harm.
- Nursing leaders, administrators, and clinicians can and must work tirelessly to apply safety science, nursing theory, nursing research, and nursing practice to achieve zero preventable harm and zero injury to patients and families served in healthcare systems.
- Nurses themselves need to make visible the incredibly important work that nurses do every day to create safety at the front line.

Addendum: Examples of Nursing Creating Safety at the Local and at the System Level

Local Example of Making Visible the Work of Nursing Creating Safety at the Front Line of Care

Situation

Manny, a new graduate nurse, is working on the medical surgical with Greta, a 71-year-old, with recent hernia repair. Greta has a surgically inserted tube into her stomach for feeding. Greta rolls over, and the feeding tube falls out. The insertion site is open and has purulent drainage. Greta is set to be transferred to a long-term care facility in 3 hours.

Manny calls the surgeon and asks that they come and reinsert the tube. The surgeon states that this is a nursing task, and they have no time to do this. Manny states that she feels uncomfortable because she has no protocol for this, the site is purulent, and the patient feels pain around the site. The surgeon comes up and reinserts the tube and states to the nurse that it is a nursing function and next time, Manny should follow their orders. During the insertion, the patient complains of pain and is very anxious. The transport for her transfer arrives and attempts to place Greta in a wheelchair. Greta refuses to get in the wheelchair and states that she is in too much pain and does not want to go. The unit is also full and needs an empty bed to allow for emergency department patients. Manny is receiving pressure to discharge Greta. The transport team attempts to force Greta into the wheelchair. Manny enters the room and asks everyone to pause for a minute, so she can discuss the situation with the patient. The patient is anxious, in pain, and distraught that her feeding tube may become dislodged again. Manny calls the surgeon again and asks for an order for an antianxiolytic, pain medication and recommends a cleaning regimen for the insertion site. She then gives the medication, assesses the response, cleans the site which also decreases the pain, and secures the tube with an effective dressing. She also calls the patient's family member and facilitates a video call to help Greta calm down. Greta is able to transfer successfully with no concerns.

Discussion

Although this example may seem like the work that nurses do constantly in the face of pressure, it is exactly the work that needs illumination to highlight the skills and expertise that nurses use to create outcomes. This is the ordinary work of nursing that is extraordinary when examined.

Safety Issues in This Example for Practice, Theory, and Research

- Nurses' role in infection control and assessing the potential for infection at every encounter with a patient.
- Intimidation and power in the healthcare organization and strategies that nurses use when confronted with such (high reliability).
- Production pressure and rushing (human factors) and how that affects safety and patient care.
- Nurses' use of critical thinking and organizing skills to achieve an outcome in the face of emergent conditions (Safety II).
- Nurse advocacy and support of patient safety as well as dignity and emotional well-being (patient advocate).
- Nurses' ability and confidence to stop the line for safety, creating an intentional pause for critical thinking and collaboration (empowerment and agency).

Every interaction between nursing and a patient is an example of advocacy and safety. This is only one of many examples that seem routine but are the fabric of what creates safety at the front line. As nursing shines light on this work through theory, practice, and research, the role of the nurse as the leader of patient safety is evident.

System Example

Nursing-Led Healthcare System Safety Initiative Improves Safety at the Front Line

Nursing is ideally situated to collaborate, coordinate, and implement system-level patient safety initiatives while fostering engagement of the interprofessional team. The following is an example of how nursing and nurses were the lynch pin in the implementation of a standardized fall prevention program to improve safety at the front line across ten hospitals in a healthcare system.

Background

The 1999 Institute of Medicine [12] report estimated that between 44,000 and 98,000 Americans die each year because of medical errors. One of the problems specifically cited in the IOM report was patient falls. Patient fall is defined as an unplanned descent to the floor with or without injury to the patient. A fall may result in fractures, lacerations, or internal bleeding, leading to increased healthcare utilization. The Agency for Healthcare Quality [47] reports that 700,000 to one million patients fall each year resulting in 250,000 injuries and approximately 11,000 deaths. Two percent of hospitalized patients fall at least once during their hospital stay; nearly 1 in 4 results in injury, with approximately 10% resulting in serious injury [48]. Each fall with injury averages 6.3 days longer hospital stay and costs approximately $14,056 [49, 50]. As of 2008, the Centers for Medicare & Medicaid Services (CMS) does not reimburse hospitals for certain types of traumatic injuries that occur after a patient fall [51].

Purpose

The Nurse Practice Council, comprised of clinical nurses from across a large healthcare system, reviewed the number of falls and falls with injury monthly. The Council noted an upward trend in the number of falls and falls with injury during the previous fiscal year. The Council requested and was granted funding by senior nurse executives to hire an expert fall prevention consultant. In December 2019, an expert fall consultant evaluated nursing fall prevention and injury management practices across the healthcare system as baseline data showed an upward trend in the number of falls and falls with injury during fiscal years 2018, 2019, and 2020. Analysis revealed standardized structure and processes for fall prevention were lacking. The consultant recommended changing nursing practice to a comprehensive fall prevention program. Healthcare system leaders commissioned the formation of a Fall Prevention Team, under the leadership of a specialty nursing director and patient safety nurse scientist, with the goal to provide clinical nurses with a comprehensive fall prevention program that was readily available and easily accessible to reduce patient injury across the healthcare system. The purpose of the safety improvement team was to decrease patient falls and falls with injury by implementing an evidence-based comprehensive nursing fall prevention program in the inpatient, emergency department, perioperative, and behavioral health settings across a ten-hospital healthcare system.

Materials/Methods

A safety improvement implementation team formed under the leadership of the nurse scientist for patient safety and a specialty nursing director. Frontline staff joined clinical nurse specialists (CNSs), clinical unit directors, patient safety managers, informaticists, director of nursing quality and analytics, data analyst, and senior healthcare system leaders including Associate Chief Medical Officer, Chief Nursing Informatics, and Quality Officer and Specialty Nursing Directors as team members. The Institute for Healthcare Improvement (IHI) Plan-Do-Study-Act (PDSA) method served as the framework for this project and assisted with engagement of nursing staff during the pilot [52].

The safety team conducted an evidentiary review over an 8-month period to determine what constitutes a fall prevention program and what is the most effective fall prevention program. Five fall prevention programs were evaluated. The team concluded that a proprietary fall prevention program was the most effective because the comprehensive program predicts patient fall risk accurately, prevents falls by catering to individualized patient needs, and sustains the program by embedding fall prevention and safety into culture.

Over the course of the next year, the team garnered support and secured funding for the proprietary program by writing a robust business case showcasing the possible fiscal benefits of a contractual agreement with the evidence-based patient safety solutions company to the healthcare system. The business case was socialized by nursing leaders throughout organizational governance structures in the system and individual entities to win support for funding the nursing practice change.

Once funding was secured and the contract signed, the safety improvement team partnered with the patient safety solutions company nursing team to work through a 6-month implementation plan. The team made clinical operation decisions, built scoring and interventions into two electronic medical record (EMR) platforms, developed reporting and super-user infrastructure, developed and deployed customized education content for RNs and RN super-users as well as content for other healthcare team members, and socialized the program throughout the enterprise. Structure metrics were the number of identified clinical nurse super-users and percent education module completion by clinical nurses across the enterprise responsible for mitigating patient falls in their discrete work settings. Post-implementation, the team continually monitored key process metrics fall risk score accuracy and intervention accuracy by auditing data collected from the EMRs, as well as percentage of clinical units in the healthcare system submitting audits. Outcome metrics are healthcare system number of falls with injury and system fall with injury rate.

End-user hesitancy to change was overcome by team members going directly to where staff worked to understand fall prevention workflows and involve frontline staff in program pre-implementation decision-making. Extensive end-user education was provided prior to and as needed following program implementation. The safety team listened to end-user preferences, designed to their needs, shared data, showed them tool customizations, and placed tools on the healthcare system intranet for easy access. Real-time follow-up to feedback helped further facilitate buy-in. A command center was manned for several days following program implementation, thus providing end-users with direct access to implementation team members. Team members answered end-user questions and adjusted tools in real time. Safety team members listened and did additional customization of resources and tools and then placed tools back on the system intranet in response to end-user feedback.

Results

Structure Metrics
One hundred percent of the 160 in scope clinical units across ten hospitals identified 10% of clinical nursing staff as super-users who all completed super-user training. All hospitals exceeded the RN education completion target of 80% with greater than 90% of healthcare system clinical staff completing customized RN training prior to program implementation. Socializing the fall prevention program throughout the enterprise educated more than 3000 assistive personnel and other healthcare team members.

Process Metrics
The percentage of clinical units across ten hospitals in the healthcare system submitting ten web-based audit forms per week averaged 95%. Average fall risk score accuracy was 76%, and average intervention accuracy was 80%.

Outcome Metrics
A 15% decrease in the number of falls with injury across the system occurred the first 6 months post-program implementation period. The number of inpatient falls with injury decreased 13%, and the number of falls with injury in emergency departments decreased 30%. The number of falls with injury across the system in the behavioral health and perioperative/procedural patient care areas did not change. The average post-implementation aggregate fall rate decreased 19% when compared to the average pre-implementation aggregate system fall rate. The average inpatient/behavioral health fall with injury rate decreased 15%, and the average emergency department fall with injury rate decreased 30% post-implementation. Perioperative/procedural areas' average fall with injury rate remained unchanged at 0%.

Discussion/Conclusions/Implications for Practice/Dissemination

The implementation of an evidence-based comprehensive standardized nursing fall prevention program, in the inpatient, emergency department, perioperative/procedural, and behavioral health settings across the healthcare system, improved patient safety. Nursing and nurses led the healthcare system transition from four different fall risk screens with generic interventions to an effective fall prevention program that incorporates patient screening and clinical assessment elements into fall risk factors, fall prevention strategies, and injury mitigation tactics for individuals deemed at highest risk for fall. Frontline staff are provided with easily accessible tools, and data is efficiently aggregated in a timely manner. Next step is to implement a similar program in the ambulatory patient care setting.

References

1. American Nurses Association. Code of ethics for nurses. American Nurses Publishing; 2015.
2. WHO (2023). Patient safety—key facts. Retrieved on November 21, 2023, at https://www.who.int/news-room/fact-sheets/detail/patient-safety.
3. Hickey JV, Giardino ER. The role of the nurse in quality improvement and patient safety. Pielęgniarstwo Neurologiczne i Neurochirurgiczne. 2019;8(1):30–6.
4. Institute of Medicine (US) Committee on Data Standards for Patient Safety. In: Aspden P, Corrigan JM, Wolcott J, Erickson SM, editors. Patient safety: achieving a new standard for care. Washington: National Academies Press; 2004.
5. Institute of Medicine (US) Committee on Quality of Health Care in America. Crossing the quality chasm: a new health system for the 21st century. Washington: National Academies Press; 2001.
6. Nightingale F. Notes on nursing: what it is, and what it is not. London: Harrison and Sons; 1859.
7. Reef C. Florence nightingale: the courageous life of the legendary nurse. Boston, MA: Clarion Books; 2017.
8. Reinking C. Nurses transforming systems of care: The bicentennial of Florence Nightingale's legacy. Nurs Manag. 2020;51(5):32.
9. Tye J. Florence Nightingale's lasting legacy for health care. Nurse Lead. 2020;18(3):220–6.
10. Kowalski SL, Anthony M. Nursing's evolving role in patient safety. Am J Nurs. 2017;117(2):34–48.
11. Harwood L, Wilson B. All-star quality improvement: keep it simple. Nephrol Nurs J. 2022;49(2):161–3. https://doi.org/10.37526/1526-744X.2022.49.2.161.
12. Institute of Medicine. To err is human: building a safer health system. Washington, DC: The National Academies Press; 2000. https://doi.org/10.17226/9728.
13. Phillips J, Malliaris AK, Bakerjian D. Nursing and patient safety. 2021. Retrieved November 25, 2023, at https://psnet.ahrq.gov/primer/nursing-and-patient-safety
14. Page A, editor. Keeping patients safe: Transforming the work environment of nurses. Washington, DC: The National Academies Press; 2004.
15. Huddleston P, Gray J. Measuring nurse leaders' and direct care nurses' perceptions of a healthy work environment in acute care settings. Part 1. J Nurs Adm. 2016a;46(7/8):373–8.
16. Huddleston P, Gray J. Describing nurse leaders' and direct care nurses' perceptions of a healthy work environment in acute care settings. Part 2. J Nurs Adm. 2016b;46(9):462–7.
17. Aiken LH, Sloane DM, Barnes H, Cimiotti JP, Jarrín OF, McHugh MD. Nurses' and patients' appraisals show patient safety in hospitals remains a concern. Health Aff. 2018;37(11):1744–51.
18. Murray M, Sundin D, Cope V. The nexus of nursing leadership and a culture of safer patient care. J Clin Nurs. 2018;27(5–6):1287–93. https://doi.org/10.1111/jocn.13980.
19. Saleh US. Theory guided practice in nursing. J Nurs Res Pract. 2018;2(1):18.

20. Nursing & Midwifery Council. Standards for competence for registered nurses; 2014. Retrieved December 3, 2023, at https://www.nmc.org.uk/globalassets/sitedocuments/standards/nmc-standards-for-competence-for-registered-nurses.pdf

21. National Patient Safety Foundation. Free from harm: accelerating patient safety fifteen years after To Err Is Human. Executive summary. Boston, MA: National Patient Safety Foundation; 2015. Retrieved December 10, 2023, at https://www.aorn.org/docs/default-source/guidelines-resources/position-statements/endorsed-documents/freefromharm_execsummary.pdf?sfvrsn=a09a1e82_1

22. Wears R, Sutcliffe K. Still not safe: patient safety and the middle-managing of American Medicine. Oxford University Press; 2019. https://doi.org/10.1093/oso/9780190271268.001.0001.

23. New England Journal of Medicine Catalyst. Lessons from health care leaders: rethinking and reinvesting in patient safety | NEJM Catalyst; 2023

24. Clapper C, Merlino J, Stockmeier C. Zero harm: how to achieve patient and workforce safety in healthcare: how to achieve patient and workforce safety in healthcare. McGraw Hill Professional; 2018.

25. Merriam-Webster. Nexus. In: Merriam-Webster.com dictionary; n.d.. Retrieved November 29, 2023, at https://www.merriam-webster.com/dictionary/nexus.

26. Weeks KR. Exploring the nexus of patient safety and patient-centered care: a study of high performing hospitals. Johns Hopkins University; 2021. Doctoral dissertation https://jscholarship.library.jhu.edu/items/77f0792f-6f29-4986-8b5a-f207acd47692

27. American Association of Colleges of Nursing. Nursing workforce fact sheet; 2023. Retrieved December 10, 2023, at https://www.aacnnursing.org/news-data/fact-sheets/nursing-workforce-fact-sheet

28. Reason JT. Human error. Cambridge, England: Cambridge University Press; 1990.

29. Mumma JM, Kazi S. Human factors engineering for reducing and recovering from error. In: Oster CA, Braaten JS, editors. High reliability organizations a healthcare handbook for patient safety & quality. 2nd ed. Indianapolis, IN: Sigma Theta Tau International, Honor Society for Nurses; 2020. p. 131–46.

30. Patient Safety Network. Human factors engineering; 2019. Retrieved December 12, 2023 at https://psnet.ahrq.gov/primer/human-factors-engineering#:~:text=In%20essence%2C%20human%20factors%20engineering,of%20error%20in%20complex%20environments

31. Junaid SB, Imam AA, Balogun AO, De Silva LC, Surakat YA, Kumar G, Abdulkarim M, Shuaibu AN, Garba A, Sahalu Y, Mohammed A, Mohammed TY, Abdulkadir BA, Abba AA, Kakumi NAI, Mahamad S. Recent advancements in emerging technologies for healthcare management systems: a survey. Healthcare (Basel). 2022;10(10):1940. https://doi.org/10.3390/healthcare10101940.

32. Institute for Health Improvement (IHI). Failure modes and effects analysis (FMEA) tool | Institute for Healthcare Improvement (ihi.org).

33. Chassin MR, Loeb JM. High-reliability health care: getting there from here. Milbank Q. 2013;91(3):459–90. https://doi.org/10.1111/1468-0009.12023.

34. Oster CA, Braaten JS, (Eds.). High reliability organizations a healthcare handbook for patient safety & quality. 2nd ed. Indianapolis, IN: Sigma Theta Tau International, Honor Society for Nurses; 2020.

35. Hollnagel E., Wears RL, Braithwaite J. From Safety-I to Safety-II: a white paper. The resilient health care net: published simultaneously by the University of Southern Denmark, University of Florida, USA, and Macquarie University, Australia;1 2015. https://www.england.nhs.uk/signuptosafety/wp-content/uploads/sites/16/2015/10/safety-1-safety-2-whte-papr.pdf

36. Hollnagel E. Safety II in practice: Developing the resilience potentials. Routledge; 2018.

37. Bos M, Schouten J, De Bot C, Vermeulen H, Hulscher M. A hidden gem in multidisciplinary antimicrobial stewardship: a systematic review on bedside nurses' activities in daily practice regarding antibiotic use. JAC-Antimicrob Resist. 2023;5(6):dlad123. https://doi.org/10.1093/jacamr/dlad123.

38. Allen D. The invisible work of nurses: hospitals, organisation and healthcare. London: Routledge; 2015.

39. McLaney E, Morassaei S, Hughes L, Davies R, Campbell M, Di Prospero L. A framework for interprofessional team collaboration in a hospital setting: advancing team competencies and behaviours. Healthc Manage Forum. 2022;35(2):112–7. https://doi.org/10.1177/08404704211063584.

40. Bochatay N, Kuna Á, Csupor É, Pintér JN, Muller-Juge V, Hudelson P, Nendaz MR, Csabai M, Bajwa NM, Mim S. The role of power in health care conflict: recommendations for shifting toward constructive approaches. Acad Med. 2021;96(1):134–41. https://doi.org/10.1097/ACM.0000000000003604.

41. Etchegaray JM, Ottosen MJ, Dancsak T, Thomas EJ. Barriers to speaking up about patient safety concerns. J Patient Saf. 2020;16(4):e230–4. https://doi.org/10.1097/PTS.0000000000000334.

42. López-Deflory C, Perron A, Miró-Bonet M. An integrative literature review and critical reflection on nurses' agency. Nurs Inq. 2023;30(1):e12515. https://doi.org/10.1111/nin.125151.

43. Booher L, Yates E, Claus S, Haight K, Burchill CN. Leadership self-perception of clinical nurses at the bedside: a qualitative descriptive study. J Clin Nurs. 2021;30(11-12):1573–83. https://doi.org/10.1111/jocn.15705.

44. Moura LN, Camponogara S, Santos JLGD, Gasparino RC, Silva RMD, Freitas EO. Structural empowerment of nurses in the hospital setting. Rev Lat Am Enfermagem. 2020;28:e3373. https://doi.org/10.1590/1518-8345.3915.3373.

45. Rangachari P, Woods L, J. Preserving organizational resilience, patient safety, and staff retention during COVID-19 requires a holistic consideration of the psychological safety of healthcare workers. Int J Environ Res Public Health. 2020;17(12):4267.

46. Hughes RG, Clancy CM. Nurses' role in patient safety. J Nurs Care Qual. 2009;24(1):1–4.

47. Agency for Healthcare Research and Quality (AHRQ). Preventing falls in hospitals, Agency for Healthcare Research and Quality. Rockville, MD; 2023. Content last reviewed March 2023. https://www.ahrq.gov/patient-safety/settings/hospital/fall-prevention/toolkit/index.html

48. LeLaurin JH, Shorr RI. Preventing falls in hospitalized patients: state of the science. Clin Geriatr Med. 2019;35(2):273–83. https://doi.org/10.1016/j.cger.2019.01.007.

49. Galbraith J, Butler J, Memon A, Dolan M, Harty J. Cost analysis of a falls prevention program in an orthopaedic setting. Park Ridge, IL: Association of Bone and Joint Surgeons; 2011. https://doi.org/10.1007/s11999-011-1932-9.

50. Haines T, Hill A-M, Hill K, Brauer S, Hoffmann T, Etherton-Beer C, McPhail S. Cost effectiveness of patient education for the prevention of fall in hospital: economic evaluation from a randomized controlled trial. BMC Med. 2013; https://doi.org/10.1186/1741-7015-11-135.

51. Inouye SK, Brown CJ, Tinetti ME. Medicare nonpayment, hospital falls, and unintended consequences. N Engl J Med. 2009;360:2390–3.

52. Institute for Healthcare Improvement. (IHI). How to improve: model for improvement. Retrieved December 11, 2023, at https://www.ihi.org/resources/how-to-improve

Printed by Printforce, the Netherlands